# Mysterious Happenings

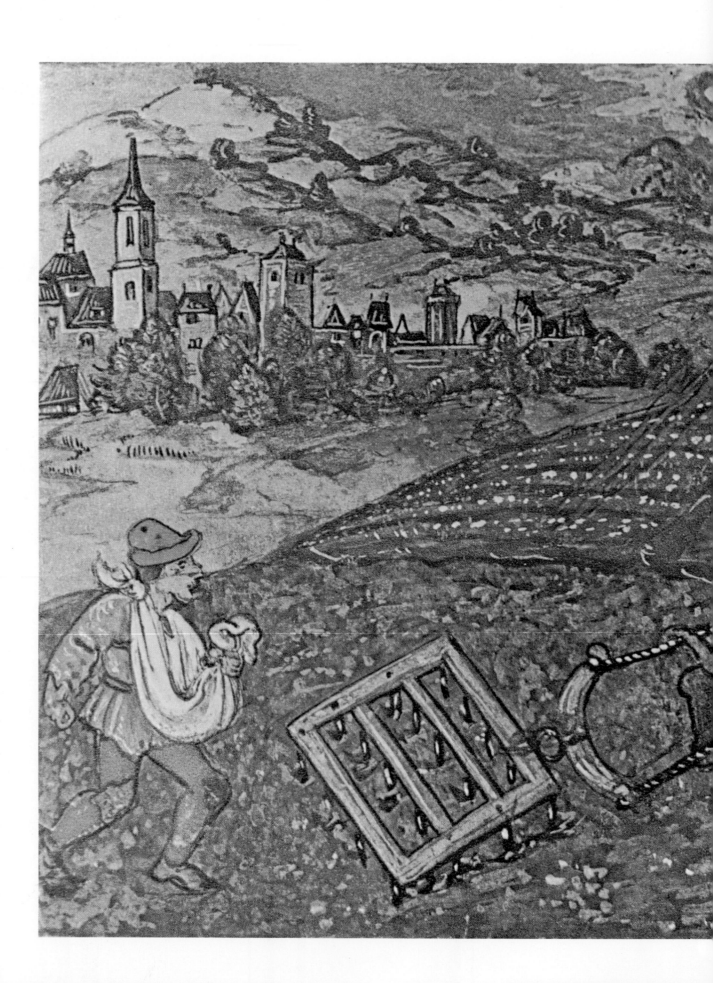

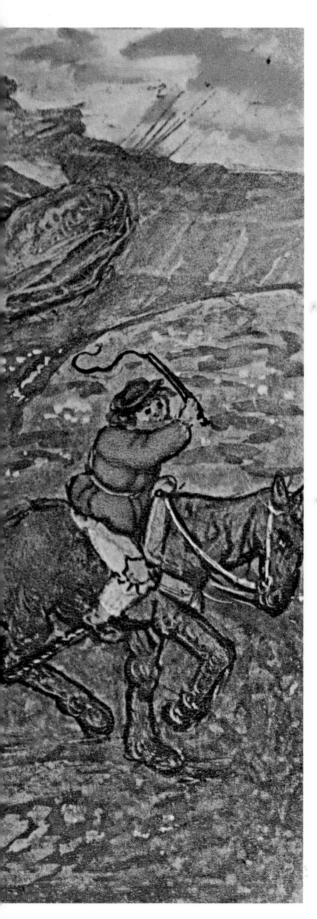

Great Mysteries

# Mysterious Happenings

## by Jeremy Kingston

Book Club Associates
London

Series Coordinator:   John Mason
Art Director:         Grahame Dudley
Design:              Ann Dunn
                     Julia Jones
Editorial:           Mitzi Bales
                     Nina Shandloff
Research:            Frances Vargo
Series Consultant:   Beppie Harrison

This edition published 1980 by
Book Club Associates
By arrangement with Aldus Books Limited
First published in the United Kingdom
in 1978 by Aldus Books Limited
17 Conway Street, London W1P 6BS

Printed and bound in Hong Kong
by Leefung-Asco Printers Limited

# Introduction

In our 20th-century conceit we usually feel we have all the answers. But do we? This book assesses a wide range of mysterious happenings which strongly challenge that confident belief. Taking as his starting point the findings of the eccentric American Charles Hoy Fort, who painstakingly collected and cataloged the unexplained and inexplicable, the author goes on to look at some of the strange phenomena that persist in human experience. They include unexpected objects that fall from the sky; unexplained disappearances, such as those of the American writer Ambrose Bierce and the British diplomat Lord Bathurst; mysterious appearances of people seemingly without a past, such as the enigmatic Man in the Iron Mask and Caspar Hauser. Other chapters examine such weird stories as the treasure of Oak Island in Nova Scotia, the evidence for jinxes and curses, and the various mysterious aspects of fire from halos to spontaneous human combustion. Three more chapters try to find rational explanations for mysterious happenings at sea, in the air, and in that infamous area of both known as the Bermuda Triangle. If present science cannot explain these phenomena, what other explanation is there for such mysterious happenings?

# Contents

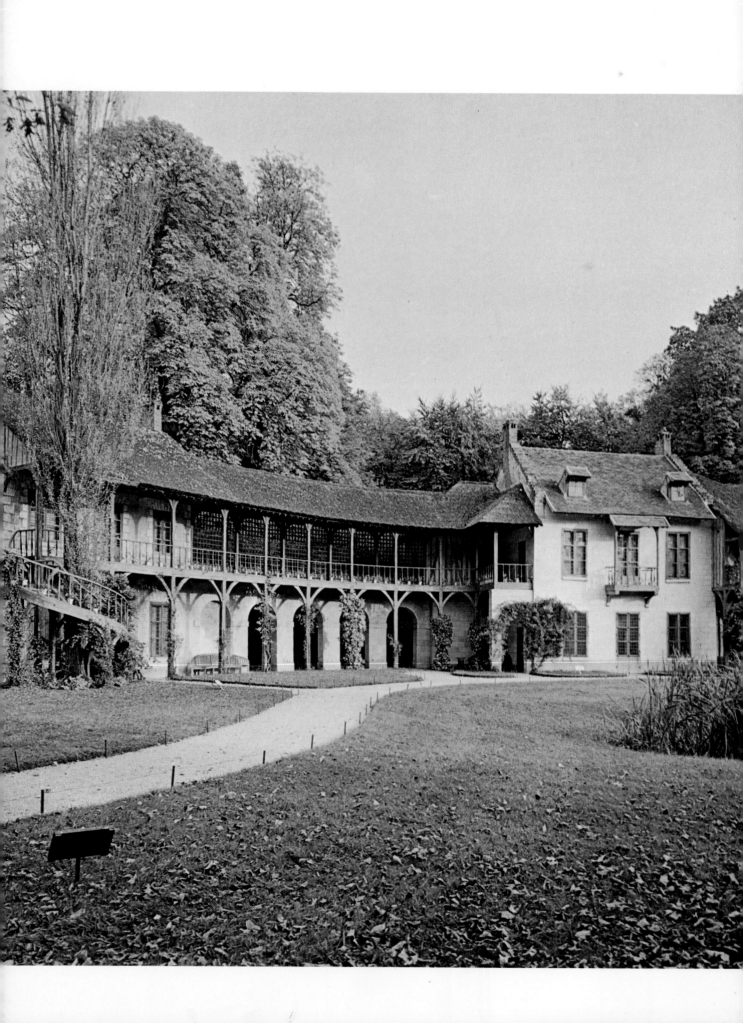

# Chapter 1 Chroniclers of the Unexplained

We often use the phrase "mind over matter" to explain psychic phenomena, but is it possible that mind and matter are not divided? How else can we explain the experience of two people who stepped 200 years back in time? Today nuclear science speaks of a particle in the brain that may communicate with other minds or with matter—and may not be hindered by space or time. Are scientists coming closer to the occult, as represented by science debunker Charles Hay Fort? Do the numerous odd occurrences he recorded indicate that there is less disparity between mind and matter than we now believe?

On the afternoon of August 10, 1901 two Englishwomen on a visit to the palace of Versailles had an extraordinary experience: they stepped back in time. The incredible happened as they walked along a shaded lane on their way to the Petit Trianon, the small secluded 18th-century mansion that had once been the private retreat of Queen Marie-Antoinette. The features of the garden, the buildings, even the people they met, obviously belonged to a time much earlier than 1901.

For Charlotte Moberly and Eleanor Jourdain, this was their first visit to Versailles, and they were puzzled by what was happening to them. They had missed the direct way to the Petit Trianon, and turned down a sunken lane that led past buildings of a domestic sort. Gradually they were overcome by an unaccountable depression, "as if something were wrong," Eleanor Jourdain recalled. They could think of no reason to account for the feeling of gloom and isolation that filled them and which they were unable to shake off. Miss Jourdain later said, "I began to feel as if I were walking in my sleep; the heavy dreaminess was oppressive."

The two women passed a stone cottage where Miss Jourdain noticed a woman handing a jug to a young girl; the old-fashioned dress of this girl struck her as odd. Then they asked the way of two distinguished looking men carrying staffs and wearing long greenish-gray coats and three-cornered hats. The men were standing near some gardening tools that included a wheelbarrow

Opposite: part of the miniature village built at the Petit Trianon for Marie-Antoinette, wife of Louis XVI. It was here in 1901 that two Englishwomen had a psychic experience which is one of the most mysterious unexplained happenings of modern times—an experience of the kind that raises all kinds of unanswerable questions about the world in which we live.

# A Strange Adventure

and a plough, and though the two women assumed they were gardeners, their dignified bearing suggested they were persons of authority. They directed the women on toward a wood where the two saw a circular kiosk, something like a small bandstand. On the steps sat a man wearing a heavy black cloak around his shoulders and a slouch hat. "At that moment," Miss Jourdain later wrote, "the eerie feeling that had begun in the garden culminated in a definite impression of something uncanny and fear-inspiring." As Miss Moberly put it: "Everything suddenly looked unnatural, therefore, unpleasant; even the trees behind the building seemed to have become flat and lifeless, like a wood worked on tapestry."

When the man turned his head they could see that his face was dark and disfigured by smallpox. His expression struck them both as "very evil and yet unseeing," and though he did not seem to be looking at them, neither of them wanted to step any closer to him. While they were hesitating, they heard the sound of running footsteps along a nearby path. The rocks separating the paths concealed the runner from their view until suddenly he was behind them and quite close. This man also wore a thick cloak and large hat, though only afterward did the two wonder at such odd clothes for a hot August afternoon. He was handsome, "distinctly a gentleman," and he called out to them in an excited manner and in oddly pronounced French that they were not to go toward the kiosk but to the Petit Trianon. Curiously, he referred to it as "la maison," the word used by Marie-Antoinette to describe her palace.

The two tourists crossed a small rustic bridge above a tiny ravine and came out into an English landscape garden that at last gave them a sight of the Petit Trianon. The windows were shuttered, but on the terrace sat a middle-aged woman wearing a light summer dress and a large white hat over her fair hair. She was sketching the trees. They could see no way of entering the building on this side, so they walked around the west corner onto a terrace looking down on the formal beds of the French garden. All but one of the windows were shuttered, but from a door in what seemed to be a separate house beyond the Petit Trianon itself, a man with the jaunty air of a footman emerged, banging the door behind him. He told them that the way to "la maison" lay through the courtyard on the other side of the kitchen, and he offered to show them the way. "He looked inquisitively amused as he walked by us down the French garden," said Miss Moberly. When he left them they at last made their way into the Petit Trianon, and followed a merry French wedding party around the rooms. Both felt lively and normal again.

Later they discovered that only Miss Moberly had seen the lady sketching and only Miss Jourdain had seen the cottage woman and the child. Neither of them could understand how the other had failed to see people so close. This discrepancy set them thinking that they must have glimpsed some sort of apparition, so they wrote down separate accounts of that afternoon in Versailles. Both were keen observers with skill in expressing themselves. Miss Moberly, elder of the two, had been for 15 years principal of St. Hugh's Hall (later College) at Oxford University; Miss Jourdain, later to be her successor at St. Hugh's, was in 1901

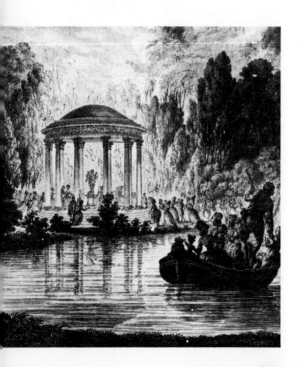

Below: this late 18th-century engraving of an evening party in the grounds of the Petit Trianon typifies the frivolous kind of entertainment which delighted Austrian-born Marie-Antoinette.

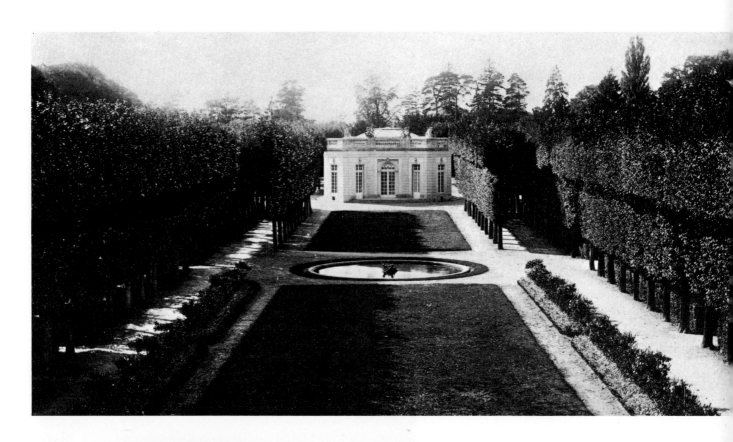

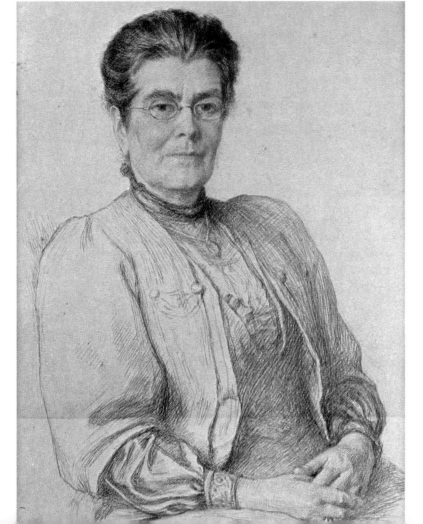

Above: the Petit Trianon, seen from the east across the English landscape garden. It was from this direction that the two tourists approached the house. On the terrace near the house they saw a middle-aged woman wearing a large white hat and a light summer dress sitting sketching the trees.

Left: Miss Charlotte Moberly, the elder of the two Englishwomen. At the time of their experience at Versailles, she was Principal of St. Hugh's College, Oxford. When the two women later compared notes, they discovered that only Miss Moberly had seen the lady sketching, while only Miss Jourdain had seen the woman handing a jug to a young girl. At this point they decided to write independent accounts of their experiences.

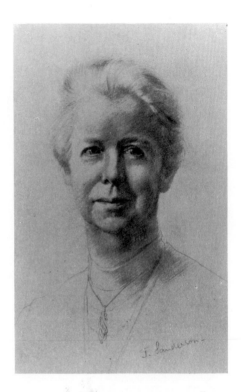

Above: Eleanor Frances Jourdain, the younger of the two Englishwomen who shared an "adventure" at Versailles in 1901 in which they apparently stepped back in time. Miss Jourdain was sufficiently impressed by their experience to go back to Versailles the next year and later both women went back.

Right: a painting of Marie-Antoinette, queen of France and wife of Louis XVI. It was her frivolous and extravagant tastes, such as the building of the elaborate gardens at the Petit Trianon, which gave rise to scandal, and eventually helped to bring about the French Revolution in 1789.

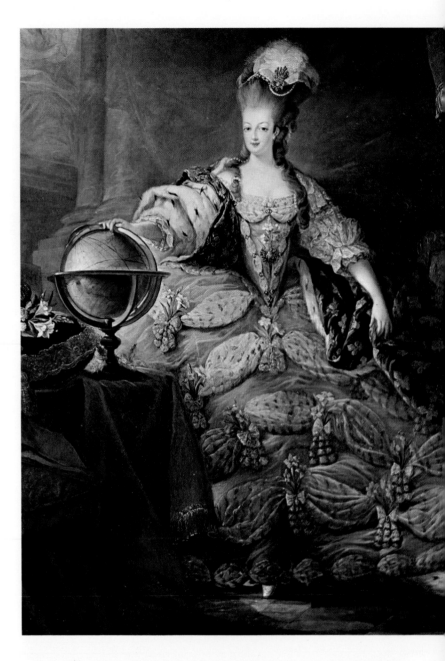

headmistress of a successful private school outside London.

The following year Miss Jourdain made a second visit to Versailles, and because of what she saw there—or rather, because of what she didn't see—she and Miss Moberly subsequently went again together. To their astonishment, derelict gates, unopened for many years, blocked the paths they had followed in 1901. No stone cottage existed, no kiosk; neither the little bridge nor the ravine it crossed could be found. In place of the rough and shaded meadow of the English garden, they saw a broad gravel sweep leading up to the terrace, and where the woman had sat sketching, they found large rhododendron bushes of many years growth. Besides these changes in the surroundings, they found numerous groups of visitors on all sides where previously they had been unpleasantly aware of being alone in that part of the garden. Miss Moberly recounted that, "Garden seats placed everywhere and stalls for fruit and lemonade took away from any idea of desolation.''

The discovery that there had been an alteration of the very scenery of the place gave an altogether more remarkable quality to their experience. They had not merely seen ghosts from the past, but in some unknown way they had entered a past where those "ghosts" were still living people, and the scenery that of their own earlier time.

The two women continued their research on Versailles in whatever hours they could spare from their academic work, and also paid further visits to the palace. They discovered that the door through which the footman had come to show them the way had been locked for many years, and the passages and stairways behind the door were all broken and unusable. When they asked an official about the green coats worn by the gardeners, they were told that green had been one of the colors of the long-vanished royal livery. No plough of the kind Miss Jourdain had seen was any longer in use at the Petit Trianon, but throughout the reign of King Louis XVI and Queen Marie-Antoinette, an old plough had been preserved there. The same sentimental view of the simple life that had prompted Marie-Antoinette to dress as a milkmaid had made her husband pose as a ploughman. The

# Travelers in Time?

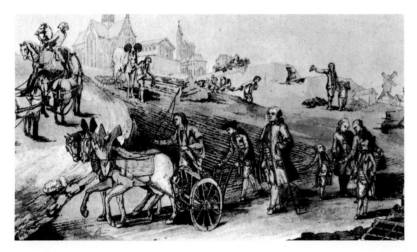

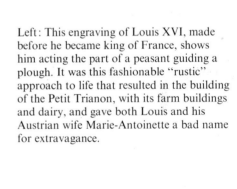

Left: This engraving of Louis XVI, made before he became king of France, shows him acting the part of a peasant guiding a plough. It was this fashionable "rustic" approach to life that resulted in the building of the Petit Trianon, with its farm buildings and dairy, and gave both Louis and his Austrian wife Marie-Antoinette a bad name for extravagance.

discovery of long-forgotten maps and paintings of the gardens confirmed the existence in the 18th century of many features seen by Miss Moberly and Miss Jourdain on August 10, 1901—but long since swept away in the aftermath of the French Revolution.

Coincidences of this kind, requiring a special knowledge neither of the two Englishwomen possessed on their first visit, seemed to confirm that they had gone back in time, and that in some incomprehensible manner the past had remained available for them to experience it. In 1911 they published a record of their experience and subsequent research, calling their book *An Adventure*. The attempt to understand their "adventure" has been continuing ever since.

Suggestions that the two tourists had interrupted a group of people rehearsing a play or making a film had been investigated at the start and proved unfounded. In *The Trianon Adventure*, a recent book on the subject, the principal author, Arnold O. Gibbons, has suggested the existence of some power, at present unknown, that enables an image of reality as it cnce existed to become available again to a living brain. The image is so vividly accurate—even to the precise details of a costume, the features of a face, and the surrounds—that those who receive the image are convinced of its reality. While the trancelike experience lasts, it entirely supplants the ordinary environment of the everyday lives of those involved.

The 18th-century person who may have been behind this image is identified by Gibbons and other contributors to the book as Antoine Richard, head gardener at the Petit Trianon from 1765 to 1795. Richard had helped save the royal garden from destruction by the revolutionary government, having carried the fight on all alone. At one point he even paid workers himself. He certainly seems a likely candidate for the role of agent, capable of triggering off a sense of reality when conditions, about which we can still merely guess, are right. An analysis of where the Moberly-Jourdain experience occurred has shown that most of the incidents happened in the neighborhood of the gardener's house. None took place inside the Petit Trianon where the memories of Marie-Antoinette, whom Miss Moberly tentatively identified as the agent, might be expected to linger. Possibly Antoine Richard was one of the authoritative-looking gardeners encountered by the two women at the start of their adventure, accompanied by his father Claude, his predecessor as head gardener.

When asked why they should have been singled out for this paranormal experience, Miss Moberly replied that she had come to think such experiences might not be so unusual. "We can imagine," she wrote, "that people, even if they suspected anything unusual, may have thought it best not to follow it up."

Until about 350 years ago paranormal experiences were accepted and appreciated in Western as in other cultures. They fitted readily with the way people pictured the universe as having

Above: a mob of revolutionary women from Paris at the palace of Versailles demanding that the king and queen should return with them to Paris. This demonstration, which took place on October 5, 1789, was the first time the revolutionaries approached the royal family at Versailles, which lies 12 miles outside Paris. That day was the last time Marie-Antoinette was to walk in the grounds of the Petit Trianon.

Right: a caricature or cartoon of the "rabbit woman of Godalming," an English example of the kind of inexplicable phenomenon, such as women giving birth to animals, which the 18th-century public were quite prepared to accept as natural abberations.

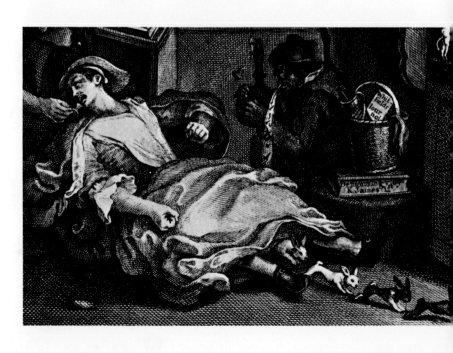

# Reality and Preconceptions

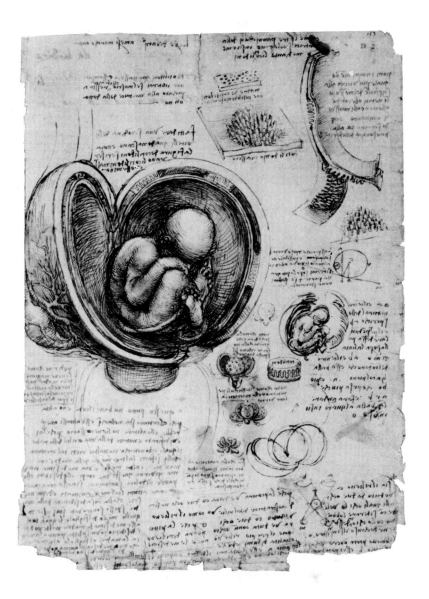

Left: this drawing by the Italian Renaissance artist and scientist Leonardo da Vinci shows the child in the mother's womb. The artist, though brilliant, has drawn the fetus incorrectly to conform to his preconceived idea about the position of the baby in the womb. This drawing is a classic in the sense that it misrepresents observable fact in favor of accepted ideas.

everything interrelated by seen or hidden affinities, called "correspondences," of color, shape, position, or mood. Supernatural beings were believed to move among the natural world and act upon it. If the consequences of mysterious happenings seemed good, they were explained as the intervention of angels; if evil, they were attributed to witchcraft.

These beliefs served to encourage credulity, and among the mysterious happenings recorded in the chronicles of earlier times are to be found reports of such impossibilities as women giving birth to puppies and cows producing lambs. The system of belief also encouraged rigidity of mind in particular areas of knowledge. For example, Flemish-born Andreas Vesalius met violent opposition when he began revising the anatomical theories of Galen, the Roman physician whose books had been the foundation of medicine for 1300 years—though much of Galen's work on anatomy was wrong. Rigidity of thought could affect even so clear-headed an observer as Leonardo da Vinci. Having dissected a woman's body to examine the position of the foetus in the womb, he still drew it according to his preconception.

# A Collector of the Unexplained

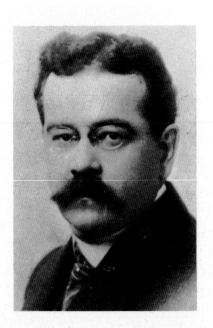

Above: the American Charles Fort, who spent his life collecting and assembling accounts of mysterious happenings and stories of inexplicable phenomena that defy the laws of rational science. Fort said that every science is a mutilated octopus—"if its tentacles were not clipped to stumps it would feel its way into disturbing contacts." Most of us have the uncomfortable feeling that there is more to the world than can be explained by conventional science.

The Renaissance and Elizabethan view of the world, then, held tight to the ancient belief that "there is one common flow, one common breathing, all things are in sympathy." The Italian humanist Pico della Mirandola neatly expresses this feeling of interdependence: "Firstly there is the unity in things whereby each thing is at one with itself, consists of itself, and coheres with itself. Secondly, there is the unity whereby one creature is united with the others and all parts of the world constitute one world."

This system of mutually supporting parts and the interplay of the natural and the supernatural had to give way as the scientific revolution began. By 1700 a mechanistic view of the world was firmly established. The bodies of living things were regarded as material objects, moving and interacting like the parts of a machine. The divorce of one area of knowledge from another began, and different sciences went their different ways. The study of the physical and chemical properties of matter, the behavior of living things, and human experiences and thoughts were cut off from one another and remained so for 250 years. Only recently has the attempt begun to draw the separate threads of knowledge together again, and to try to fashion an understanding of the unity that underlies our existence. Paranormal events are now studied by physicists, biochemists, mathematicians, and other scientists. Many scientists admit that no picture of our existence can be considered complete if it deliberately ignores what we now call the paranormal and the mysterious—but which at some future date may well be seen as normal and everyday.

An implacable opponent of all scientists who held strong mechanistic views was Charles Hay Fort, intellectual rebel and recluse who died in New York in 1932 at the age of 57. He made it his life work to painstakingly collect and catalog thousands of inexplicable events that scientists had either ignored or dismissed as of no importance.

Fort's father was a wealthy businessman who ruled his family with autocratic severity, often beating young Fort with a dog-whip. An intelligent and strong-willed child, Charles grew up with a passionate hatred of authority and stupidity. In his teens he decided to be a writer, but his one published novel was a failure, perhaps because of his style of writing which is a series of brief statements, often without verbs; he also darts from one idea to another without any particular order. To say that his style lacks flow and readability is an understatement.

From an early age Fort had been obsessed by the mysterious and the unexplained. He devoured books on the lost continent of Atlantis, the hollow earth theory, and the mystery of the pyramids. One of his earliest books, which he simply named *X*, argued that our civilization was controlled by Mars. Subsequently he wrote a book titled *Y* and planned another titled *Z*. He wrote *X* and *Y* with tongue in cheek, but later he attempted a reasoned statement of his beliefs in *The Book of the Damned*, published in 1919. By "damned" he meant phenomena that had been discredited and excluded by orthodox science. Here is a typical Fort entry:

"Extract from the log of the bark *Lady of the Lake*, by Capt. F. W. Banner:

"That upon the 22nd of March 1870 at Lat. 5*47′N., Long.

27*52′W., the sailors of the *Lady of the Lake* saw a remarkable object, or cloud, in the sky. They reported to the captain.

"According to Capt. Banner, it was a cloud of circular form, with an included semicircle divided into four parts, the central dividing shaft beginning at the center of the circle and extending far outward, and then curving backward.

"Geometricity and complexity and stability of form: and the small likelihood of a cloud maintaining such diversity of features, to say nothing of appearance of organic form . . .

"Light gray in color, or it was cloud-color.

"That whatever it may have been, it traveled against the wind.

"For half an hour this form was visible. When it did finally disappear that was not because it disintegrated like a cloud, but because it was lost to sight in the evening darkness."

This might make the reader think at once of a flying saucer, especially since Captain Banner's description sounds like many other UFO sightings. But Fort recorded this account in 1919, 30 years before the start of the UFO craze, and he was quoting from the *Journal of the Meteorological Society*, an eminently respectable publication. He makes no attempt to draw conclusions from the report. It is simply one of hundreds of similar mysterious occurrences that he quotes at length and in detail.

Fort's contemporaries regarded him as mildly insane, and it

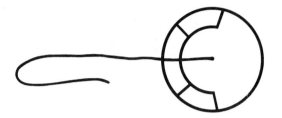

Above: this drawing from one of Fort's books represents in diagram form a sighting by Captain Banner of the *Lady of the Lake* of a kind of unidentified flying object (UFO) in the year 1870.

Below: one of the more recent photographs of a UFO. This one was taken in Oklahoma in 1965 by Alan Smith, who was then a newsboy. Most skeptical investigators into the subject of UFOs have agreed that some expert observers seem to be genuinely convinced that they saw something in the sky. Is the same true of Captain Banner?

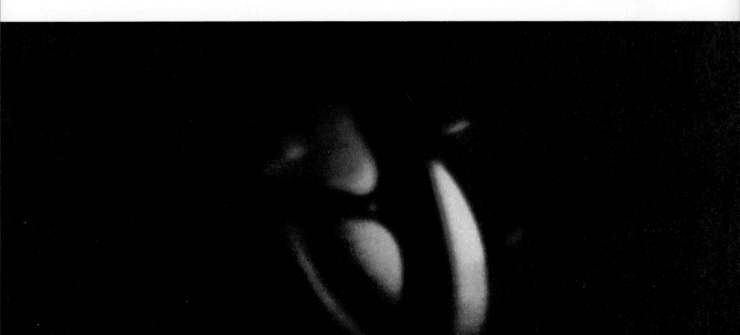

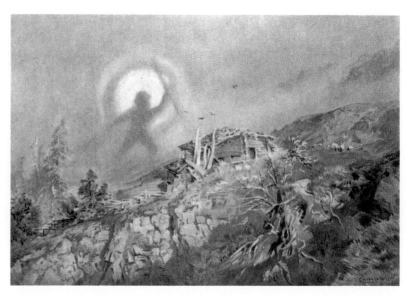

Above: photograph of the so-called "Brocken Specter," an effect observed when the sun is in a position to throw a shadow of the observer onto a cloud. This phenomenon is now accepted by scientists as a normal result of certain conditions.

Above right: an artist's impression of a "Brocken Specter" from the 19th century. Once a subject of superstitious horror, the "Specter" is now accepted by scientists. Is it possible that other Fortean phenomena could similarly be accepted one day?

is easy to understand why. He spent 30 years of his life in the New York Public Library, searching through piles of old newspapers and magazines for items like the one quoted. He was particularly fond of tales of odd things falling from the sky—frogs, fish, blood, stones, or two-feet-square snowflakes. He collected reports of sudden floods, vanishing ships, strange lights in the sky, luminous birds, people who disappeared into thin air, children who came from nowhere. In his third book *Lo!*, he wrote, "I labor, like workers in a beehive, to support a lot of vagabond notions. But how am I to know? How am I to know but that sometimes a queen-idea may soar to the sky, and from a nuptial flight of data, come back fertile from one of these drones?"

Fort's intuition told him there was something wrong with the neat and orderly universe as pictured by science, and that it was a thousand times stranger than even the most brilliant scientists of his day could imagine. It was this intuition that rang a bell when he read the flying saucer story and dozens more like it. Toward the end of his life he put forward some highly personal theories to account for the phenomena he had recorded, but generally he was not concerned with explanation. He felt there could be any number of possible explanations, all equally at variance with scientific thinking, all equally exciting and fruitful.

"Newtonism is no longer satisfactory," he wrote. "There is too much that it cannot explain.

"Einsteinism has arisen.

"If Einsteinism is not satisfactory, there is room for other notions."

Fort had no patience with scientific experts because of cases like the Valparaiso earthquake. Among the many records he collected of "fires in heaven" that had been seen before or accompanying earthquakes, is a reference to the one in Valparaiso on August 16, 1906. "Chile lit up," he wrote. "Under a flaming sky, the people of Valparaiso were running from the smashing city . . ." He goes on to remark that 136 reports of illuminations in the sky were examined by Count De Ballore, a noted seismologist, who dismissed them all as indefinite or impossible.

" 'The lights that were seen in the sky,' said De Ballore, 'were very likely only searchlights from warships. Or the people may have seen lights from streetcars.' " Fort comments: "It does not matter how preposterous some of my own notions are going to seem. They cannot be more out of accordance with events upon this earth than is such an attribution of the blazing sky of a nation to searchlights or to lamps in streetcars."

Astronomers fared no better at his hands than seismologists. In a flash of barbed wit, he compares the slit in the dome of an observatory with the fixed grin of a clown. To show he had good historical reasons for his criticism, he gives an account of how astronomers long disbelieved in meteorites.

"About one hundred years ago, if anyone was so credulous as to think that stones had ever fallen from the sky, he was reasoned with:

"In the first place there are no stones in the sky:

"Therefore no stones can fall from the sky."

# "Fires in Heaven"

Below: a contemporary illustration of the streets of Valparaiso during the earthquake of 1906. Charles Fort was intrigued by reports of mysterious lights in the sky at the time.

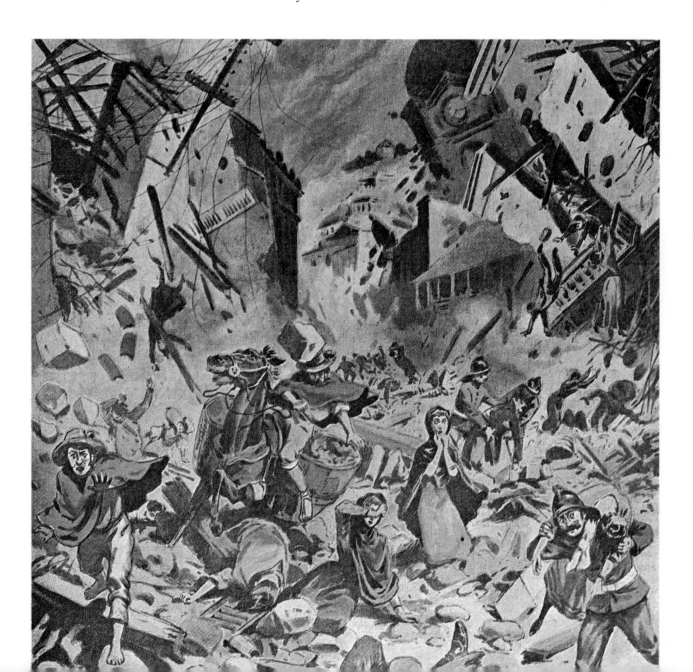

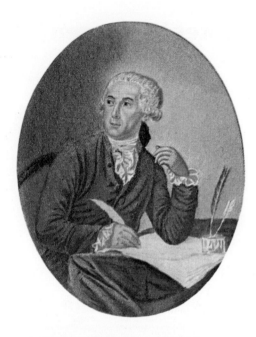

Above: the 18th-century French scientist Antoine Lavoisier. His theory that a particular meteorite was simply the effect of lightning upon rocks was dismissed with typical Fortean sarcasm: Lavoisier, he said, "absolutely proved that there were no meteorites with this explanation."

Below: Lavoisier working in his laboratory. The French scientist, who appears to be involved in an experiment connected with his work on oxygen, is seen here with his wife taking notes at a small table at the right of the picture.

He goes on to tell about a report in 1772 that a blazing stone had fallen from the sky at Luce, France. One of the members of the committee appointed by the French Academy to investigate the report was the distinguished scientist Antoine Lavoisier, who wrote the first modern chemistry textbook, among other achievements. But where meteorites were concerned, Lavoisier took the conventional line of his time. The object that fell at Luce, like any meteorite, showed signs of fusion as a result of its passage through the earth's atmosphere. Lavoisier explained this by saying that a stone on the ground had been struck by lightning, which heated and melted it. As Fort sarcastically put it, Lavoisier "absolutely proved" that there were no meteorites with this explanation.

After Lavoisier's time, an increased flow of data and fresh theories about the earth's place in the universe led to a new understanding of meteorites. Perhaps it is not a full understanding, but at least the luminous objects are no longer incorrectly thought to be stones struck by lightning or boulders flung out by volcanoes. Fort hoped that by accumulating data concerning other strange phenomena, a body of information could be built up to help future thinkers reconsider other accepted theories about life on earth. He kept a meticulous record of his sources of information in newspapers and journals.

As could be expected, most of Fort's contemporaries ignored him; but he also ignored them. Even when he was recognized he did not respond. On the launching of a Fortean Society in his honor by the writer Tiffany Thayer, Fort firmly declined to become a member. He may have feared that his disciples would try to pin him down to a definite set of ideas and beliefs, and he had no intention of being pinned down.

Day after day and year after year, he continued his obsessive search through the world's publications, making endless notes on slips of paper that he kept in shoe boxes. After *The Book of the Damned* came *New Lands*, then *Lo!*, and finally *Wild Talents*. He became more and more of a hermit. Almost his only recrea-

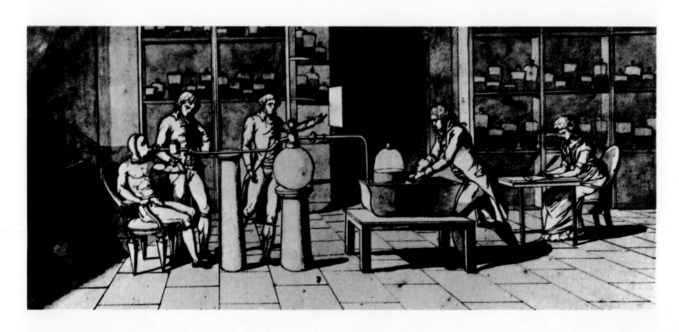

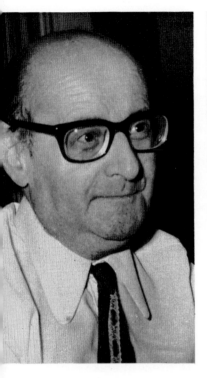
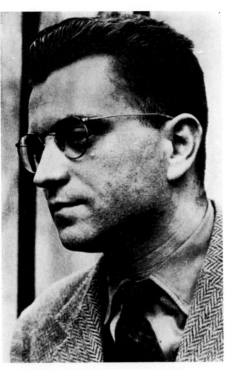

## The Fortean Revival Today

Far left: Jacques Bergier, the French writer on scientific matters, who with fellow Frenchman Louis Pauwels (left), are well known for their book *The Morning of the Magician*. First published in 1960, it contained a chapter on Fort and, by becoming an immediate best-seller, helped to rekindle interest in the American recluse.

tion was going to the movies, and he said he did that only to keep his wife company. For himself, most films "bored him to death."

While finishing *Wild Talents* Fort's health began to break down—understandably in view of his dreary existence. He finally became so weak that his wife had to send for an ambulance to take him to the hospital. When his publisher brought a copy of *Wild Talents* to him he was too weak to hold it. He died later the same day.

Fort was ignored in death as in life. Although the Fortean Society continued, it was composed of a small group of eccentrics who admired his fierce individualism. So far as the general public was concerned, his lack of style and unsystematic organization of material kept his books unread and almost forgotten for a quarter of a century after his death.

He was resurrected in France in the mid-1950s by two ardent admirers: Jacques Bergier and Louis Pauwels. Bergier had been trained as a chemist, but was fascinated by alchemy and the occult. Pauwels was a successful journalist and student of the paranormal. After pooling their talents they produced the book Fort had tried to write all his life. They called it *The Morning of the Magicians*. First published in 1960 it became an immediate success, and has been a best-seller in many languages. Pauwels and Bergier, like Fort, are critical of the mechanistic views of 19th-century science. They devote a chapter to Fort's life, quoting extensively from his works and drawing attention to his call for a revision of the very structure of our knowledge. "He sees science," they explained, "as a highly sophisticated motor car speeding along on a highway. But on either side of this marvelous track, with its shining asphalt and neon lighting, there are great tracts of wild country, full of prodigies and mystery. Stop! Explore in every direction! Leave the high road and wander!"

# Scientists Probe the Paranormal

With the international success of their book, interest in Fort revived along with interest in all studies of the paranormal and the nonmechanistic. All Fort's books were reissued and translations appeared all over the world. Recognition had finally arrived.

Ironically, assistance to this contemporary surge of interest in the paranormal has come from science, in particular from that branch of science devoted to probing the atom. Very mysterious states of being occur within the atom, and to understand them nuclear physicists have become increasingly daring in their hypotheses. Matter has become progressively dematerialized. A single electron has been made to pass through two holes in a screen at the same time—a feat, it has been said, that not even a ghost can manage! The Nobel Prize-winning British physicist Paul Direc has suggested that interstellar space is not empty, but filled by a bottomless sea of electrons with negative mass. Does this not begin to sound like Fort's Super-Sargasso Sea? Fort theorized that many strange objects falling from the sky came from this Super-Sargasso Sea, which he described as a "region somewhere above the earth's surface in which gravitation is inoperative."

Experiments of investigators into the paranormal have become more sophisticated and scientific. The card-guessing and dice-throwing experiments pioneered by J. B. Rhine at Duke University in North Carolina gave place to the advanced electrical equipment of his successor, Helmut Schmidt. In Schmidt's first precognition experiment in 1969 subjects were asked to predict

Right: British physicist Paul Dirac (center with folded arms) and his wife at a presentation in 1963. Dirac's idea that interstellar space is filled by a bottomless sea of electrons with negative mass gives credence to Fort's theory of a Super-Sargasso Sea, a "region somewhere above the earth's surface in which gravity is inoperative."

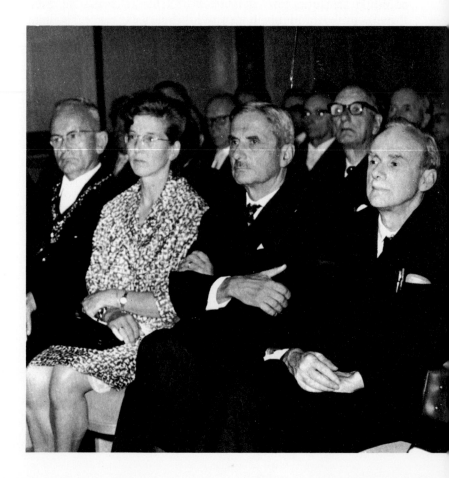

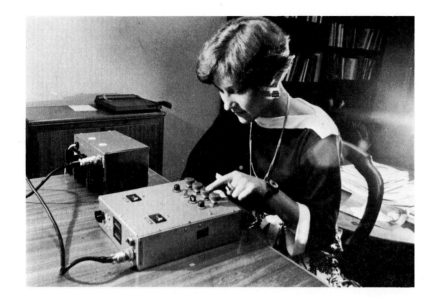

Left: one of the tests carried out by Dr. Helmut Schmidt at Duke University, North Carolina. The test is aimed at finding out whether subjects could influence events by thought control or psychokinesis (PK). Here the subject tries to predict which of four test buttons will light up next. The machine automatically counts the "hits" and "misses."

Below: leading brain scientist Sir John Eccles, whose own work in the field of brain activity, together with the results of tests like the one above, has provided him with evidence for his own theory concerning the power of mind over matter.

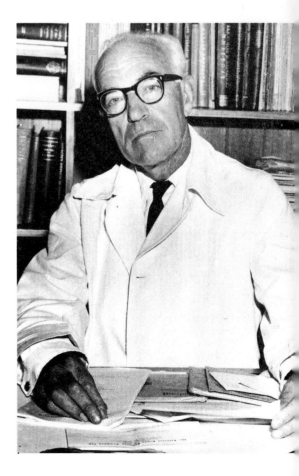

the order in which four colored lamps would be lit. The lamps were lit in an entirely random sequence provided by the discharge of electrons from radioactive strontium-90. In a series of nearly 74,000 trials, the subjects gave about 900 more correct guesses than would be expected by chance. This is a very high achievement by the laws of probability.

In 1970 Schmidt designed an experiment to see if subjects could influence events on the subatomic scale by means of thought—that is, by psychokinesis. Subjects were seated in front of a circle of nine lamps that could light up in either a clockwise or a counterclockwise direction. The direction depended on which of two numbers was produced by the Random Number Generator, and this in turn was governed by the decay of radioactive strontium-90. The subjects were asked to select a particular direction and try to cause the lamps to go on lighting up in that direction. In a run of 30,000 trials, 300 more occurred in the direction desired than could be accounted for by chance. In fact, the odds against such a score by chance over so long a run are 1000 to one. The conclusion that interested physicists and parapsychologists alike was that the emission of the electrons had been effected by human thought to some degree.

Sir John Eccles, winner of a Nobel Prize in 1963 for his work on the transmission of nerve impulses in the brain, regards such experiments as evidence for the power of mind over matter. Several physicists have suggested the existence of certain particles —variously named mindons, psychons, or psitrons—that might carry information between mind and matter and between mind and mind. Even the vast distances of interstellar space and the passage of time—for example, between the 18th and the 20th century—might be no hindrance to these particles.

Insights along these lines may help to explain the constantly puzzling phenomenon of coincidence. When the mechanistic view of the world was fully accepted, very little consideration was given to coincidence. If two strangers met and discovered they shared the same birthday, it meant nothing more than the workings of blind chance. It was argued that the year contained

365 days; people met strangers all the time; sooner or later, by the laws of chance, two people whose birthdays were on the same day would meet. Any person claiming to be scientific who devoted any further time to the matter was branded as superstitious.

In the course of the 20th century this attitude has altered, though it is still to be met with in many branches of science and among people who pride themselves on their rationalist approach to existence. It took a remarkable coincidence in the life of Arthur Koestler, Hungarian-born author and historian of scientific ideas, to change his attitude toward the paranormal.

During the 1930s Koestler had the misfortune of being arrested and imprisoned by both the Fascists and the Communists. In 1937 during the Spanish Civil War, he was imprisoned for three months and threatened with execution by the Franco regime as a suspected spy.

"In such situations," he recalled, "one tends to look for metaphysical comforts, and one day I suddenly remembered a certain episode in Thomas Mann's novel *Buddenbrooks*. One of the characters, Consul Thomas Buddenbrook, though only in his forties, knows that he is going to die. He was never given to religious speculation, but now he falls under the spell of a 'little book' in which it is explained that death is not final, merely a transition to another, impersonal kind of existence, a reunion with cosmic oneness."

The "little book" was an essay by the 19th-century German philosopher Schopenhauer, *On Death and its Relation to the Indestructability of our Essential Selves*. Remembering the passage gave Koestler, as it had given the Consul in the novel, just

Right: the Hungarian-born author and science historian Arthur Koestler. An experience of coincidence during the Spanish Civil War in the 1930s had a profound effect upon his thinking and in particular his attitude to the paranormal. While under threat of execution by Franco supporters, he remembered a passage in a book he had recently read which referred to a "little book" which gave comfort to one of the characters. This "little book" was an essay by the German philosopher Arthur Schopenhauer.

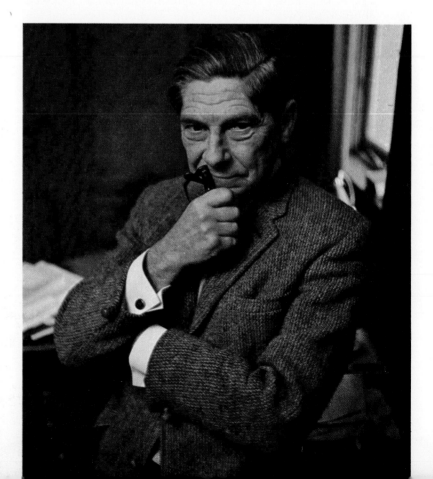

the comfort he needed. The day after his release from prison he wrote to Mann, whom he had never met, thanking him for the help he had derived from the book. Mann's reply reached him a few days later in London. Mann explained that he had not read Schopenhauer's essay since writing *Buddenbrooks* 40 years before; but the previous day, sitting in his garden, he had felt a sudden impulse to read the essay once more. He went indoors to get the volume from his library. At that moment there was a ring at the door and the mailman handed him Koestler's letter.

Perhaps this coincidence is simply an impressive demonstration of the powers of telepathy. But what is to be made of the following incident, quoted by Koestler in his book *The Roots of Coincidence*? It was recounted by the psychologist Carl Jung, who kept a logbook of coincidences. Jung writes:

"A young woman I was treating had, at a critical moment, a dream in which she was given a golden scarab. While she was telling me this dream I sat with my back to the closed window. Suddenly I heard a noise behind me, like a gentle tapping. I turned around and saw a flying insect knocking against the windowpane from outside. I opened the window and caught the creature in the air as it flew in. It was the nearest analogy to a golden scarab that one finds in our latitudes, a scaraboid beetle, the common rose-chafer (*Cetonia aurata*), which contrary to its usual habits had evidently felt an urge to get into a dark room at this particular moment."

Koestler asks, "What does this scarab at Jung's window mean?"

In our present state of knowledge, all answers are obliged to be

# An Incredible Coincidence?

Below: the German novelist Thomas Mann. It was his novel *Buddenbrooks*, first published in 1900, which Koestler remembered when under sentence of death. When Koestler later wrote to Mann telling him of the incident, Mann, whom he had never met, replied that immediately before receiving Koestler's letter he had felt a sudden impulse to reread the essay by Schopenhauer.

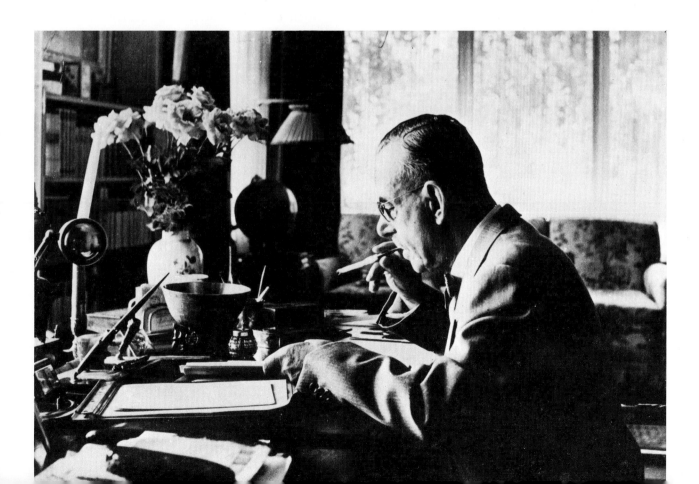

# "Everything is Interrelated"

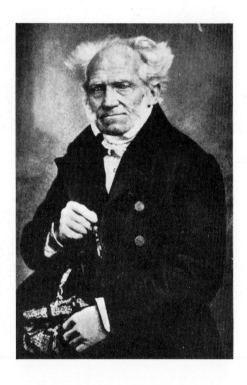

speculative but Koestler suggests that the right approach to an answer lies in considering once more the views of the universe held by thinkers before the mechanistic revolution: "There is one common flow, one common breath, all things are in sympathy." Schopenhauer set his thinking firmly against the prevailing mechanistic views of his age. Where they insisted that physical cause must precede physical effect, he believed that there was also a metaphysical realm, a kind of universal consciousness, so that the events in a person's life existed at one and the same time in the reality of ordinary, everyday perceptions and in a greater reality. Each person is the hero of his or her own drama while simultaneously figuring in a wider drama. "Thus everything is interrelated and mutually attuned," said Schopenhauer. In his view, a coincidence is a single event occurring in two different realities.

This profound interrelationship is accepted in nuclear physics. "What we call an isolated particle," writes Dr. F. Capra, "is in reality the product of its interaction with its surroundings. It is therefore impossible to separate any part of the universe from the rest."

The 300-year-old division of the universe by science into "mind" and "matter" shows signs of coming together as the matter of the atom is disclosed to be a form of energy. The relationship between this energy and the human mind is still far from clear, but a readiness to consider the relationship now exists.

Schopenhauer believed that existence was "a great dream" dreamed by an entity he termed "the Will to Life." Others who have followed him in calling the universe a dream or a thought have done so not from any temptation toward mysticism, but as the outcome of their scientific thought. The kind of scientist against whom Charles Hay Fort pitted himself no longer holds undisputed sway.

Above: the German philosopher Arthur Schopenhauer. It was Schopenhauer who challenged the mechanistic, cause-and-effect approach to natural phenomena of 19th-century science. "Everything," he wrote, "is interrelated and mutually attuned." He went on to express the view that a coincidence is a single event occurring in two different realities.

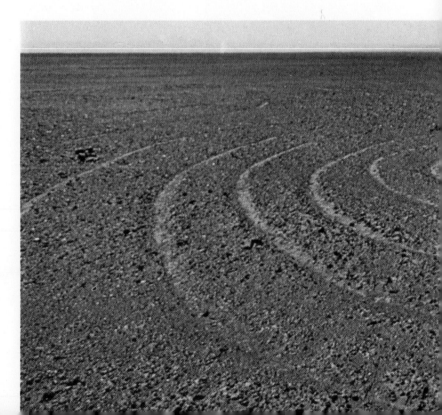

In spite of this new approach, however, an explanation may never be found for some of the mysterious happenings of the past. For example, in August 1887 peasants of the small village of Banjos, Spain, saw two young children walk out of a cave. Their clothes were unfamiliar and they could speak no Spanish, but even more extraordinary, their skin was green. Where they came from no one has ever discovered. There have been other sudden appearances—and sudden disappearances—equally unexplained. David Lang, a farmer of Texas, vanished from the middle of a field in full view of four witnesses. No one is ever likely to find out what happened to him.

Shall we ever solve the mystery of crewless ships like the *Mary Celeste*? Will we discover who planned and built some of the mysterious structures in the world? Our increasing knowledge of our surroundings can solve some puzzles that baffled our ancestors. Black rain, showers of blood, fish, and other creatures falling from the sky: we think we know their true nature. Further study may bring the answer to the perplexing problem of the Bermuda Triangle, that weird area of the Atlantic where planes and ships still vanish today. But will we find the explanation to the gruesome deaths of certain people by spontaneous combustion? What about objects that seem cursed? Their evil reputation may be the effect of imagination; but could there be some innate property in the objects that brings death to those associated with them? Science has become more concerned with probing such mysteries, and today seems less the full opposite of the paranormal.

Fort once said that every science is a mutilated octopus. "If its tentacles were not clipped to stumps, it would feel its way into disturbing contacts." Half a century after his death, at least some of those tentacles have been allowed to grow. It seems that we may at last be entering the age of "disturbing contacts."

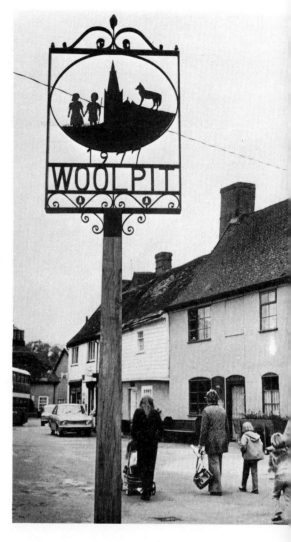

Above: this inn sign in the English village of Woolpit commemorates the strange appearance of two extraordinary children who walked out of a cave near the village in the 11th century. Both children were normal in every way, except that they were green. The boy died, but the girl lived on to learn English, and explained that they had come from a land where there was no sunlight. A similar story is told of two green children who appeared in Spain in 1887.

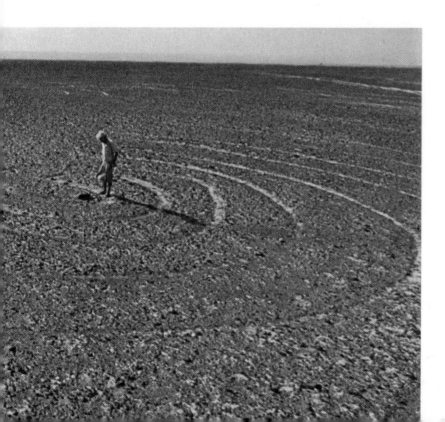

Left: German mathematician and geographer Maria Reiche, who has made it her life's work to interpret the extraordinary marks on the vast Nazca Plain in Peru. Because the huge figures can only be seen properly from the sky, it has even been suggested that they are landing signals for ancient UFOs.

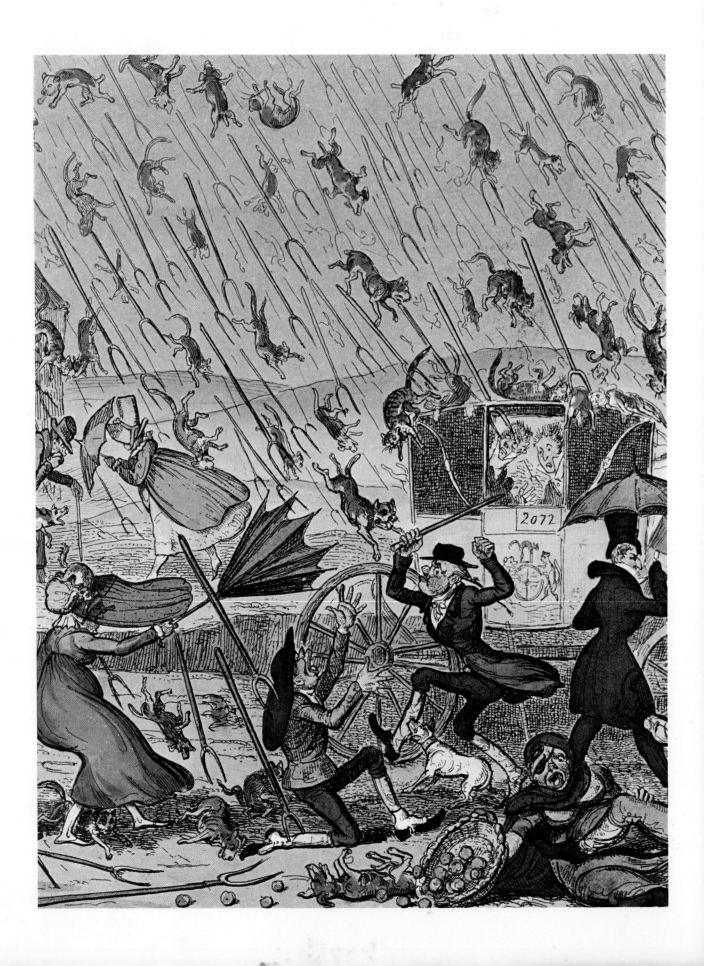

# Chapter 2
# Curious Rain

Of all the strange happenings on record, one of the most common is unnatural rain. Frogs, periwinkles, jelly—these and more have poured out of the skies. What causes such falls? What about the unusual colored rains of yellow, black, or red, or the strange blankets of color-tinted dry frogs? Charles Fort tied odd rains in with his theory of an extraterrestrial source for life on earth. Strangely enough, recent analyses of meteorites have shown them to contain certain substances necessary to living cells. Is there something to the idea that life as we know it originated outside of earth?

We use the phrase "raining cats and dogs" to describe a downpour. But rains of many kinds of living creatures have actually been reported from earliest times and all over the world. On May 28, 1881 during a thunderstorm on the outskirts of Worcester, England, tons of periwinkles and small hermit crabs fell on Cromer Gardens Road and the surrounding fields. They came down out of the sky in a broad band extending for about a mile. When news of this amazing fall reached the center of Worcester, a town 40 miles from the sea, many people hurried to Cromer Gardens Road carrying pots, pans, bags, and even trunks. One garden alone yielded two sacks of periwinkles; 10 sacks of them altogether were taken back to the markets of Worcester for sale.

Showers of fish, frogs, and many other animals are rare but have long been known of. Like comets and shooting stars, they were frequently interpreted as omens of calamity. Such an attitude is understandable. People need an ordered environment if they are to feel at home in the world, and fish falling from the sky is a clear sign of disorder. In the 18th and 19th centuries many rationalists overreacted to what they took to be the superstitions of earlier ages, and denied altogether the possibility of such marvels. So the case of the Worcester periwinkles was explained as the result of a fish dealer who abandoned his stock on the road before the storm. Two people were found who reported that they had seen the periwinkles on the ground before they came down from the sky. It is hard to understand why a fish dealer would

Opposite: "Very Unpleasant Weather," a 19th-century cartoon illustrating the old saying "It's raining cats, dogs, and pitchforks." Charles Fort was fascinated by the many reports of objects of all kinds falling from the sky. Could the saying have arisen from an actual rain of animals and even implements?

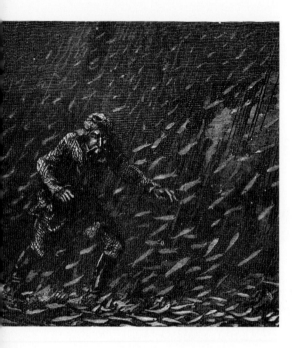

Above: a 19th-century engraving of a fall of fish. Fort in his *Book of the Damned* lists five such occurrences one after another and gives his own explanation "that the bottom of a super-geographical pond had dropped out."

Right: the cover of *Lo!*, Fort's third book. One of Fort's few friends, Tiffany Thayer, suggested the title, "because in the text the astronomers are forever calculating and then pointing to the sky where they figure a new star or something should be and saying '*Lo!*'—and there's nothing whatever to be seen where they point." Fort agreed to the suggested title at once.

want to get rid of his winkles when, as was pointed out, they would sell at a high price in Worcester that day. This unseen merchant, then, introduces a solution as unlikely as the idea that periwinkles and small crabs somehow managed to get into the air and later fell out of it.

About 20 years earlier, on February 16, 1861, a weird shower had been reported from Singapore. An earthquake had been followed by three days of incessant rain, in the course of which great numbers of fish were found in the puddles of streets throughout the city. Local residents reported that the fish had fallen from the sky. One writer of an account in *La Science pour Tous* stated that he himself did not see any of the fish falling—adding that the deluge of rain was so heavy that sometimes he could not see more than three yards ahead of him. But he specifically mentioned that some of the fish had been found in his courtyard, which was surrounded by high walls. The explanation generally accepted, however, was that overflowing streams had left the fish on the land after the waters receded.

Occasionally there is some truth in the explanation that objects said to have fallen from the sky were on the ground all the time. Showers of frogs and toads have been reported many times, frequently in Italy in both ancient and modern times. Arguments regularly broke out as to whether the animals had originated on the earth or in the clouds. Some witnesses reported that they had seen the frogs fall. Other witnesses said that they had seen them only close to the walls of houses, which could mean that they had slipped down from the gutters of the roofs. A German naturalist writing in 1874 observed that frogs said to have been rained down but not seen to fall were seldom dead, lamed, or bruised because, he implied, they had been on the ground all the time. "The appearance of the frogs after a rain is easily accounted for by the circumstance that during a long-continued drought they remain in a

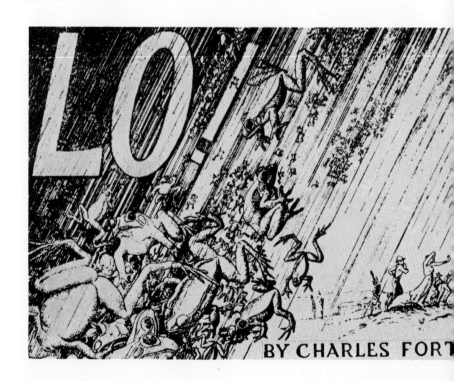

BY CHARLES FORT

state of torpor in holes and coverts, and all that the rain does is the enlivening of them, giving them new spirits, and calling them forth to enjoy the element they delight to live in."

Thomas Cooper, a popular 19th-century lecturer on Christianity, witnessed the phenomenon of raining frogs during his boyhood in Lincolnshire, England. "I am as sure of what I relate as I am of my own existence," he declared. He said that the frogs were alive and jumping, and that they "fell on the pavement at our feet, and came tumbling down the spouts from the tiles of the houses into the water tubs." It is interesting that in most of the reports of frog showers, the size of the frogs is always very small.

There seems no reason to doubt that showers of frogs occur from time to time—which is not to deny that at other times the frogs simply emerge from holes in the ground when the first raindrops enliven them. It seems hasty to conclude either that frogs seen after a rainstorm have always fallen from the skies, or that frogs seen after a rainstorm were always on the ground beforehand. The evidence seems to show that sometimes frogs fall from above and sometimes they don't.

The scientifically accepted explanation for a frog rain is that they have been carried in the air, sometimes for great distances, from a pool or stream where they were sucked up by sudden strong winds. Charles Hay Fort, the cataloger of phenomena who was rejected by science in his day, regarded this as unlikely. But Fort was also guilty of error, and not above altering the evidence when it suited his argument. In *The Book of the Damned* he wrote: "After one of the greatest hurricanes in the history of Ireland, some fish were found as far as 15 yards from the edge of the lake." In these words he implied that an unprecedented hurricane is required to move a fish a few yards, because he wanted to cast doubt on the likelihood of the wind moving any object a matter of miles—for instance, periwinkles 40 miles from the mouth of the nearest river to Worcester, or the enormous number of eels that fell in Coalburg, Alabama, on May 29, 1892.

The power of the wind is enormous. On August 19, 1845 a whirlwind in France uprooted 180 large trees in a few seconds in Houlme, and destroyed three mills in Monville, dropping planks from the factory buildings half an hour later on the outskirts of Dieppe 20 miles (32 kilometers) away. Though it takes a whirlwind to transport planks, a far less violent wind can bear away small frogs, periwinkles, and eels.

So many eels fell in Coalburg that farmers came into town with carts and took them away to use as fertilizer for their fields. Eels also fell in Hendon in the northeast of England on August 24, 1918. Hundreds of them covered a small area about 60 by 30 yards. Hendon is a coastal town, but the eels were probably carried in the air for some time and from another part of the coast because, according to witnesses, "the eels were all dead, and indeed stiff and hard, when picked up, immediately after the occurrence."

Fish that fall in showers generally are dead. Lunged creatures are frequently alive, making it difficult to say how long they have been in the air. Live lizards fell on the streets of Montreal, Canada, on December 28, 1857. Snails fell in such quantities in Redruth, England, on July 8, 1886, that people were able to

# Unbelievable Phenomena

Below: the plague of frogs which was the second of the plagues of Egypt described in the Book of Exodus in the Old Testament. Was this strange phenomenon just another of the strange rains that Fort describes but never attempts to explain away?

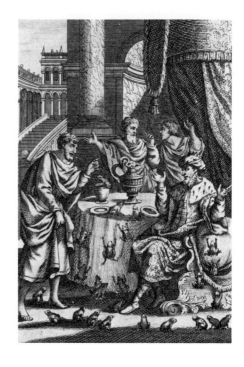

# What Causes Them?

gather them up in hatfuls. A yellow cloud appeared over Paderborn, Germany, on August 9, 1892, and a torrent of rain from it brought hundreds of mussels. More recently, on September 28, 1953 a shower of toads fell on Orlando, Florida, in the middle of the afternoon.

An uncommon shower of live fish descended on Mountain Ash, Wales, on February 11, 1859. The vicar of the neighboring town of Aberdare interviewed John Lewis, an employee of the sawmill in Mountain Ash. Said Lewis: "I was getting out a piece of timber for the purpose of setting it for the saw, when I was startled by something falling all over me—down my neck, on my head, and on my back. On putting my hand down my neck I was surprised to find they were little fish. By this time I saw the whole ground covered with them. I took off my hat, the brim of which was full of them. They were jumping all about. They covered the ground in a long strip of about 80 yards by 12, as we measured afterward." These fish fell in two showers, with an interval of about 10 minutes, each shower lasting about two minutes. Some people, thinking they might be sea fish, placed them in salt water, whereupon they instantly died. Those that were placed in fresh water thrived well, and were later identified as sticklebacks.

Showers of living objects fall over a relatively small area, but other kinds of unnatural rain can sometimes cover an entire country. Yellow rain has been reported from all parts of the world, and because of the Christian link-up between brimstone and hell, the yellow has been popularly identified as sulfur and regarded as a warning from on high. Although yellow rain does not look different while it is falling, the ground is afterward found to be covered with a fine yellow dust. This dust burns easily, encouraging the belief that it is sulfur, but in the majority of cases the accepted explanation is that the yellow is pollen from trees. A forest of hazelnut trees coming into flower in April, or beeches in May or June, or pine trees from midsummer onward,

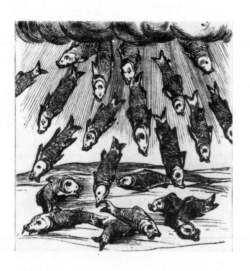

Above: one of the many unexplained showers of fish that have occurred around the world. One of the most recent was in Wales in 1859, and another in Singapore in 1861. Fort suggested that "a whole lakeful of fish had been shaken down from the Super-Sargasso Sea."

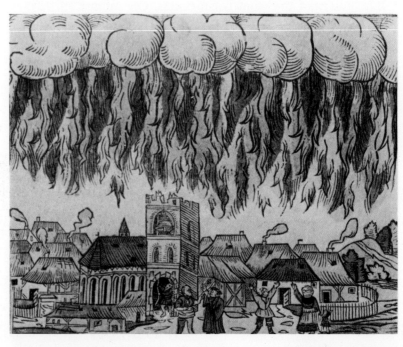

Right: woodcut of an unexplained rain of fire which occurred near the town of Forcheim, Germany, in 1560. Large, long flames of fire came down from the sky, and after an hour or so the heat became so great that an alarm was raised. Many people saw the fire, but almost as many ideas were put forward to explain it.

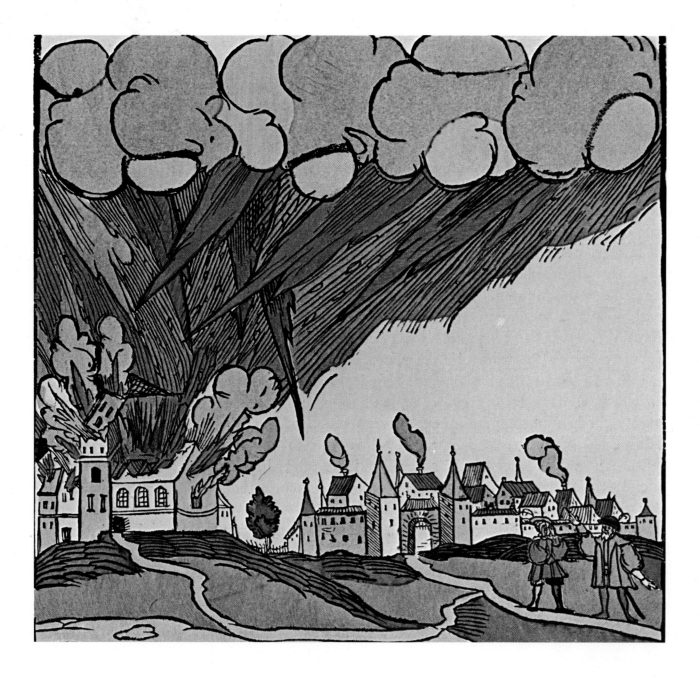

can produce a vast amount of fine pollen—and a strong wind following a spell of tranquil weather can bear away enormous quantities, which may subsequently fall down with rain.

Sometimes a yellow substance falls in the absence of rain. On February 27, 1877 in Peckloh, Germany, a golden-yellow fall was found to contain four different kinds of organisms. Their shapes resembled microscopic arrows, coffee beans, horns, and disks, and none was identified as pollen.

Another unnatural shower often reported is black rain. The blame for this has usually been placed fairly on smoke belching from factory chimneys in an industrial area somewhere along the path of the wind. But on August 14, 1888 there was a heavy downpour of black rain on the Cape of Good Hope, a part of South Africa then remote from any large concentration of industry. Could the blackness have come from a forest fire? This was the explanation given to account for the celebrated Canadian black rain 69 years before the Cape Hope incident, when it had been said that the rainclouds had been stained by the dense smoke of forest fires south of the Ohio River. In the case of the Cape of Good Hope, however, the direction of the prevailing wind makes

Above: this terrible storm took place over Germany in 1555. In the late evening there was such a spectacle of sheet lightning and thunder that it was taken to be a sign from God that all Christians should repent of all their sins, and take such a demonstration of divine wrath to heart.

# Rains of Blood

it unlikely that fires in the forest region could have been the cause. Nor would smoke have produced a rain so black as to be described as "a shower of ink."

What was not realized in the past was how enormous a quantity of material the wind can carry, and how vast the distances it can carry the burden. Concentrations of dust in major storms have been estimated to reach as much as 200,000 tons per square mile of land surface. In February 1903 large areas of Western Europe were covered by a dark sand blown from the Sahara Desert. It varied widely in color, different reports describing it as reddish, yellowish, gray, and the color of chocolate. In one place it was described as "sticky to the touch and slightly iridescent." A quantity amounting to about 10 million tons is calculated to have fallen on England alone. A similar fall occurred in the south of England and Wales on June 30, 1968, when storms broke after the hottest day for 11 years. The following morning a fine sandy dust was found coating parked cars, greenhouses, windows, and washing. The dust was yellow, pink, or bright red, and analysis established that it had originated in the Sahara.

Red rain—popularly mistaken for showers of blood—has in the past understandably spread more alarm than rain of any other color. Homer tells of showers of blood that fell upon the Greek heroes at ancient Troy as an omen of their approaching death in battle. References to similar showers in Roman times mention the terror they caused among the populace. St. Gregory of Tours, the 6th-century historian of the Franks, recorded that in A.D. 582 in the Paris region "real blood rained from a cloud, falling on the clothes of many people, and so staining them with gore that they stripped them off in horror."

A long list of unnatural rainfalls was compiled by the French astronomer and writer Camille Flammarion, who died in 1925. He was fascinated with anything to do with the heavens, and in the chapter entitled "Prodigies" in his book *The Atmosphere*, he listed over 40 references to "showers of blood" before 1800 and a further 21 that had been reported in the 19th century. The reports cover a wide area, from Brussels to Baghdad, from Hungary

Below: this extraordinary shower of what appeared to be blood occurred in the city of Lisbon in 1551, where it not surprisingly terrified the city's inhabitants.

Below right: blood-red rain that fell in England and Wales during the night of June 30, 1968, seen here on the windshield and hood of a car. Meteorologists explained it as being the result of fine sand being picked up in the Sahara in dust storms and carried northward in the upper air. It was calculated that 10 million tons of sand fell in thundery rain that night.

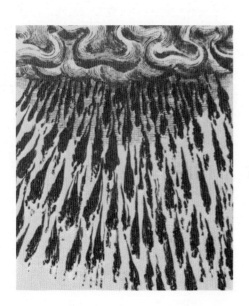

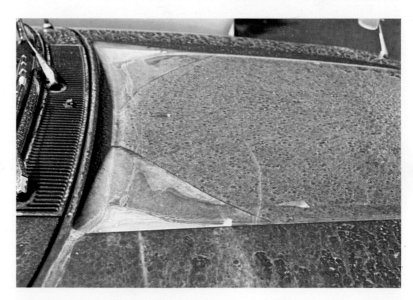

to Lisbon. When the reaction of the populace is given it is invariably one of panic. Supernatural signs were sometimes reported as accompanying the showers. During a red rain that fell
on France and Germany in March 1181 a luminous cross was
observed in the skies. Frequently the showers were said to be the
warning of death; when showers of blood persisted intermit-
tently for three days and nights in Brescia, Italy, they were
followed by the death of Pope Adrian II on the fourth day.

One of the first to attempt to find a cause for these fearful
showers was a Mr. de Peiresc. When numerous red spots had
been discovered on the walls and stones on the outskirts of Aix-
en-Provence in July 1608, the local priests attributed them to the
influence of the Devil. Mr. de Peiresc examined the spots carefully and concluded that they were not of blood—the Devil's or
otherwise—but the secretions of a butterfly. He pointed out that
the species now known as the Large Tortoiseshell, which has a
red secretion, had been seen in unusually large numbers that

Below: a contemporary representation of an
apparently inexplicable shower of blood
near Aix-en-Provence in France in 1608. On
this occasion, a certain M. de Peiresc
pointed out that the red spots were simply
secretions of the large tortoiseshell butterfly,
which had been seen in unusually large
numbers that year.

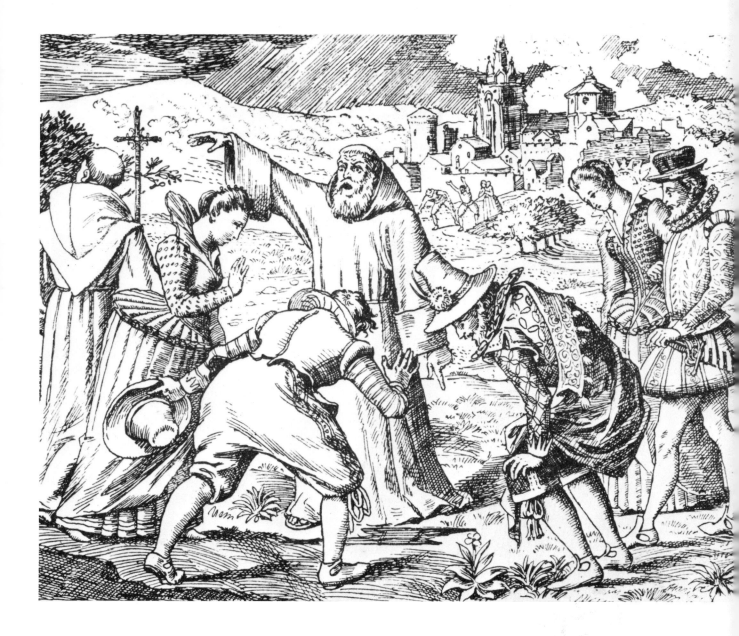

# The Showers of Cruciform Hail

month. Moreover, red spots were absent from the center of the town, where the butterflies had not made an appearance, and had been found on the higher parts of the buildings, about the level to which they flew. However, the citizens of Aix preferred to believe that the Devil was the culprit.

In general, the cause of rains of blood is, like that of yellow rain, dust originating in a desert region. Signor Sementini, professor of chemistry at Naples, was ahead of his time when in 1813 he accurately identified as dust the red shower that fell on Gerace, Italy, on March 14 of that year. He also recorded a vivid impression of the event. "The wind had been westerly for two days," he wrote, "when at 2 p.m. it suddenly became calm, the atmosphere grew cloudy, and the darkness gradually became so great as to

Right: a contemporary illustration of an extraordinary collection of objects seen in the sky over Nuremberg, Germany, in 1561. The objects included blood-red streaks, crosses, rings around the sun, and two large cylinders. All these fell to the ground, at which point an enormous spear appeared in the sky.

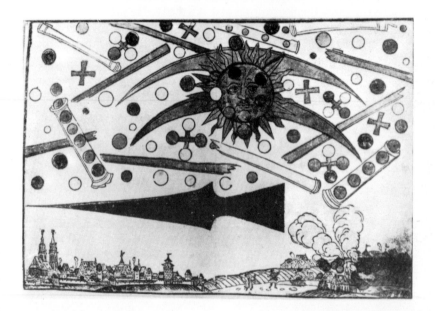

render it necessary to light candles. The citizens, alarmed by the obscurity, rushed in a crowd to the cathedral to pray. The sky assumed the color of red-hot iron, thunder and lightning continued for a considerable length of time, and the sea was heard to roar, although six miles from the city. Large drops of rain then began to fall, which were of a blood-red color."

The rain deposited a yellow powder and had a slight earthy taste. Sementini analyzed it and concluded that it was a terrestrial dust of some kind, but could not guess where it came from. It is now difficult to establish if it had blown from the Sahara since one account states that the wind was westerly while another gives it as easterly. Such a basic error, made at a time when accurate observations were being attempted, throws serious doubts on earlier reports, made when natural phenomena were unquestioningly regarded as direct communications from God, and reported in that light.

In this category must be included showers of crosses. In France in the year 764 crosses were said to have appeared on men's clothes during a shower of blood. In 1094 crosses are reported to have fallen from heaven, alighting on the garments of priests. In 1501 crosses rained down in Germany and Belgium during the week before Easter, and left marks on clothes, skin, and bread.

In the annals of unusual rains, "the Miracle of Remiremont" holds a unique position. On the afternoon of May 26, 1907 the Abbé Gueniot was snug in his library as a hailstorm battered down outside. Suddenly his housekeeper called to him to come see the extraordinary hailstones. She told him that images of Our Lady of the Treasures were printed on them. The Abbé later described the event like this:

"In order to satisfy her, I glanced carelessly at the hailstones, which she held in her hand. But, since I did not want to see anything, and moreover could not do so without my spectacles, I turned to go back to my book. She urged, 'I beg of you to put on your glasses.' I did so, and saw very distinctly on the front of the

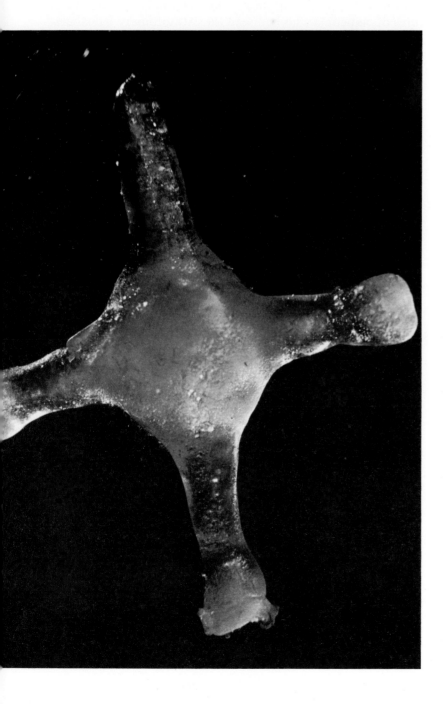

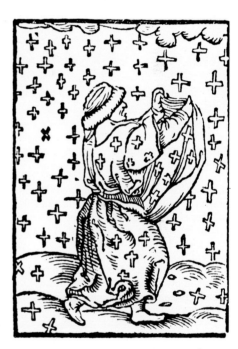

Above: a rain of crosses reported in 1094, shown here in a contemporary woodcut. Fort found and recorded several accounts of falls of tiny crosses. He adds, "But some are Roman crosses, some St. Andrew's, some Maltese."

Left: this photograph of a hailstone in the shape of a cross that fell in the United States perhaps provides the explanation for the many accounts of cruciform hailstones. Moreover, it has been suggested by scientists that there is nothing mysterious about showers of hailstones of a particular shape or size.

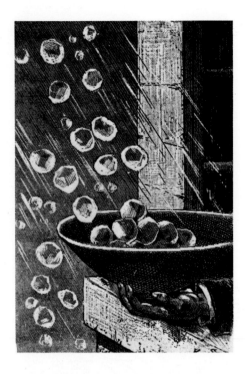

Above: a 19th-century illustration of a shower of hailstones "as large as oranges." There are plenty of accounts of showers of this kind, or even larger in size. In 1831, in the city now known as Istanbul, hail fell in stones weighing more than a pound apiece and as large as a man's fist. If this is true, then can we doubt the truth of an account from the time of Charlemagne of a fall of hailstones 15 feet long and 6 feet wide, nor even of an account from 18th-century India of hailstones the size of elephants?

Right: this extraordinary photograph shows men clearing hail from an inn yard in Camelford, Devon, England, where an intense fall of rain was accompanied by unusually heavy hail.

hailstones, which were slightly convex in the center, although the edges were somewhat worn, the bust of a woman, with a robe that was turned up at the bottom, like a priest's robe. I should, perhaps, describe it more exactly by saying that it was like the Virgin of the Hermits. The outline of the images was slightly hollow, as if they had been formed with a punch, but were very boldly drawn. Mlle. André asked me to notice certain details of the costume, but I refused to look at it any longer. I was ashamed of my credulity, feeling sure that the Blessed Virgin would hardly concern herself with instantaneous photographs on hailstones."

Nonetheless, the Abbé picked up three of the hailstones to weigh them and found they weighed between six and seven ounces. One was perfectly round and had a seam all around it, as though it had been cast in a mold. Later he collected the signatures of 50 people who had seen the extraordinary hailstones.

There seems little doubt that the hail that fell on Remiremont that afternoon bore strange markings. The Secretary of the French Academy wondered whether lightning might have struck a medal of the Virgin and reproduced the image on the hailstones. Other reports state that the print was found on the inside of the hailstones after they had been split. The key to the mystery probably lies there. When hailstones are formed, they are frequently tossed up and down between layers of cold and less cold air, in the process accumulating several layers of ice that show as rings on a cross-section of the individual hailstone. The circumstances of hail formation at Remiremont may have been such as to allow an irregular layering of ice that was then seen to resemble the appearance of the Virgin. It is worth mentioning that a few days

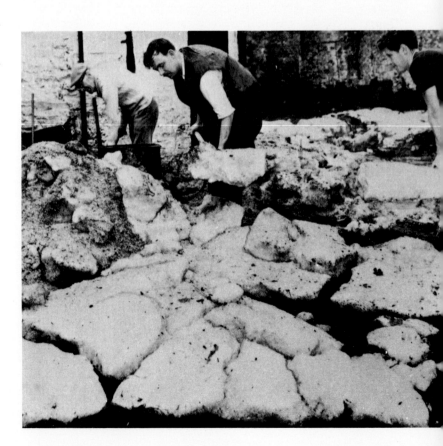

before the storm, the local government had forbidden a religious procession through the town and this had created a high degree of agitated excitement among the devout—an atmosphere conducive to the occurrence of a miracle.

Showers of a liquid looking like milk have been reported at various times in Italy. In one such rain, coins and copper pots exposed to the downfall became silvered, and kept this appearance for three days. This suggests that the rain contained mercury, although it is hard to imagine the circumstances under which this would be possible.

In the Silesian province of what is now Poland, at a time of great shortage of wheat, a violent storm broke over the countryside—and afterward the ground was covered with small round seeds. The country folk at first believed their prayers had been answered and that the skies had rained millet. Unfortunately, the seeds proved to be from a local species of the herb speedwell. In 1804, however, a real wheatfall took place in parts of Andalucia in southern Spain. What happened was that a hurricane removed the grain from a threshing floor in Tutua on the Moroccan coast, carried it across the Straits of Gibraltar, and dropped it on the amazed and grateful Spanish peasants.

Fort gives his own eccentric possibilities for these phenomena:

"Debris from interplanetary disasters.

"Aerial battles.

"Food-supplies from cargoes of super-vessels, wrecked in interplanetary traffic."

In the spring of 1695 dwellers in the Irish counties of Limerick and Tipperary experienced showers of a greasy substance having a "very stinking smell." This grease, which the local people called "butter," fell in lumps an inch in diameter, and was soft, clammy, and dark yellow in color. The Bishop of Cloyne called it "stinking dew." Fort says, "We'll not especially wonder whether these butter-like or oily substances were food or fuel . . ." and goes on to suggest that they fell from "a super-construction, plying back and forth from Jupiter and Mars and Venus."

Fort's achievement in tracking down many thousands of strange happenings—and urging people to think about them—is undermined by the weird theories he put forward to account for them. It is as though he were still a little boy deliberately pasting wrong labels on cans, as he used to do in rebellion when working in his father's store. In his rebellion against autocratic science, did he sometimes deliberately apply a wrong label? In any case, his view of the universe was something like a store out of which he pulled a variety of goods.

For example, sometimes he imagined that a circle of ice surrounded the earth, that fragments break off and fall to the earth as hail, and that we see the stars through the resulting gaps. Other times he felt that the earth is ringed with a gelatinous substance, and that globs of this jelly also fall down. He talks of a "super-geographical pond" above the earth—his Super-Sargasso Sea.

Fort may not have believed all these fanciful theories—or at least not all of them at the same time—but the space probes of the 1960s and 70s have exposed them as nonsense. Nowadays it is difficult to read any of Fort's books without finding a foolish and disproved theory on every page, including the gelatin ring.

# The Flying Hay

Below: a well-documented case of flying hay in the neighborhood of Wrexham, Wales, in the 1860s. According to newspaper accounts, the haymakers who saw the hay said it was flying higher than they had even seen a crow fly, and though there was a slight wind, it was flying in the opposite direction. As one account added, "it caused much consternation while passing over the town."

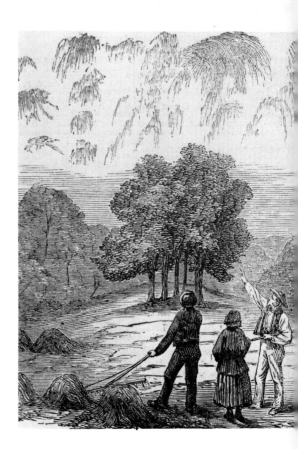

# Manna Explained?

Opposite: a 15th-century Flemish painting of the Israelites picking up the manna as it fell from heaven during their wanderings in the Sinai desert, as described in the Book of Exodus.

Below: among the numerous rational explanations for the miraculous fall of manna, one is that the Israelites were blessed with a shower of the secretion of an insect which sucks the sap of the tamarisk, small drops of which fall to the ground as sticky honeydew. The Bedouin of today still collect this sweet substance, which they regard as a great delicacy.

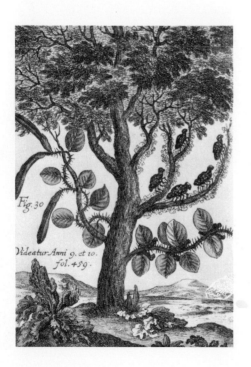

But can there be a fall of jelly? In Massachussetts on the night of August 13, 1819 a bright light was seen moving above Amherst, and a sound was heard that was described as being as loud as an explosion. Next morning, in the front yard of a professor, was found a substance "unlike anything before observed by anyone who saw it. It was a bowl-shaped object, about eight inches in diameter, and one inch thick. Bright, buff-colored, and having upon it a fine nap. Upon removing this covering, a buff-colored pulpy substance of the consistency of soft soap was found, of an offensive, suffocating smell. A few minutes of exposure to the air changed the buff color to a livid color resembling venous blood. It absorbed moisture quickly from the air and liquefied."

No explanation of this strange object was put forward at the time, but a few years later a similar one was found near the same place. It was shown to Professor Edward Hitchcock, who pronounced it to be a gelatinous fungus. He said similar fungi might spring up within the next 24 hours, and sure enough two others had done so before nightfall.

The moving light and the loud sound remain unexplained, but the fungus was probably of the kind called nostoc. Natural appearances of nostoc in unusual places presumably gave rise to the reports of more jellylike falls in several other parts of the United States over the years. Lumps of jelly looking like coagulated white of egg have been found in Rahway, New Jersey. A mass like boiled starch was reported from West Point, New York. The flakes of a substance that looked like thin slices of beef floated down from a clear sky at Olympian Springs, Kentucky. This was a thick shower, but fell only on a narrow strip of land about 100 yards long and about 50 yards wide.

Nostoc—a word first coined by the 16th-century German physician and alchemist Paracelsus—is usually considered, like frogs, to have been on the ground all the time when said to have fallen from the sky. But there is no reason why it should not occasionally, again like frogs, be borne in the air by winds and fall to the ground when the wind drops. A primitive alga, nostoc is thought to be one of the world's oldest organisms. In dry periods the common form of nostoc can shrivel into paper-thin strands, swelling up again after rain or in the presence of moisture. Practically invisible when dry, the fungus colonies can take in water and enlarge quickly to the size of a grapefruit. These sudden appearances have often given rise to the idea that they dropped from the sky.

Some varieties of nostoc are eaten by South American Indians, and one of its species may have been the substance called manna in the Bible. Manna, which provided food for the Israelites during their wanderings in the Sinai desert, cannot now be identified with any certainty. The sweet globules produced by the lichen *Lecanora esculenta* are thought to be one of the most likely sources, although this lichen is not now found in Sinai. Another possibility is the secretions of an insect that sucks the sap of the tamarisk, small drops of which fall to the ground as sticky honeydew. At the beginning of Chapter 16 of Exodus, Moses tells the Israelites that the Lord will rain bread from heaven, but the belief that the manna would come from above is linked to the old and widespread idea that dew falls from the sky. "In the morning

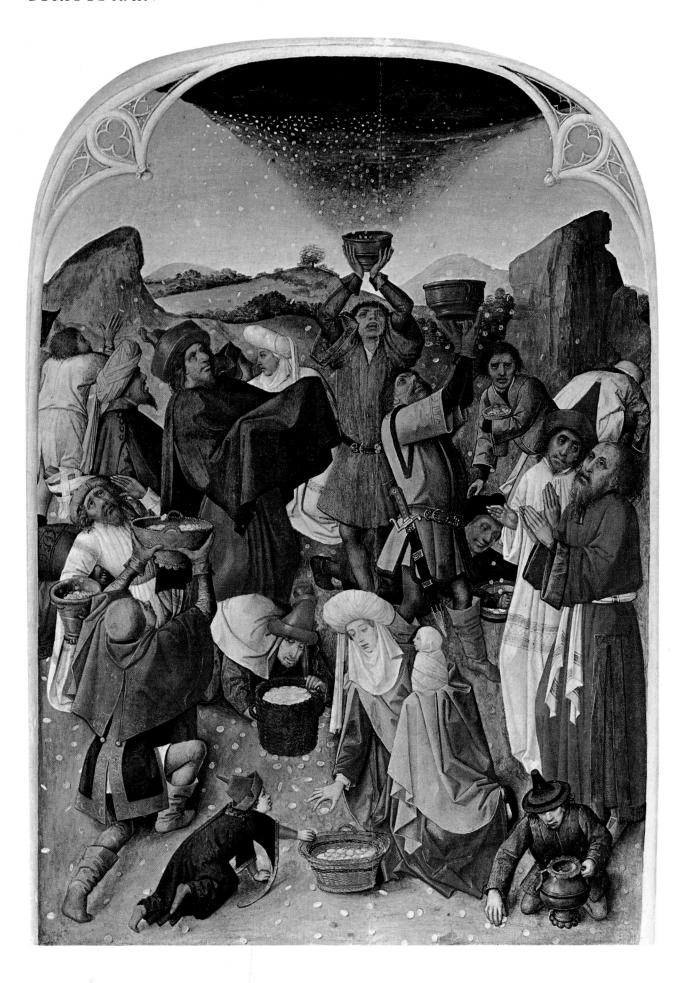

# Miraculous Meteorites

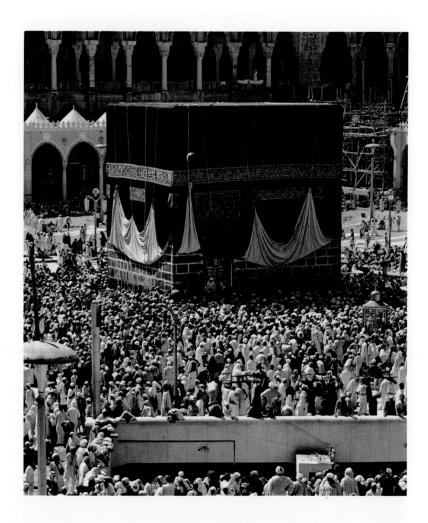

Right: the Kaaba at Mecca was a sanctuary and a religious center for the nomadic Arabs centuries before the time of Muhammed. Today it is a sacred shrine which every Moslem pilgrim to Mecca must kiss. Built into one corner of the Kaaba is a large meteorite which fell to earth at about the time of Muhammad, and which has understandably added to the religious importance of the shrine.

the dew lay round about the host. And when the dew that lay was gone up, behold, upon the face of the wilderness, there lay a small round thing, as small as the hoar frost on the ground."

It is now known that dew is not a precipitation like rain, but is formed on the ground as a deposit of water vapor. But the idea that dew drops from the sky is persistent. Schoolchildren in France in the early years of this century were still being taught that it dropped. At an earlier period pearls were thought to be congealed dew. It was said that oysters rose to the surface of the sea during the night and caught the falling dewdrops, which in time hardened into pearls.

Although Charles Fort is mistaken in most of his theories, he is not entirely wrong in suggesting that certain mysterious happenings are extraterrestrial: meteorites, for example. Their seemingly supernatural origin has frequently led to them becoming objects of worship. One that fell in Arabia about the time of Muhammad is still preserved in Mecca, built into a corner of the sacred shrine known as the Kaaba; every pilgrim must kiss it in the course of his visit to the city. The Roman Emperor Heliogabalus had a black meteorite carried in solemn procession through streets strewn with gold dust. Even when not worshipped, the fallen meteorite was long regarded as a miraculous object. The oldest authenticated meteorite in a museum is the one that fell on the Swiss town of Ensisheim in 1492. The local church records give a good contemporary account of the event:

"On the 16th November 1492 a singular miracle happened: for between 11 and 12 in the forenoon, with a loud crash of thunder and a prolonged noise heard afar off, there fell in the town of Ensisheim a stone weighing 260 pounds. It was seen by a child to strike the ground in a field near the canton called Gisgaud, where it made a hole more than five feet deep. It was taken to the church as being a miraculous object. The noise was heard so distinctly at Lucerne, Villing, and many other places that in each of them it was thought that some houses had fallen. King Maximilian, who was then at Ensisheim, had the stone carried to the castle: after breaking off two pieces, one for the Duke Sigismund of Austria and the other for himself, he forbade further damage, and ordered the stone to be suspended in the parish church."

Not all visiting objects that arrive from beyond the earth come as stones. The strange dry fogs that at long intervals blanket wide parts of the globe may occur when the earth passes through the vast clouds of dust that are believed to occur in the depths of

Below: the world's oldest authenticated meteorite fell on the town of Ensisheim, Switzerland, in November 1492. It made a crater in the ground over 5 feet deep and was later found to weigh 260 pounds. Local church records tell how "it was taken to the church as being a miraculous object."

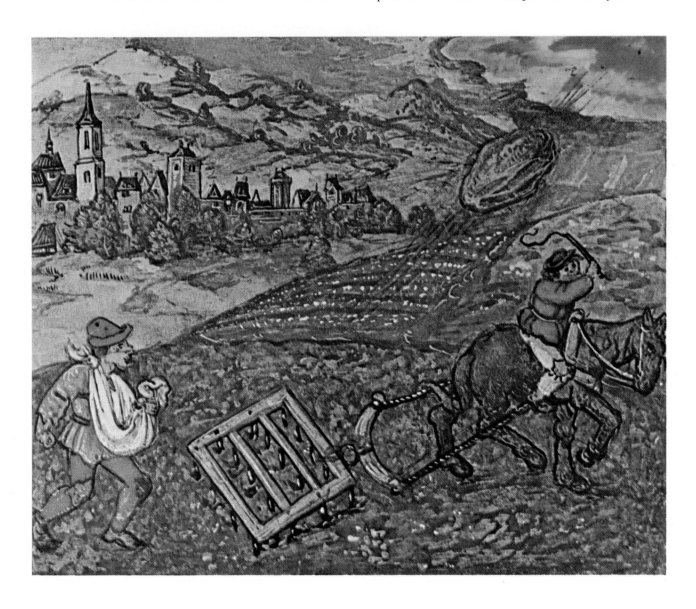

Right: comatose citizens of London, in an illustration from Sir Arthur Conan Doyle's story *The Poison Belt*. First published in 1912, it describes realistically what happens when the earth passes through a cloud of "ether," or interstellar gas, bringing death and fire in its vaporous path.

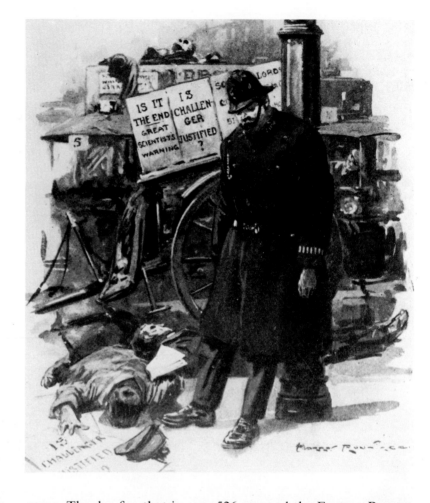

Below: a shower of meteors seen over the Mississippi in 1833. This phenomenon occurs fairly regularly in different parts of the world, and is believed to consist of the fragments of comets that are steadily disintegrating and scattering their substance along their orbits.

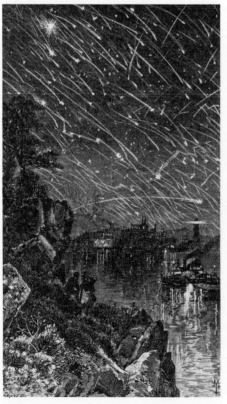

space. The dry fog that in A.D. 526 covered the Eastern Roman Empire with a reddish haze may have been caused in this manner. So also with the blue fog that hung over much of the northern hemisphere for most of the summer of 1783. It began at Copenhagen on May 24, and by June had extended to Germany, France, and England. Eventually it spread eastward as far as Syria and westward over a large part of North America. It showed no trace of humidity and was unaffected by rain or wind. The pale blue haze was sometimes so dense that visibility was reduced to half a mile, and the sun only became visible when it stood 12° above the horizon. The fog had a strong, disagreeable odor, and caused severe catarrh in humans and animals as long as it lasted. Another strange feature of the blue fog was the peculiar phosphoric gleam that accompanied it, and made reading possible at night, even small print. The same gleam came with a haze in 1831, when the sun appeared tinged with green.

Many people thought such an extraordinary event must mean the approaching end of the world. Sir Arthur Conan Doyle may have had such fears in mind when he wrote *The Poison Belt*, a story in which the earth passes into a cloud of interstellar gas, bringing death and widespread fire in its inexorable progress across the globe.

Whether or not meteoric dust brings about the end of civilization, it seems certain that meteorites helped to get it going. Of the three main types of meteorite, one is almost entirely composed of pure iron, a crucial metal in the development of civilization. Iron occurring naturally on earth is invariably combined with other elements and gives no indication of its special properties. But meteoric iron found by primitive mankind was literally "a pure gift from heaven," needing no more attention than softening by fire and hammering to a convenient shape. The Eskimos have long used meteoric iron for spears, axe heads, and knives. Fragments of such iron have been found in the burial mounds of the prehistoric Hopewell Indians of North America.

Even Fort's theory of an extraterrestrial source for life on earth has received support from the recent chemical analysis of meteorites. In 1969 the British chemists J. Brooks and G. Shaw examined the meteorite that had fallen at Murray, Kentucky, in 1950 and discovered that it contained sporopollenin, a highly complex biological substance that forms the outer coating of pollen grains. In another meteorite the quantity of sporopollenin was found to be four percent of the total weight.

When an enormous fireball swept over the countryside of Victoria, Australia, on September 28, 1969, it exploded near the town of Murchison and showered the area with fragments. Examples sent to the NASA Research Center in Ames, California, revealed large quantities of five of the 20 amino acids found in living cells. The presence of these chemicals is considered to be essential before life can originate on a planet. Experiments have shown that they could have been generated by the action of lightning on the gases that composed our earth's primitive atmosphere—ammonia, methane, water vapor, and hydrogen. But an extraterrestrial origin for life on earth cannot be ruled out.

# The Meaning of the Meteorites

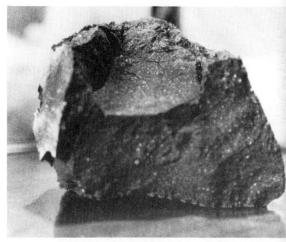

Above: a fragment of the enormous fireball which swept over Australia in September 1969, eventually exploding over the town of Murchison, scattering fragments such as this one over an area 5 miles long by 1 mile wide. A specimen was rushed to the NASA Research Center at Ames, California, where sophisticated tests found traces of five of the 20 amino acids normally found in living cells. Is this the proof scientists have been looking for that life exists in outer space in a form similar to our own?

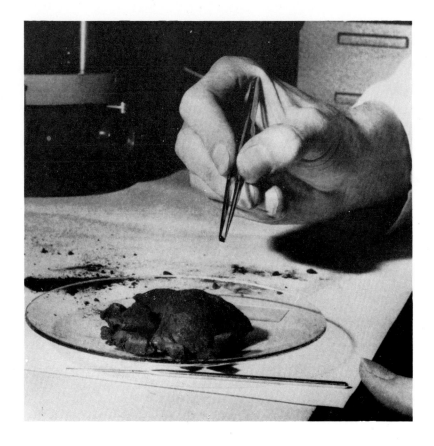

Left: examining particles of the Murchison meteorite in a laboratory at Melbourne University.

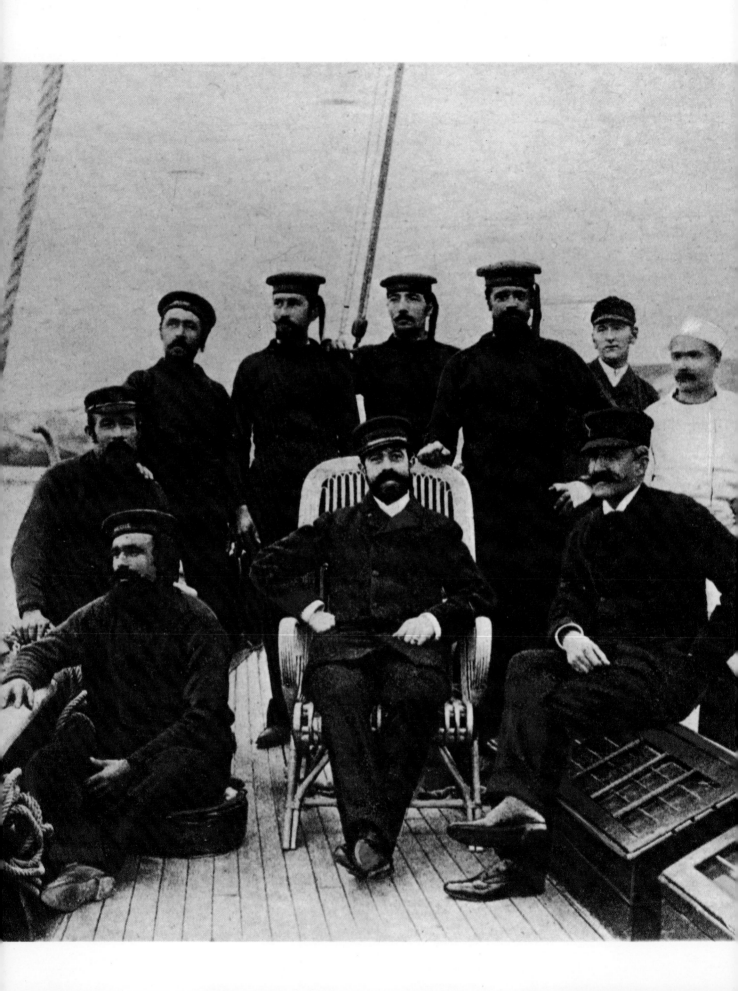

# Chapter 3
# Strange Disappearances

A man running along the road in sight of three witnesses vanishes without trace . . . a well-known journalist is lost in puzzling circumstances while on an assignment . . . three lighthouse keepers are seemingly swallowed up by the air or the sea. What could have happened to them and others who have mysteriously vanished? Sometimes there seems to be a logical and possible explanation for disappearances, but the absence of a body always creates and sustains a doubt that there is any rational reason. Is it because the explanation is, in fact, supernatural?

James Burne Worson was a hard-drinking man, a shoemaker who lived in Leamington, England. When under the influence of liquor, he would boast of his great athletic skill, and would often make foolish wagers involving some trial of strength. On September 3, 1873 he made a sizeable bet that he could run all the way to Coventry and back, a distance of something more than 40 miles. He set out at once. The man with whom he made the bet—whose name is not remembered—and Barham Wise, a linen draper, and Hamerson Burns, a photographer, followed him by cart.

Worson did very well for several miles, going at an easy gait without apparent fatigue, for he genuinely had great powers of endurance. The three men in the cart kept a short distance in the rear, occasionally calling out friendly encouragement or teasing him, as the spirit moved them. Suddenly, in the very middle of the road not a dozen yards from them, and with their eyes right on him, Worson seemed to stumble, pitched headlong forward, uttered a loud cry—and vanished! He did not even fall to the earth, but simply vanished before touching it. No trace of him was ever discovered.

This account, somewhat compressed, is taken from an article entitled "Mysterious Disappearances" by the American journalist and writer Ambrose Bierce. Toward the end of his life, this master of the vitriolic pen, scourge of corruption in high places and of incompetency in all places, made a collection of such un-

Opposite: John Orth, originally an Austrian archduke, with the crew of his three-masted schooner the *Santa Margherita*. This ship, complete with crew, vanished on a voyage from Buenos Aires, Argentina, to Valparaiso, Chile in the summer of 1890. This photograph was taken just before the schooner set out on her last mysterious voyage.

# The Mysterious Ambrose Bierce

Below: Ambrose Bierce, the American writer who disappeared mysteriously in Mexico in 1913 at the age of 71. Bierce had for a long time been fascinated by strange disappearances and had written factual accounts of several. Charles Fort noted that another man named Ambrose Small also disappeared at about the same time, and Fort came up with the theory that some "daemonic" force was collecting Ambroses.

explained vanishing acts. Their matter-of-fact tone is strikingly different from the ghoulish excitement of his celebrated ghost stories. They have more in common with the tales he set in the Civil War, tales that drew upon his real-life experiences as a soldier fighting on the Union side.

At this late date it is impossible to say whether Bierce was trying to create an effect by writing about make-believe events in a straightforward style. In any case, he provides factual details for even the most ghostly of these accounts, which is that of Charles Ashmore's disappearance. This 16-year-old boy set off from the family farmhouse one snowy winter evening, apparently to fetch water from the nearby spring, Bierce relates. When he failed to return his father and sister went to search for him. They found that his footsteps in the snow stopped short about halfway along the path to the spring. Young Ashmore never reappeared, though his voice was heard in the immediate area of the spring for several months after. Even that sign of his presence ended by midsummer.

Bierce's interest in disappearances becomes all the more fascinating in view of the most famous of his mysterious disappearances —in this case it happened to be his own.

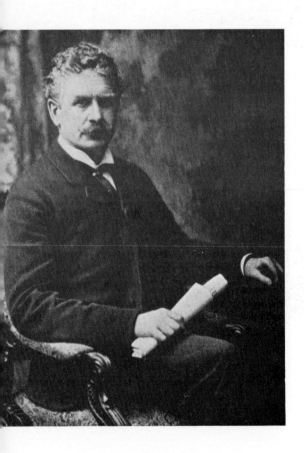

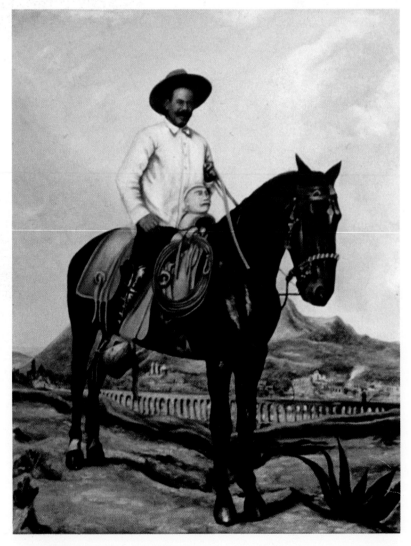

Right: the Mexican revolutionary general Pancho Villa. Bierce's last letter from Mexico said that he expected to be sent with Villa's troops to join a siege 125 miles north of Chihuahua City. One story describes how Bierce became one of Villa's officers, quarreled with him, and was shot.

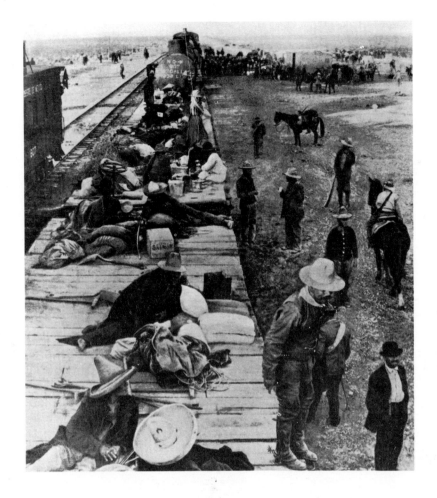

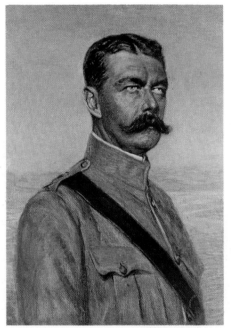

Left: a troop train in Mexico during the 10-year civil war that began in 1910. The war made conditions chaotic, and it seems hardly surprising that the disappearance of one lone American journalist went unnoticed.

Above: the British Field-Marshal Lord Kitchener of Khartoum. One of the wilder theories about the disappearance of Ambrose Bierce was that he joined Lord Kitchener as an adviser in World War I and was drowned with him when the cruiser *Hampshire* in which he was sailing to Russia sank after hitting a mine in June 1916.

In November 1913 Ambrose Bierce crossed the border into Mexico where a civil war had broken out. He was granted credentials as an observer with the revolutionary army of Pancho Villa, and in a letter postmarked Chihuahua City and dated December 26, he said he expected to be sent with Villa's troops to join the seige of Ojinaga, 125 miles to the northeast. That letter proved to be his last, for nothing more was ever heard from him.

Because of the chaotic conditions in a country torn by civil war, it was some time before the United States government could persuade the Mexicans to search for the missing writer. No hard evidence ever emerged from the investigation, but wild rumors circulated from the start. One of these maintained that Bierce had joined Villa as a staff officer, quarreled with him, and was executed. Some versions of this persistent rumor had it that Villa personally shot Bierce after discovering he wanted to travel with the other side. In another variant, Bierce was said to have gone over to the more-or-less legitimate government of General Carranza and, when Villa's troops came upon Bierce accompanying an ammunition train, had been shot on the spot. Some people believed he had managed to cross Mexico and sail for England where, they said, he became an adviser to Lord Kitchener on the conduct of the Great War, dying at Kitchener's side when the ship carrying the British general sank in the autumn of 1916.

When it seemed likely that Bierce would not return, his secretary Carrie Christiansen left their apartment in Washington and

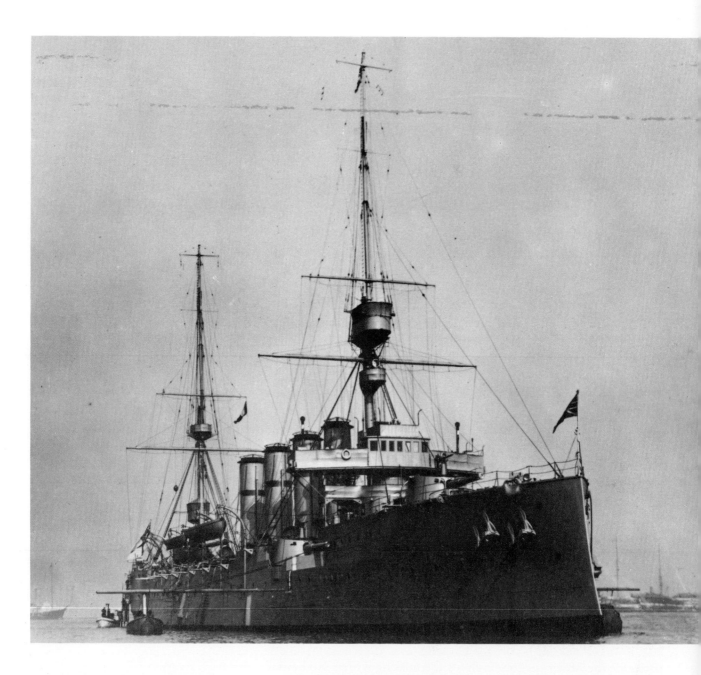

Above: H.M.S. *Hampshire*, in which Lord Kitchener was drowned when it struck a mine and sank in the North Sea in June 1916. Mystery in any case surrounds the circumstances of the sinking of the *Hampshire*, which was allowed to sail in a stretch of sea that had not been swept for mines and without an escort of destroyers which was allowed to turn back because of bad weather. However, the theory that the cruiser also carried Ambrose Bierce to his death seems highly far-fetched.

settled in Napa, California, where she had first met Bierce some years before. Because there happened to be a state hospital for the insane in Napa, her arrival started a rumor that Bierce had gone mad and was confined in the Napa institution.

Interested in Bierce by the publicity surrounding his disappearance, people began to read his books, none of which had sold well during his lifetime. They searched for clues in his caustic volume, *The Devil's Dictionary*, where among hundreds of cynical definitions are to be found such shocking statements as:

*Birth*—the first and direst of all disasters.

*Worm's-Meat*—the finished product of which we are the raw material.

The hints to Bierce's disappearance probably lie in the record of his life. He grew up in a poor farming community without any formal education. At the age of 19 he was one of the first to volunteer for the Civil War, and his experiences in that conflict turned him from a discontented youth stirred by unformulated longings into a bitter man determined to make his mark. A brave and efficient soldier, he was commissioned as an officer in the field, eventually becoming a brevet major. Visits to headquarters gave him ample opportunity to study the Union generals, most of whom seemed to him reckless opportunists, who were willing to sacrifice the lives of the men under their command in order to score over their rivals. What little respect Bierce possessed for men in authority was eroded.

After the war Bierce went to San Francisco and began writing for the newspapers. His phenomenal powers of invective quickly brought him notoriety, and he continued to write his bitterly humorous columns for a variety of publications with scarcely a break until he finally retired from journalism over 40 years later.

By that time he had lived through an unsatisfactory marriage and family tragedy. His eldest son died at 20 in a ludicrous

# Bierce the Man

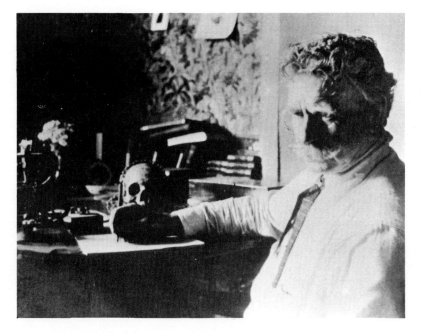

Left: Ambrose Bierce the writer. Bierce was a deeply unhappy man, and also feared old age. There seems to have been a touch of desperation in his decision to go down to Mexico in the middle of a civil war. A short time before he left he said to his daughter: "In America you can't go east or west any more, or north; the only avenue of escape is south."

attempt to kill his rival for a girl's love. His second son died of drink and pneumonia. His daughter took to religion, something that always drew Bierce's fiercest scorn. In middle age he began to write psychological stories about sons who kill their fathers, fathers who kill their children, sons who sleep with their mothers, and criminals who escape the legal consequences of their crimes but come to a dreadful end brought on by remorse or by the ghosts of their victims. For all his aggressive manner, "Almighty God Bierce," as he had sometimes been called, was undoubtedly a tormented man. His *Dictionary* entry for *ghosts* is unusually earnest. It says, "the outward and visible sign of an inward fear."

What did he fear? Loneliness, certainly. Many of his Civil War tales tell of soldiers cut off from their fellows by the vicissitudes of battle. Yet in the last summer of his life Bierce deliberately destroyed several friendships of long standing by sending his

# How Did He Die?

friends a brutal letter. He feared old age, and he knew he was out of step in a greatly changed United States. For a lifelong journalist this realization must have been particularly troubling. In the summer of 1913 he said to his daughter, "Why should I remain in a country that is on the eve of prohibition and women's suffrage? In America you can't go east or west any more, or north; the only avenue of escape is south."

One of the last letters he wrote was from Washington to his nephew's wife. It suggests that he would not be surprised if this "avenue of escape" turned into a one-way street.

"Good-bye—if you hear of my being stood up against a Mexican stone wall and shot to rags please know that I think that a pretty good way to depart this life. It beats old age, disease, or falling down the cellar stairs. To be a Gringo in Mexico—ah, that is euthanasia!"

Ambrose Bierce is thought to have reached Ojinaga with Pancho Villa's rebel troops. He was then 71 and far from well. Years of hard drinking and bouts of asthma had taken their toll of his once legendary stamina. What happened to him during the

Right: a military execution during the Mexican civil war. It has often been said that this is the most likely way in which Bierce died. He even wrote himself in one of his last letters: "Good-bye—if you hear of my being stood up against a Mexican stone wall and shot to rags please know that I think that a pretty good way to depart this life." Perhaps his words were prophetic.

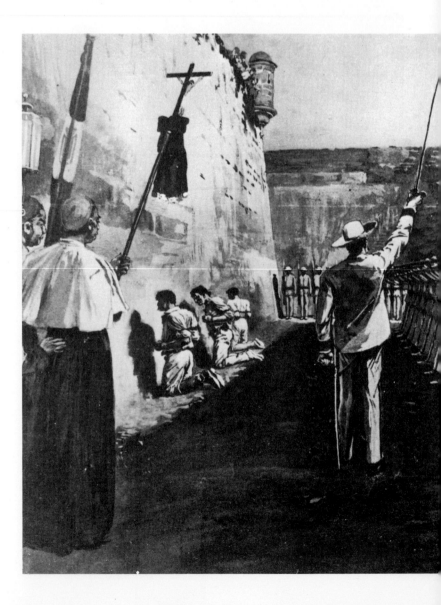

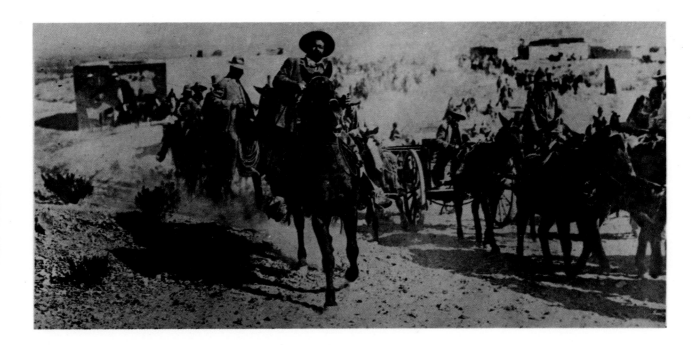

ensuing campaign will never be known, but the most likely suggestion was made by Edwin H. Smith, who interested himself in Bierce's disappearance. He wrote in 1927: "My own guess is that he set off to fight battles and shoulder hardships as he had done when a boy, somehow believing that a tough spirit would carry him through. Wounded or stricken with disease, he probably lay down in some pesthouse of a hospital, some troop train filled with other stricken men. Or he may have crawled off to some waterhole and died, with nothing more articulate than the winds and stars for witness."

Bierce would probably have preferred the stone wall, but however his end came, such evidence that exists suggests he chose it for himself. Could he also have planned to make it a mystery?

The disappearance of Bierce, even though shrouded in mystery, permits of a rational explanation. No explanation has ever been forthcoming for the disappearance of the three lighthouse keepers of the Eilean Mor lighthouse on the Flannan Islands off the west coast of Scotland.

These desolate rocks are situated on the outermost fringe of the British Isles. The nearest land is the island of Lewis in the Outer Hebrides 20 miles to the east; westward the Atlantic Ocean stretches uninterrupted across to North America. The islands are small—Eilean Mor, the largest, is only 500 feet across. They have the reputation of being haunted, and though Hebridean farmers might sometimes leave their sheep for fattening on the fine green turf of the tiny isles, nothing would persuade them to remain overnight themselves.

Four retired seamen looked after the lighthouse, working three at a time in shifts of six weeks on the island followed by two weeks leave on the mainland. Every two weeks the supply vessel *Hesperus* arrived with mail, oil, and food. The boat brought one man back from his two weeks off, and left with another due for his two weeks away.

On December 6, 1900 it was the turn of Joseph Moore to be

Above: Pancho Villa photographed leading his men. It seems certain that Bierce reached Villa's rebel troops at the besieged town. What happened after that remains a mystery.

# The Riddle of the Lighthouse Men

relieved. When the skipper of the *Hesperus* asked him if he was looking forward to his shore leave, he replied, "Aye," and added, with a nod to the tiny island fading out of sight behind them, "'Tis pretty lonely there sometimes."

The lighthouse was just one year old. Moore and the others—Thomas Marshall, James Ducat, and Donald McArthur—had served through one long winter. None of them looked forward to their second experience of it. The living quarters of the lighthouse gave them shelter from the howling winds, but there was little to do to pass the time except read and reread newspapers and books, play checkers, and stare out at the gray restless sea. Moore had noticed how the four of them were speaking less to each other. The natural conviviality of the mariner had given place to long periods of solitary brooding.

On December 21 Joseph Moore again boarded the *Hesperus* to return for his period of duty on Eilean Mor. The weather had been unexpectedly calm during his two weeks of leave, but a severe storm blew up soon after the boat left port. For three days the *Hesperus* rode the storm off the Hebridean coast, and it was only on the 24th that it was able to approach the Flannan Isles. Moore was alarmed to see that the 140,000-candlepower light of the lighthouse was out, but anxious though he was to land and find out what was wrong, it was two more days before the *Hesperus* could safely approach the island's east dock.

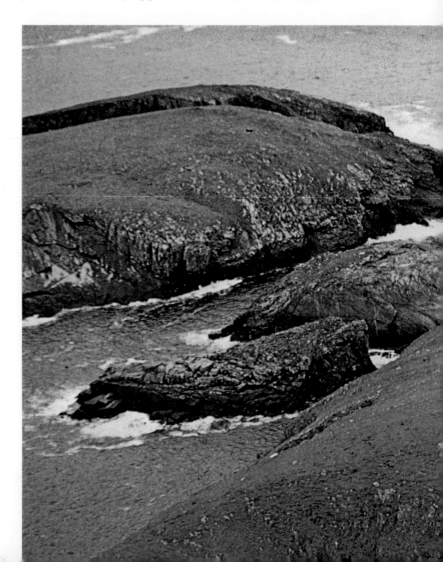

No preparations had been made for their arrival. There were
no empty packing cases or mooring ropes on the jetty. Repeated
blasts on the foghorn brought no one from the lighthouse. A boat
was let down and Joseph Moore was the first ashore. The entrance gate and the main door of the lighthouse were closed.
Moore went inside and shouted. There was no reply. The place
was cold and empty, and the clock on the shelf had stopped.
Moore ran back to the jetty for help, afraid that he might find
the keepers dead in the lighthouse turret. Two men climbed the
stairs with him to investigate, but there was no sign of life. The
entire lighthouse was empty, but everything was neat and in
order. The wicks of the lanterns had been cleaned and trimmed,
and the lamps filled with oil ready to be lit after dark. The last
entry on the record slate had been made on December 15. The
only unusual thing was that two of the three sets of oilskins and
seaboots belonging to the men were missing.

Sailors from the *Hesperus* searched the island. They found no
trace of the missing men, but came upon some clues that at first
suggested an answer to the mystery. The west dock had suffered
extensive storm damage. On a concrete platform 65 feet above
the water stood a crane with ropes trailing down from it. These
ropes were usually stored in a tool chest kept in a crevice 110 feet
above sea level. Had some tremendous storm, with waves over
100 feet high, battered this island and carried away the chest,

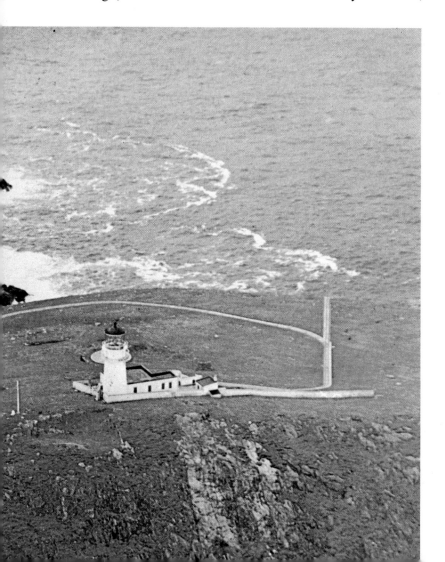

Left: an aerial view of the Eilean Mor
lighthouse on the Flannan Islands off the
west coast of Scotland. It was from this
lighthouse that three keepers vanished so
inexplicably on what appears to have been
a calm day in 1900.

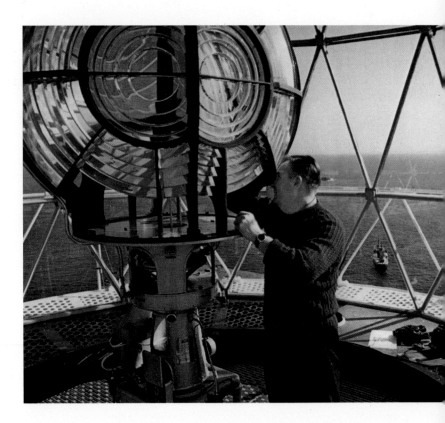

Right: a keeper tending for the last time the great light on the Eilan Tor lighthouse. Today the lighthouse is operated mechanically as an unmanned lighthouse, but until the last few years, three keepers continued to carry out duties on the isolated island.

draping its ropes over the crane? Had it also swept the three men to their deaths? This was unlikely because such exceptionally high waves are extremely rare. Besides, experienced lighthouse keepers would hardly have been so foolish as to venture onto a jetty during a storm, but if they had, all three oilskins would have been missing instead of two.

Meanwhile Moore was examining the log with the captain of the *Hesperus* at his side. Thomas Marshall had written the log, and from his brief entries sprang the image of an unnameable terror that had overwhelmed the men on their isolated rock. The log said:

"December 12: Gale, north by northwest. Sea lashed to fury. Stormbound. 9 p.m. Never seen such a storm. Waves very high. Tearing at lighthouse. Everything shipshape. Ducat irritable."

Moore and the captain glanced at each other. On December 12 no storm had been reported at Lewis, 20 miles away. The reference to Ducat's temper was also unusual.

The next entry had been written the same day at midnight:

"Storm still raging. Wind steady. Stormbound. Cannot go out. Ship passing sounding foghorn. Could see lights of cabins. Ducat quiet. McArthur crying."

Again Moore and the captain stared at each other. What extremity could have caused the veteran seaman Donald McArthur to weep? They read on.

"December 13: Storm continued through night. Wind shifted west by north. Ducat quiet. McArthur praying."

Yesterday McArthur had been crying; today he prayed.

"12 Noon. Gray daylight. Me, Ducat, and McArthur prayed."

When Moore spoke before the board of inquiry that investigated the disappearance, he stated that he had never known any of his companions to pray. Fear of the storm was unlikely to have made them do so since all had experienced many storms during their long years on the high seas.

One last entry remained in the log:

"December 15: 1 p.m. Storm ended. Sea calm. God is over all."

There was no entry for December 14. Why? It will probably never be known, just as what happened after the final log entry remains a mystery. At the inquiry it was reported that on the night of December 15 the *SS Archer* narrowly escaped running onto the rocks of Eilean Mor because no light was visible. It can be presumed that all three men were gone by then.

Could a freak storm, undetected elsewhere, have broken over the island? Could Ducat and McArthur have gone down to the west dock and been swept away? It seems more likely that the men went out in calm weather after the storm to inspect it, especially since Marshall's last entry reports the end of the storm. No one can say what happened next. One suggestion that gained wide acceptance is that one of the three went insane, killed his two companions and then himself. Although hammers, knives, and axes were all untouched in their proper places, the attacker could have used a rock as a weapon. He could have pushed their bodies into the sea, plunging after them to his own death.

Did some overmastering religious mania come upon one of the men? Did he see visions, as St. Flannan, a hermit on the island long ago, is said to have seen God? Could the raging storm of the log entry have been in his mind only? After all, the damage to the dock could have been caused by the storm that delayed the *Hesperus*, after the unknown events of the lighthouse had taken place. Whatever happened during those terrible days and nights, the rocks of Eilean Mor have kept their secret.

Some disappearances are so baffling that people have been tempted to put forward supernatural explanations. Even so pronounced a skeptic as Ambrose Bierce was tempted by a theory — very much ahead of its time — that there are voids or holes in the visible world that exist "as caverns exist in the earth, or cells in a Swiss cheese." In such a cavity, Bierce suggests, "there would be absolutely nothing. Through one of these cavities light could not pass, for there would be nothing to bear it. Sound could not come from it; nothing could be felt in it. . . . A man inclosed in such a closet could neither see nor be seen; neither hear nor be heard; neither feel nor be felt; neither live nor die. . . . Are these the awful conditions (some will ask) under which the friends of the lost are to think of them as existing, and doomed forever to exist?"

As an attempt to explain the phenomenon of disappearances this bears a striking resemblance to the theories advanced by physicists of the present concerning the so-called "black holes" in space. These conjectural objects are regarded as the final relics of massive stars that have consumed all their fuel and have collapsed in on themselves. Becoming even smaller and denser, they generate a gravitational attraction so unimaginably powerful that no matter, light, or other radiation can ever escape from them; hence the term "black hole." Anything falling into a black

# What Happened?

Below: inside the lighthouse. Most of the furniture is still the same as that used by the vanished men, and the room looks much as it did that day when the three walked out on the mysterious errand from which they never returned.

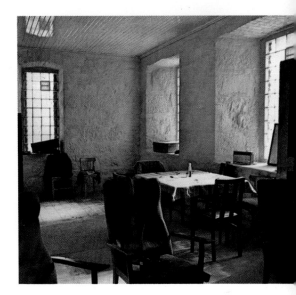

hole will never get out again. Any spaceship or planet that finds itself being sucked into such a whirlpool of destruction has no hope of escape.

Of course nothing like a collapsed star can exist on earth, but occasionally strange events are reported that make one wonder if there is a terrestrial version of a black hole. An extraordinary incident that could lead to the conclusion of a black hole on earth occurred in Bristol, England, early in the morning of December 9, 1873.

Police were called to the railroad station where a married couple had been found, quaking with fear. They were clad in only their nightclothes. When the police discovered that the man had been firing a pistol, the couple was arrested. At the police station the man, who proved to be Thomas B. Cumpston, was still so excited that he could hardly express himself, although there was no indication that either he or his wife had been drinking. He told the police that he and his wife had arrived the previous day from Leeds, and had taken a room in the Victoria Hotel. Early in the morning the floor had suddenly opened up and Cumpston had found himself being dragged down into the opening. His wife had managed to pull him back after a desperate struggle. Both of them were so terrified that they had jumped out of the window and had run to the station for safety. Cumpston insisted that he was telling the truth.

Mrs. Cumpston's testimony added a few details. She said that both of them had been alarmed by sounds earlier in the evening

Below: an artist's impression of a "black hole"—a collapsed star in space. The hot radiating gas glows red as the star implodes into the black hole, producing a gravitational field so powerful that even light would not escape from it. Scientists seem convinced that such phenomena exist in outer space: could their existence here on earth explain some mysterious and otherwise inexplicable disappearances?

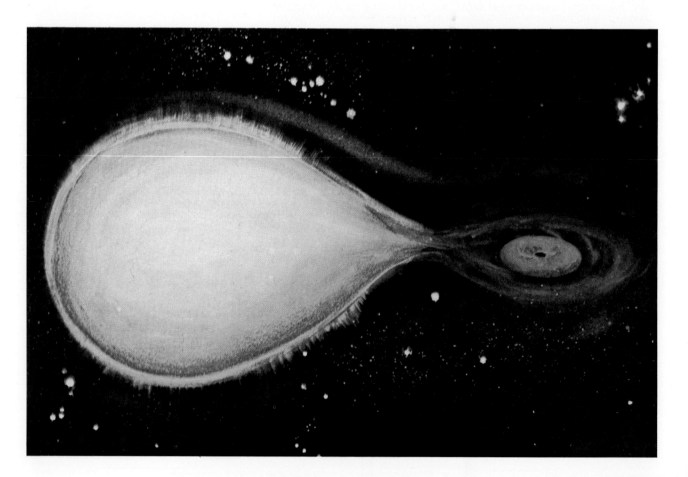

but had been reassured by the hotel manager that they meant nothing. At three or four in the morning, she said, they heard the sounds again, jumped out of bed onto the floor, and felt it giving way under them. When they cried out, their cries were repeated, but they were not sure if by other voices or by an echo of their own voices. The floor had opened up, and only with great difficulty had she been able to stop her husband from disappearing into the hole.

When the hotel manager was contacted, she confirmed that sounds had been heard but she was unable to describe them clearly. Police examined the hotel room and found nothing out of the ordinary. Mr. and Mrs. Cumpston continued to believe that they had been exposed to extreme danger, but they were regarded as victims of a collective hallucination.

Is there a simple and rational explanation based on the fact that the Cumpstons were elderly people in a strange town and in unfamiliar beds? Could the story go like this? The couple slept in an awkward position that interfered with the supply of blood to their legs. If they woke abruptly and stepped onto the floor without thinking, their legs would have collapsed under them, giving a strong sensation that the floor was in motion or no longer there.

What if this is not the explanation, however? Might one of Bierce's "caverns" have opened up beneath their hotel room? The Cumpstons are not alone in reporting the phenomenon of a powerful force, usually operating inside a building, that drags a person away from companions who have to exert all their strength to effect a rescue. But no consistent pattern can be found for these various disappearances.

Take this mystery, for example. Owen Parfitt, a former soldier and tailor, disappeared from the chair in which he was sitting in the doorway of his cottage. The door opened directly onto a busy road along which people, carts, and wagons were passing all the time. When his sister discovered that he was gone, she raised the alarm and within a short time parties of men searched the neighborhood for several miles around. He was never found. That was in 1768 in the small English town of Shepton Mallet.

Not much in that story to arouse interest, perhaps, after more than 200 years—until one further fact is added. Parfitt, aged 70, had been a bedridden cripple for years; he could not move his body an inch without assistance.

His sister, older than himself but still active, and a young girl of the town, Susannah Snook, had lifted the old man from his bed that afternoon and carried him downstairs to the door. When they left him he was settled in his invalid chair, wearing his nightdress and an old greatcoat he used against the cold he felt even in July.

His sister was away making his bed for less than a quarter of an hour. When she returned the old man was gone from his chair, his greatcoat lying beside it. She called out, "Owen, where are you?" but no answer came. And no answer ever came.

One witness reported that a noise had been heard at the time of the disappearance. It was the single meager clue to a puzzle that has never been solved. Brooks were dragged, and woods and fields searched as far as the cathedral city of Wells, six miles away.

# A Whirlpool of Destruction

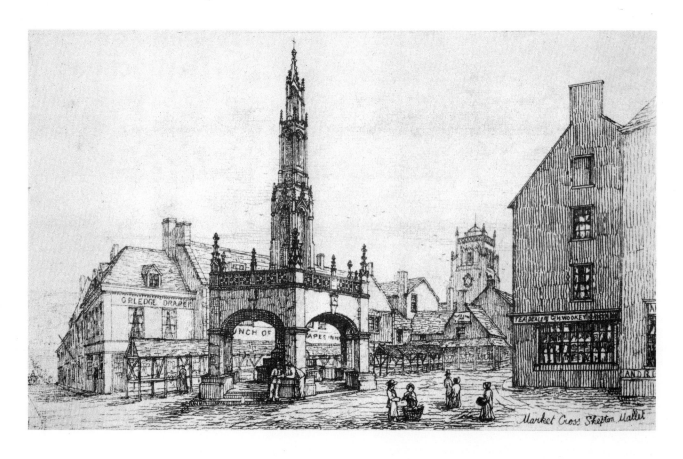

Above: an early 19th-century drawing of the town center of Shepton Mallet, in the southwest of England. It was in this town in 1768 that a crippled old man of 70, bedridden for many years, simply vanished from outside the doorway of his cottage where his sister had placed him in the sun to watch the passers-by.

That Parfitt had been seriously crippled for a long time is beyond doubt. Many people in the town had come to him for tailoring work until his growing paralysis forced him to give the work up. Susannah Snook said that "he could not move at all without aid of someone else." As for his character, a neighbor said of him, "He was not a very good or a very bad man." In his youth he had lived a wild life, soldiering in the New World and Africa. But if a longing to roam once more came over him in old age that warm July day, how could he have moved from his chair? If he had managed to move, why didn't the haymakers working on both sides of the road see him along the way? How could he have been missed by the search parties that were out looking for him within minutes?

Perhaps, it was said, a passing cart took him away. If so, he probably did not go willingly considering he only wore his night clothes without the greatcoat he had had around his shoulders. A man who had known him well said later, "Many folk round here at the time believed that Owen Parfitt had been spirited off by supernatural means."

Forty years afterward a skeleton was found buried in a garden a field away from where Owen Parfitt's cottage had stood. The skeleton, which lay face downward as though it had been thrown down hastily, was covered with two feet of soil. It was thought that the mystery of old Owen's disappearance had been solved until an anatomist established that the bones were those of a young woman.

Shepton Mallet is an old sheep trading settlement dating back to Saxon times. Many remarkable incidents must have taken

# Leaving No Trace

place there, but few could have been stranger than the vanishing of an old invalid that warm summer day in 1768.

Another celebrated case in which a man vanished while people were close by is that of Benjamin Bathurst, British envoy to Vienna during the Napoleonic Wars. In November 1809 this handsome and youthful diplomat, a cousin of Britain's foreign minister, was returning to England with important dispatches. Napoleon had recently defeated Austria at the Battle of Wagram, and had imposed a peace treaty on the conquered country. French spies were active throughout Europe, and Bathurst had to follow a circuitous route. He went by way of Berlin, where he obtained false passports for himself and his Swiss servant, and then made for the still independent city of Hamburg along roads bristling with French troops. On Saturday November 26, when the coach had covered about half the distance, Bathurst stopped in the small Westphalian town of Perleberg for a change of horses. The four occupants of the coach—Bathurst, his servant, and two other travelers—dined in the post house, and at 9 o'clock went out to the coach to continue their journey. While their belongings were being packed, Bathurst stepped behind the coach for some unknown purpose—and vanished. The others waited for him, looked for him, called for him, all in vain.

Finally Bathurst's servant went to Captain Klitzing, the Prussian Governor of the town, and acquainted him with what had occurred. Klitzing already knew of the presence of the travelers because one of them, possibly Bathurst himself, had asked for protection during the stay in Perleberg. Two soldiers had been sent to the post house for that purpose, and had remained there until 7 o'clock when one of the travelers—which one is not known—sent them away. On learning of the disappearance, Klitzing arranged for the others to be accommodated in the Gold Crown Hotel, assigned a detachment of guards, and ordered all the belongings of the missing man to be brought to him.

At that stage the disappearance was being treated as a straightforward case of abduction, possibly murder, for the sake of the money the vanished man was presumed to be carrying. A fur cloak of sable, trimmed with violet velvet, was found to be missing from his belongings. This was eventually discovered in a woodshed of the post house, covered up with firewood. The wastrel son of the family who ran the post station was later arrested for theft and briefly imprisoned, but the reappearance of the cloak threw no light on the disappearance of the man.

The town's four magistrates were roused from their sleep, and searched the taverns and coffee houses of the area until far into the night. The next Sunday a fisherman was instructed to explore the Stepnitz River that passes through and around the town. He discovered nothing. Also on Sunday the Governor left town, for an unannounced destination—perhaps Berlin, perhaps one of the French garrisons that had been placed at strategic positions throughout Prussia. On his return the following day he seems to have become aware that Bathurst was a diplomat trying to elude the French, and that the missing man's valuables consisted of his dispatches. What these contained was never to be known.

Klitzing's loyalties seem to have been for his own nation rather than for the French, but whatever the precise nature of his senti-

# The Ambassador Who Disappeared

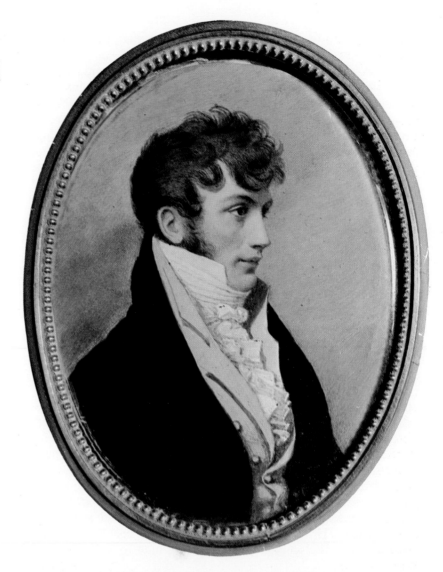

Right: Benjamin Bathurst, British envoy to Vienna during the Napoleonic Wars. In 1809, on his way from Vienna via Berlin to Hamburg, following a circuitous route to avoid French troops in the area, Bathurst stopped at the small town of Perleberg to change the horses on his coach. Bathurst walked behind the coach for some unknown reason—and vanished just as completely as if the earth had opened up and swallowed him.

ments, he was forced to act carefully. Gamekeepers and huntsmen were sent out to search the entire countryside with hounds. The river was dammed so that the bed could be examined. Was he just going through the formalities? Did he know that none of this activity would be productive?

One of Bathurst's other two fellow travelers turned out to be a British courier. He was allowed to return to Berlin accompanied by his servant. Bathurst's own servant remained in Perleberg, however, and so was on hand when a female laborer gathering brushwood in a remote beech forest discovered a pair of Bathurst's trousers on a lonely path. They had been turned inside out and placed on the ground as though someone had intended them to be found, she declared. The trousers had been perforated by two pistol balls fired at them after they had been removed from their wearer. In one of the pockets was found a scrap of dirty paper on which Bathurst had scribbled a letter to his wife. In this he expressed his fear that he would not see her again, and blamed his perilous situation on a certain Comte d'Entraigues. There was no way of telling whether he had written this letter while at the post house or after he had vanished.

When the British government learned of their envoy's disappearance, they offered a reward of £1000. Bathurst's influential family offered a similar sum. In spite of this, no news was forthcoming. In the spring of 1810 Bathurst's young wife traveled to Perleberg and then throughout Germany and France, having obtained a passport from Napoleon himself, in search of information concerning her missing husband. She heard from one source that he had escaped to the north coast of Germany and drowned in the Baltic, from another that he had been drowned while trying to cross the Elbe, from a third that he had been killed by a disgruntled servant. More significantly, she learned that the governor of Magdeburg prison had been overheard to say, "They are looking for the English ambassador, but I have him up there," pointing to the fortress in which prisoners were kept. When Mrs. Bathurst faced the governor with his words, he did not deny uttering them but explained that he had been mistaken in the identity of his prisoner. Her comment on this reply was, "I thought that governors of state prisons do not make mistakes." In spite of all her efforts, however, she was unable to learn more of Magdeburg's mysterious prisoner.

Back in England, Mrs. Bathurst had a visit from Comte d'Entraigues, the man mentioned as a danger in her husband's last note to her. Mrs. Bathurst treated his approach with great caution—wisely, as it proved, because d'Entraigues was a double agent. He told Mrs. Bathurst that her husband had indeed been taken to Magdeburg. Since she did not know whether to believe him or not, she asked for proof and he agreed to obtain it. Whether he actually tried to is unknown because a few days later he met the not unusual fate of double agents: death by assassination. He and his wife, who was privy to all his secrets, were stepping out of their house in Twickenham when a newly hired French servant plunged a dagger into her bosom and she fell dead on the spot. The count ran back to his bedroom for his pistols, followed closely by the man. Two gun shots were heard. When the other servants ran into the room, both the count and his assailant were dead. After these sensational deaths no further clues to Bathurst's whereabouts were uncovered. His wife accepted the fact that he had been killed, but his mother never gave up hope of his return.

It is presumed that Bathurst's disappearance was arranged by the French, but how remains a mystery. If French spies or soldiers overpowered him as he walked behind the coach, it is remarkable that his fellow travelers—only too conscious of the perils of their situation—heard or saw nothing. A German chronicler of the events writes, "The disappearance of the English ambassador seems like magic. It is just as if the ground had opened itself under his feet and swallowed him up, closing itself upon him without leaving the least trace behind."

It is not only during wars that nations have disposed of troublesome individuals by causing them to disappear. Such is thought to have been the fate of Rudolf Diesel, inventor of the type of engine that bears his name.

On the night of September 29, 1913—10 months before the outbreak of World War I—Diesel and two friends embarked at Antwerp, Belgium, on the steamer *Dresden* for the overnight trip to Harwich, England. He was due in London to meet naval

Below: a painting by an unknown artist of Bathurst's mother and sisters. His entire family were tireless in their efforts to trace what had happened to Bathurst, and his wife even traveled to Germany with the express permission of Napoleon to search for evidence. She finally accepted the view that her husband had been killed by French agents, but his mother never gave up hope that he would return. He was never seen again, nor was his body ever found.

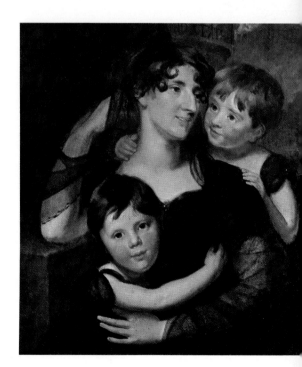

officers and industrialists interested in his latest invention. A man of 56, of German nationality though born in Paris, he had found it difficult to get enough backing to develop the engine he claimed was the most efficient in the world. The German firm of Krupps had originally underwritten him, but Diesel had run foul of certain American firms, and by 1913 his personal and business finances were in bad shape. The forthcoming discussions in London were therefore very important to him, and he hoped they would lead to a change in his financial situation. As the *Dresden* steamed across the North Sea, he dined with his companions Georg Carels, a fellow director, and an engineer named Luckmann. After dinner they took a stroll around the deck, and at 10 o'clock retired to their cabins.

The next morning Diesel did not appear. A search in his cabin revealed that his bed had not been slept in, although his belongings were arranged as though he had intended to go to bed. For example, his watch had been placed in a high position so that he

Right: Rudolf Diesel, the German engineer and inventor best known for the pressure-ignited heat engine that bears his name. His disappearance from the steamer *Dresden* one night in September 1913 has been variously explained. One theory is that his affairs were in bad shape and that he took his own life in a sudden fit of deep depression. Another suggests that Diesel was pushed overboard while taking a late-night stroll on deck to prevent his taking important secrets to the British in those tense months before the outbreak of World War I. No body was ever picked up, and it seems likely that we shall never know the truth.

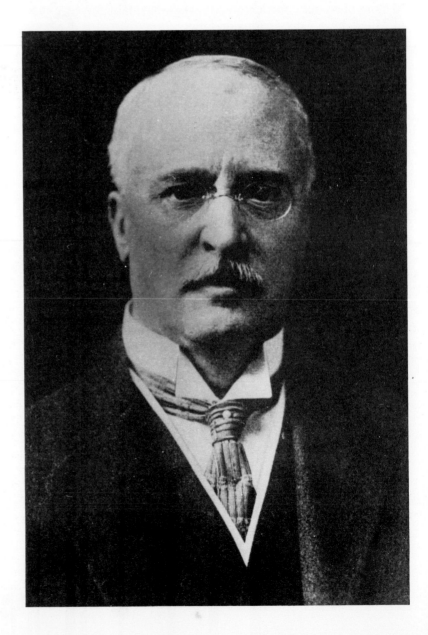

could see it from where he lay in bed. Since Diesel suffered from insomnia, and in recent weeks had seldom slept for more than two hours a night, it was assumed that he had gone for a walk on deck and fallen overboard. Even though the deck was surrounded by a rail four feet high, no other explanation seemed possible. Accidental death was presumed when his two companions said he had been in excellent spirits at dinner and showed no sign of mental breakdown or thoughts of suicide.

Ten days later a fishing crew off the coast of The Netherlands observed a body floating in the water. For some reason the fishermen were unable to bring the body ashore, but they retrieved certain articles from it including a diary and an eyeglass which Diesel's son recognized as belonging to his father. The family offered a reward for the recovery of the body, but it was never seen again. Was the body that of Diesel? The failure to bring it ashore and the removal of identifiable objects from it look most suspicious. In addition, the body had been described as being in an advanced state of decomposition, which is surprising after so short a time in the water.

In 1915 a German prisoner-of-war is said to have revealed that he was instructed by the German secret service to follow Diesel and push him overboard to prevent him from passing the secret of his invention to the British. With suicide or accident highly implausible, murder seems the most likely explanation for Diesel's disappearance. The prisoner's story could not be checked, however, so whatever happened to Diesel on board the *Dresden* that night remains unknown.

Some people have deliberately planned their disappearance in order to be free of the ties and responsibilities of their old life and start a new one elsewhere. The American detective William J. Burns recalled the case of a New York toy maker, cursed with a shrewish wife, who vanished while on his way to his factory carrying $10,000 meant as wages for his workers. He left a note in the back of his car saying, "Has been bumped off. Look for

# Pre-planned Disappearances

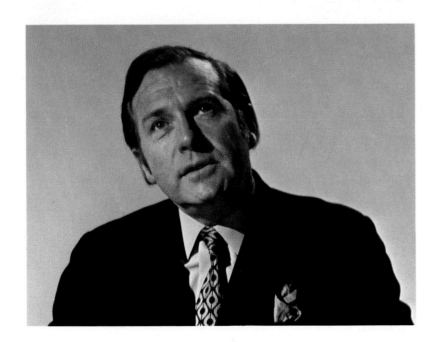

Left: John Stonehouse, the British member of Parliament who, in December 1975, faked his own disappearance by leaving his clothes in a beachside changing room in Miami, Florida and taking a flight under a false name to Australia. There he was later found and extradited to stand trial in Britain. Stonehouse is the latest in the list of people who have planned their own disappearance in order to be free of the ties and responsibilities of their old life and to start a new one elsewhere. In his case, the new life led to a sentence of seven years in prison for a number of criminal acts, including forgery.

# Where Do They Go?

Right: Victor Grayson, British member of Parliament, addressing a Labor Party rally in 1906. Grayson, a powerful speaker on all questions of social injustice, appeared to have a promising future when in 1920 he took a night train from Liverpool to Hull, England. When the train arrived, Grayson was simply not on it. He had vanished completely, and no one has yet come up with a feasible explanation for his disappearance. Grayson's is one of the most mysterious cases of disappearance of all time.

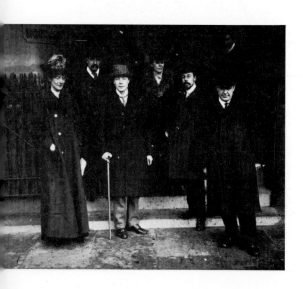

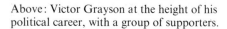
Above: Victor Grayson at the height of his political career, with a group of supporters.

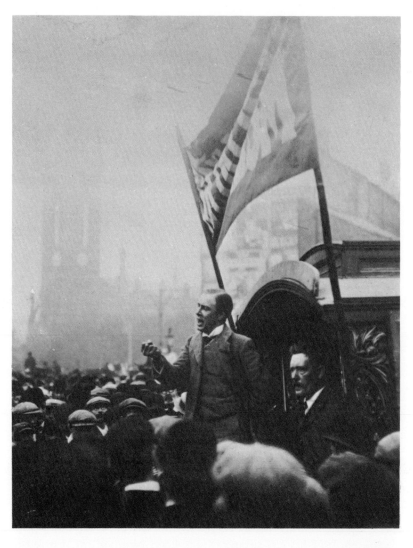

body in the river." The message would hardly fool anyone, however, since the river was icebound at the time! Eight years later the man was seen by chance and recognized in a park 1500 miles away. He had been living a new life in contentment the whole time.

Perhaps a wish to start life afresh also accounts for the disappearance in 1920 of Victor Grayson, a former British Labor politician. Born the son of a carpenter in 1882, he became the Member of Parliament for Colne Valley, Yorkshire, at the age of 25. Much in demand as a public speaker, particularly on matters of social injustice, he was once suspended from the House of Commons for his inflammatory language. After being defeated in 1910 he became a journalist, married an actress, and accompanied her to New Zealand on a tour. There he joined the New Zealand Army, returned to fight in France in World War I, and was wounded at Passchendaele.

In August 1920 he boarded a night train from Liverpool, England, to Hull, where he was due to make a political speech. When the train arrived, Grayson was not on it. Later his bag was found in a London hotel, having been left there, said the manager, by a man whose head was bandaged and whose arm appeared to be injured. The man never occupied his room nor collected the bag.

Over the following years there were several reports that Grayson had been seen by people who had known him. In 1924 and again in 1928 he was thought to have been recognized in England. In 1932 a political colleague, G. A. Murray, was convinced he saw Grayson from the top of a London bus. He looked fit and well-dressed, but though Murray quickly descended the stairs of the bus to go after the missing man, he was gone by the time he reached the street.

Another former colleague believed he saw Grayson on the London Underground, but realized it too late to challenge him. He was accompanied by a woman who called him "Vic," and when the couple left the train near Parliament, the man had said with a laugh, "Here's the old firm." There were persistent reports that he had gone to Australia, one of these as late as 1957 when Grayson would have been a man of 75.

If the person seen on these occasions really was Victor Grayson, he had managed to stay hidden in his own country for years. If those who thought they recognized him were mistaken, he probably disappeared in 1920 on a train between Liverpool and Hull or in London. Either way his end is a mystery that has never been cleared up.

When adults disappear, there is always the possibility that they have done so voluntarily, but this is hardly true of children. When a 12-year-old girl vanishes, as Eliza Carter did in January 1882, the first thought is of abduction. When she never reappears, the mystery deepens. When she is one of a number who disappear from the same area, the mystery defies solution.

Eliza Carter was one of the first to vanish in a 10-year series of such happenings known as the "West Ham Disappearances," so called because most of them occurred in the West Ham sec-

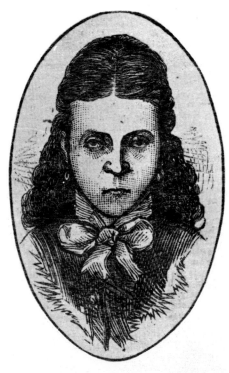

Above: Eliza Carter, the 12-year-old girl from West Ham, London, who disappeared in January 1852. She was the first victim of the so-called "West Ham Disappearances." Below: a contemporary newspaper account of the disappearance of Amelia Jeffs, another of the children who vanished during the 10-year period of the West Ham disappearances. However, as can be seen from this account, her fate was tragic but mundane.

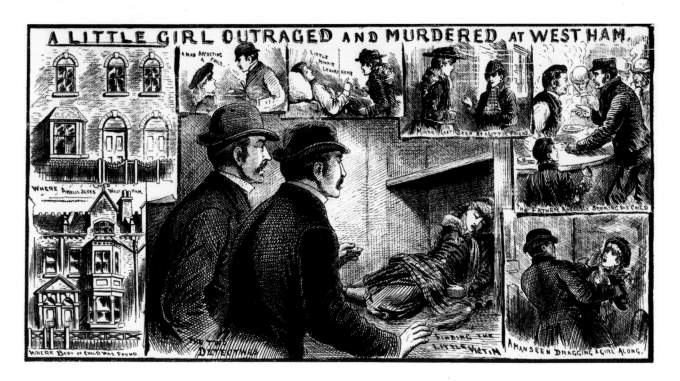

# "Never Believe That I Am Dead"

Below: Colonel Percy Fawcett, the middle-aged Englishman who in 1925 set off into the Matto Grosso in the Amazon Basin of Brazil to search for a lost city. Some weeks after setting out he wrote to his wife. Then Fawcett vanished without trace.
Below right: the "Flying Duchess," the British Duchess of Bedford, being helped into her flying suit by her pilot, Flight-Lieutenant Preston in August 1936. After achieving two record flights, to India in 1929 and to South Africa in 1930, the Duchess finally vanished completely on a solo flight over the North Sea in 1937, the year after this photograph was taken.

tion of London's East End. After a visit to her sister, Eliza failed to return home. When later seen in the street by some of her schoolgirl friends, she was in a state of fear. They urged her to return to her family, but she said she could not. "*They* wouldn't let me," she said. At 11 p.m. she was seen in the company of a middle-aged woman; then she disappeared for good. The only trace was her dress, found in the football stadium of neighboring East Ham. If some harm had come to her, why did her body never show up? What about all the other West Ham residents who vanished? Where were their bodies, and why was an ordinary working class area of town the scene of such unexplained events?

An interesting case of someone who disappeared and reappeared before making a final disappearance was that of Private Jerry Irwin of the United States army. He was not to be found anywhere for a time, then turned up at camp again. Not long afterward he disappeared again, but reappeared once more. Neither time was the soldier able to say where he had been. On August 1, 1959 he disappeared for good.

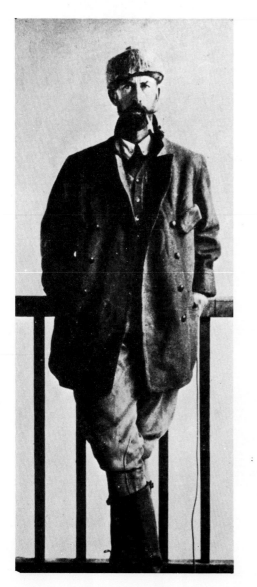

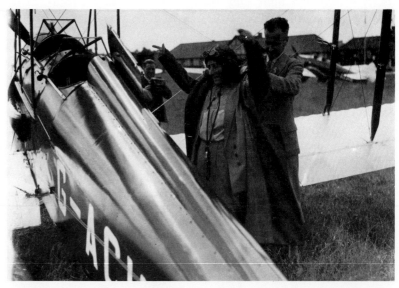

The disappearance of the explorer Colonel Fawcett in the Brazilian jungle in 1925 and of the Duchess of Bedford—the "Flying Duchess"—on a solo flight in 1937 were sensations in their time. So was the disappearance of the Austrian Archduke Johann Salvator in 1890 following the climax of a series of quarrels with his cousin, Emperor Franz Josef. The archduke renounced his rank, became a commoner, and took the name John Orth. Having bought a three-masted schooner, he and his wife sailed to Buenos Aires, Argentina. There he took on a new crew and a cargo, and set sail for Valparaiso, Chile. The ship was never seen again.

His mother and brothers were reluctant to believe him dead, especially because on his last visit to them before leaving Austria he had said, "Never, never believe that I am dead; for I will return one day, and we shall meet again and talk of this." It was rumored that he had not sailed with the ship, but had staged a

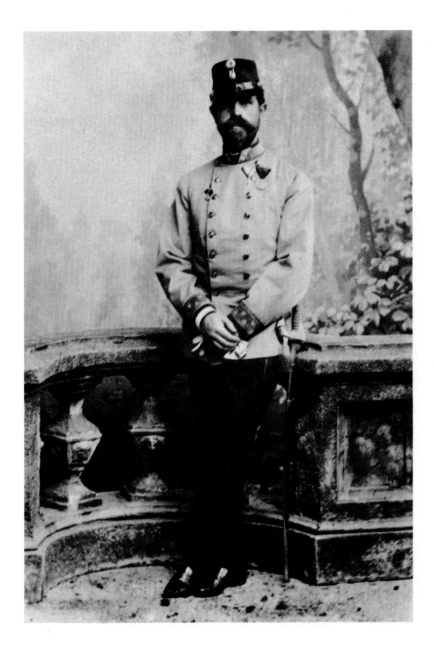

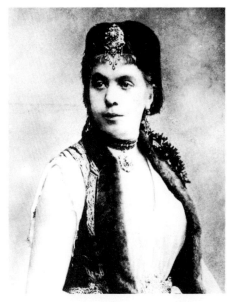

Left: John Orth, previously Archduke John Salvator of Tuscany, a member of the Hapsburg family. After numerous quarrels with his cousin, the Emperor Franz Josef of Austria, he gave up his title, became a commoner, and took the name John Orth. In the same year of 1889 he married Milly Stubel, a dancer at the Viennese Opera, and set out on a world tour which ended apparently with their complete disappearance on a voyage from Argentina to Chile. Did he really go down with the ship, the schooner *Santa Margherita*? Or did he simply stage a disappearance in South America in order to live a private life of peace? We shall probably never know the true answer.

Above: the dancer Milly Stubel, whom the reluctant archduke first met romantically on a hunting trip in the forest outside Vienna. They proved a devoted couple.

successful disappearance in South America in order to live a private life in peace. But his family never heard from him again. Did he go down with his ship in the treacherous waters around Cape Horn? We may never know. Likewise, although we may assume that Colonel Fawcett was killed by cannibal Indians, and that the plane of the Flying Duchess crashed into the desert or the ocean, we cannot solve these mysteries for sure.

Sudden disappearances are always intriguing, particularly when the vanished person is someone in the public eye. Generally the disappearance proves to have a rational, if sometimes complicated, explanation; but an element of doubt always persists. It is the absence of a body that keeps the flame of doubt glowing at the back of our minds, no matter how rational and persuasive the arguments for natural death may be. In this respect we show ourselves still close in habit to primitive people: anxious to have our dead buried properly so that their spirits can rest in peace.

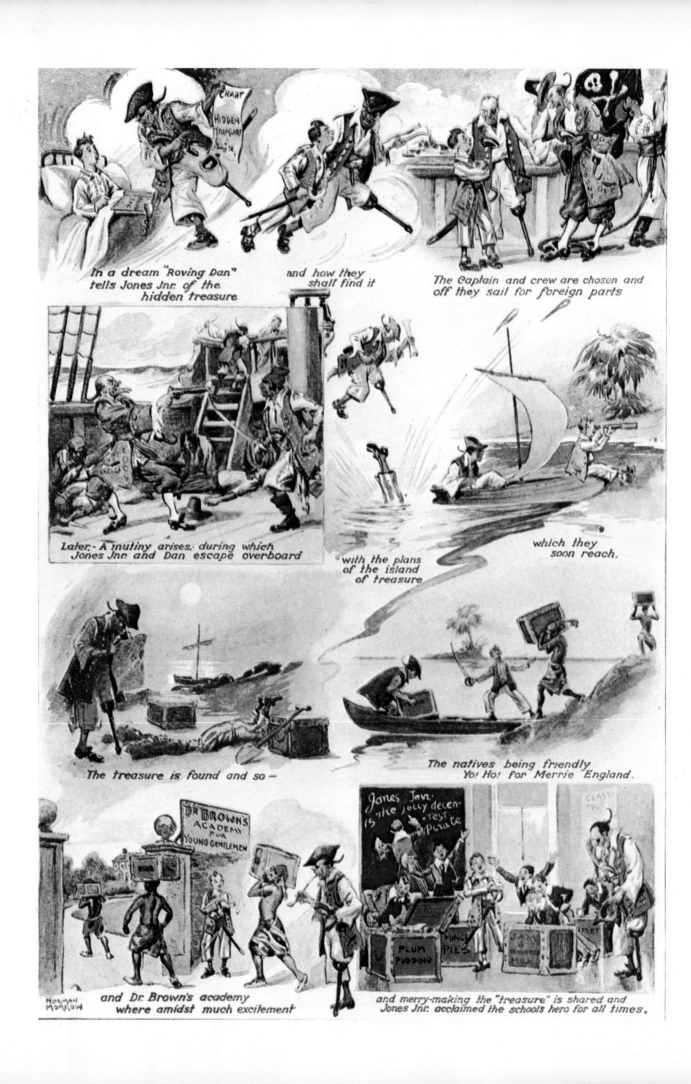

In a dream "Roving Dan" tells Jones Jnr. of the hidden treasure

and how they shall find it

The Captain and crew are chosen and off they sail for foreign parts

Later:- A mutiny arises, during which Jones Jnr. and Dan escape overboard

with the plans of the island of treasure

which they soon reach.

The treasure is found and so —

The natives being friendly Yo! Ho! for Merrie England.

and Dr. Brown's academy where amidst much excitement

and merry-making the "treasure" is shared and Jones Jnr. acclaimed the schools hero for all times.

# Chapter 4
# The Puzzle of Oak Island

Is there a buried treasure in the Money Pit on Oak Island, Nova Scotia? For nearly 200 years, hopeful prospectors have tried to unearth one. All have been defeated by the ingenious construction that floods the shaft when a certain depth is reached—and a fortune in money and five lives have been lost in the treasure hunt. Did Captain Kidd bury his rich hoard in a seemingly bottomless pit on this insignificant island? Could the unknown engineering genius who built the structure have long ago retrieved whatever was buried? The mystery still remains unsolved today.

Buried treasure is like a magnet to many who get wind of it. They immediately imagine untold wealth, like that described by the French writer Alexandre Dumas in his adventure novel *Count of Monte Cristo*: "Three compartments divided the coffer. In the first, blazed piles of golden coin; in the second, bars of unpolished gold were ranged; in the third, Edmond [Dantès] grasped handfuls of diamonds, pearls, and rubies, which as they fell on one another sounded like hail against glass . . ."

In one real-life treasure hunt, the mere vision of gleaming gold and sparkling gems has kept several generations of hopeful prospectors on the search. But no evidence has ever emerged to link the site of suspected buried treasure with any objects of value. Undeterred by this discouraging record, modern treasure hunters have brought increasingly sophisticated machinery to the task of wresting its secret from the earth. In the nearly 200 years since its chance discovery, an estimated $1½ million has been spent in finding . . . nothing.

The site is on an island, but hardly one associated with dangerous reefs and sharks as popularly imagined for hidden treasures. Oak Island in Mahone Bay on the southern coast of Nova Scotia has long been used by residents on the surrounding mainland simply as a pleasant place for a picnic. It owes its fame to a long-ago excursion for that innocent purpose. In the summer of 1795, 16-year-old Daniel McGinnis was paddling his canoe across the bay, intent on going to one of the innumerable uninhabited and

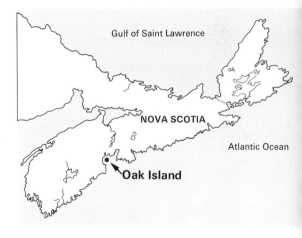

Opposite: the idea of hunting for—and finding—buried pirates' treasure has fascinated and attracted people for many centuries. This cartoon illustrates the idea with tongue firmly in cheek.

Above: the exact location of Oak Island is pinpointed on this map of Nova Scotia.

# First on the Scene

unexplored islands. The one he picked was Oak Island, which owed its name to the luxuriant growth of red oaks that thickly covered both ends of it. In shape, the mile-long Oak Island resembled a slightly distorted hourglass, with an area of low swampland linking the two halves.

Daniel beached his canoe in the wide cove on the island's southeastern shore and made his way into the trees. He had not wandered far when he came upon a clearing, in the center of which stood a gnarled and ancient oak. Fifteen feet above the ground one of the branches had been cut short, and the remaining stump showed the marks of scoring by rope and tackle. Directly under the stump the youngster noticed a circular depression in the ground some 12 feet in diameter. In the clearing a good deal of wood had been cut down, and new growth was springing up to take its place.

Daniel forgot his picnic. He hurried away from the island, convinced that he had stumbled upon the site of buried treasure. Like all the boys on that coast, he had been brought up on tales of pirates. Even the name of the bay is thought to have come from the French word *mahonne*, a swift, low-lying ship much used by pirates in the Mediterranean. Back in his home town of Chester on the eastern shore of the bay, Daniel shared his discovery with two friends, John Smith, aged 20, and Anthony Vaughan, aged 13. The following day the three of them rowed to Oak Island with picks and shovels and began to dig beneath the tree.

Their excitement mounted when they discovered that they were digging down into a circular shaft with walls of hard clay that clearly bore the marks of picks. Four feet down they found a layer of flagstones, of a kind not found on Oak Island. Ten feet down they came upon a platform made of solid oak logs six inches thick. These extended the full width of the shaft and were embedded firmly in the clay walls. The boys hauled the wood out and resumed digging. At 20 feet they encountered a second oak platform similar to the first, and at 30 feet still another. The earth had settled for about two feet between the platforms.

With the tools at their disposal the three boys could go no deeper. They left sticks to mark the point they had reached, and returned to the mainland to seek help.

This proved more difficult than they expected. Many local people believed the island to be haunted. A woman whose mother was one of the original settlers in the neighborhood recalled that strange lights and fires used to be seen on the island at night. A boatload of men had once rowed to the island and never returned. Not until nine years later, in 1804, did the three treasure seekers manage to persuade someone to come to their aid. By that time John Smith had bought the area surrounding the site. Over the next 30 years he acquired more lots until he owned the entire east end of the island.

The person they had interested was Simeon Lynds, a well-to-do young man who formed a syndicate of friends "to assist the pioneers in the search after the treasure and to complete it." A quantity of mud had settled in the pit during the intervening years, but when this was cleared away the diggers came upon the sticks left in the mud by the three discoverers, and they were satisfied that the site had not been interfered with since then.

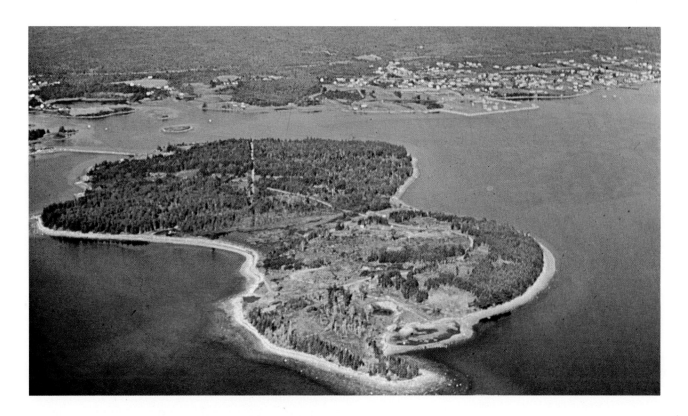

As the level of the shaft was lowered, a succession of oak platforms was uncovered, some of them reinforced with other
materials. There is some confusion as to the exact sequence of
platforms, but one version gives it like this: at 40 feet, a platform
of oak sealed with putty; at 50 feet, plain oak; at 60 feet, oak
sealed with coconut fiber and putty; at 70 feet, plain oak; at 80
feet, oak sealed with putty. So much putty was brought to the
surface that the amount set aside for reuse served to glaze the
windows of 20 houses around Mahone Bay.

At 90 feet a flat stone was uncovered. Measuring three feet
long and one foot wide, it was of a material not found in Nova
Scotia. Roughly cut letters and figures were observed on the
underside, but the treasure hunters could not make sense of
them. They seem to have paid little attention to what could have
been a valuable clue. Smith fitted it at the back of the fireplace in
the house he had built on Oak Island, and there it remained for
at least half a century. Some time in the 1860s it was taken to
Halifax and displayed in the window of a bookbinder's shop to
help attract people to contribute money for a further search for
the treasure. Time and Smith's fireplace had rendered the markings still less legible, although a professor of languages interpreted them to read "Ten feet below two million pounds." Some-
time in the 20th century the stone disappeared. In 1935, however,
a very old employee of the bookbindery described the stone as
resembling "dark Swedish granite, or fine grained porphyry,
very hard, and with an olive tinge," adding, "we used the stone
as a beating stone and weight."

The searchers of 1804 didn't see any significance in the stone,
and ignored it. They pushed a crowbar into the earth, which was
by then becoming so waterlogged that they had to remove one

Above: this aerial view of Oak Island shows
how numerous excavations have been torn
away at the corner of the island where the
so-called "Money Pit" is situated.

# The First Shaft

cask of water to every two of earth, and struck something hard and unyielding that seemed to stretch across the width of the shaft. All those present agreed it was wood; some said it must be a chest.

This discovery was made near nightfall on a Saturday. The treasure seekers climbed out of the shaft, convinced that their goal lay but a few inches farther down. They occupied the evening happily working out how to divide the treasure. They could not work on the Sunday, so it was Monday morning before they returned—only to find the shaft flooded with water to within 33 feet of the top. They bailed out the water with buckets, but no matter how much they removed, the level of water remained constant. A pump was obtained and lowered into the shaft. When it burst, work was abandoned for the year.

In the spring of 1805 the treasure seekers returned and attempted to drain the flooded shaft by digging a second one alongside. At 110 feet they tunneled sideways toward the first shaft. Suddenly there was a thunderous roar and a surge of water overwhelmed them so rapidly that they were lucky to escape with their lives. The old shaft had collapsed, and water soon filled the second shaft to within 33 feet of the top.

The syndicate had used up its capital, and all there was to show for it was two flooded holes and a large quantity of oak logs. Writing to a friend, Smith said, "Had it not been for the various mischiefs nature played us, we would by now, all of us, be men of means." He did not know that this mischief was not of nature's doing, because the incredibly cunning design of the Money Pit, as it came to be called, remained unguessed for many years to come.

No other attempt was made to excavate the Money Pit until 1849, when a group of investors from another part of Nova Scotia formed the Truro Syndicate. There was continuity with

Below: this view of Oak Island, the site of the so-called "Money Pit," is from the mainland, and was probably taken at the time of the operations of the Oak Island Treasure Company formed by Frederick Blair in the early 1900s. In the prospectus for this new company, Blair wrote that this time he intended to "use the best modern appliances . . . such an attempt will be completely successful."

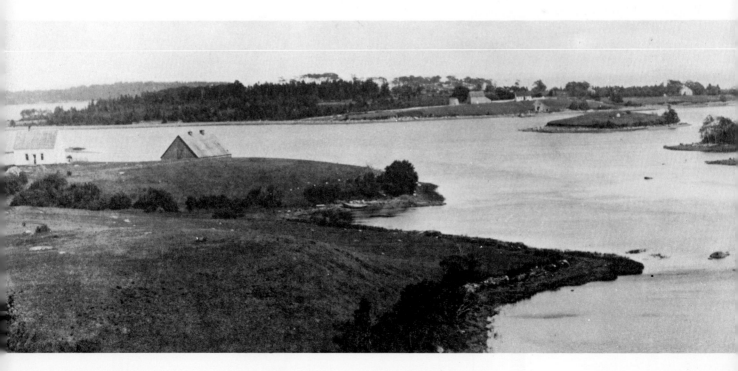

the group of 45 years before, however. Dr. David Lynds was a relative of Simeon Lynds, head of the first syndicate. Anthony Vaughan, one of the three original discoverers, was then in his late 60s; he helped the new syndicate locate the site of the Money Pit. Of the other discoverers, McGinnis was dead and Smith, who lived until 1857, seems to have taken no active part in the new search.

Both the shafts had caved in, but after 12 days of work on the original shaft, a depth of 86 feet was reached. Flooding no longer appeared to be a problem. Once again work came to a halt on a Saturday night. The next day the men were relieved to see that hardly any water had seeped into the pit, but at two o'clock they returned from church "and to their great surprise found water standing in the pit, to the depth of 60 feet, being on a level with that in the bay."

On Monday, disappointed but not discouraged, they began bailing out the shaft. Soon they realized that "the result appeared as unsatisfactory as taking soup with a fork," in the words of a contemporary account. They decided to find out what lay in the depths by employing a pod auger, a horse-driven drill that brought up samples of whatever material it passed through, then used in mining operations. A platform was erected above the water and five holes were bored to a depth of 106 feet. The first two holes were drilled to the west of the center of the pit and brought up nothing but mud and stones. The statement from the man who directed the drilling shows what was found by the first borings east of the center:

"After going through the platform [at the level reached by the crowbar in 1804] which was five inches thick, and proved to be spruce, the auger dropped 12 inches and then went through four inches of oak; then it went through 22 inches of metal in pieces; but the auger failed to bring up anything in the nature of treasure, except three links resembling the links of an ancient watch chain. It then went through eight inches of oak, which was thought to be the bottom of the first box and the top of the next; then 22 inches of metal, the same as before; then four inches of oak and six inches of spruce, then into clay seven feet without striking anything."

The second bore struck the upper platform as before but missed what was thought to be some boxes, although the jerky motion of the rotation chisel suggested that it might be striking the outer edge of a box. Splinters of oak were drawn up with a quantity of what appeared to be coconut fiber. These borings certainly suggested that the Money Pit contained two oak chests, one on top of the other. The nature of the "metal in pieces" is not recorded as being known. One member of the syndicate later referred to the "links of a watch chain" as "a piece of gold chain," but this looks like pure embellishment.

The last boring became an event of the greatest importance. The foreman, James Pitblado, was told to carefully remove every scrap of material brought up to the surface so that it could be examined by microscope. What happened next is confused. Pitblado was accused of taking something out of the auger, studying it closely, and putting it in his pocket. When asked to produce it, he refused, saying he would show it to the next meeting of the

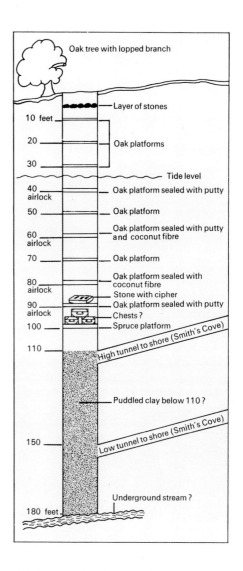

Above: this diagram shows the various levels of the Money Pit on Oak Island as they appeared to the ever-confident treasure hunters as they worked and invested away. The high flood tunnel, the low flood tunnel, and the levels at which they were found are clearly shown.

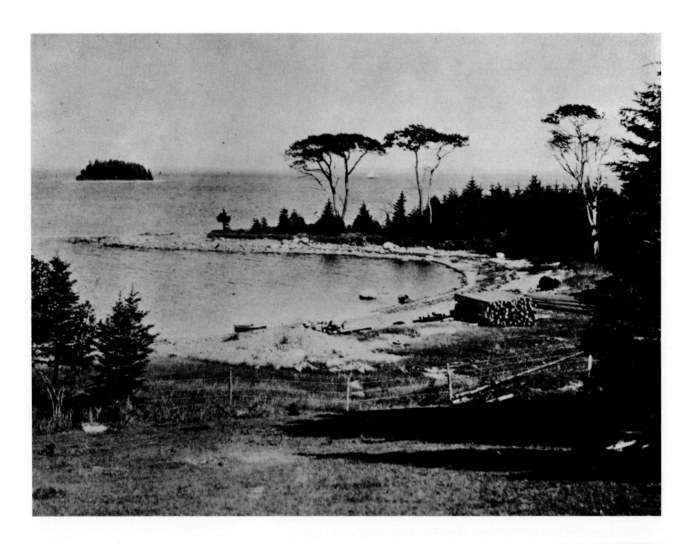

Above: Smith's Cove on Oak Island, where the treasure hunters discovered the source of the cunningly built engineering device that flooded the pit with salt water when the tide came in, thus ensuring that, each time the investigators reached a certain depth, water broke through from below and flooded the shaft.

directors of the syndicate. Surprisingly, no attempt was made to search him—and he never appeared at the board meeting. Apparently he had had a talk with a local businessman who then made a determined, though unsuccessful, bid for the east end of Oak Island. What happened to Pitblado is uncertain, but tradition has it that the object he removed from the auger was a jewel.

The Truro syndicate was convinced that two chests of treasure lay in the Money Pit. The problem still was how to get at it. In 1850 they sank a third shaft to the west of the pit and dug through hard clay to a depth of 109 feet without meeting any water. Like their predecessors in 1805 they tunneled sideways toward the Money Pit, but before they reached it a flood of water burst in upon them, and once again the workmen were lucky to escape with their lives. Within a few minutes, the new shaft was more than half filled with water.

Only then did someone think of trying to find out where all the water might be coming from. Legend has it that one member of the syndicate fell into the shaft and discovered that the water was salty. Whether or not this really happened, someone at last got around to tasting it and determined that it was sea water. Watching the flood level in the shafts thereafter, they observed that it rose and fell with the tide in the bay. Since there was no possibility of seepage through the impermeable clay soil, the only alternative was that a man-made tunnel connected the Money Pit with the waters of the bay. They hastened to the nearest shore, a beach known as Smith's Cove, 500 feet to the northeast, and there the amazing theory was confirmed. As the tide ebbed, the sand "gulched water like a sponge being squeezed."

They dug into the beach and at a depth of three feet found a two inch layer of the same coconut fiber that had been discovered in the Money Pit. Beneath this fiber came a four or five inch layer of eel grass or kelp, and beneath this had been placed a quantity of flat stones. For 150 feet along the beach between high and low water marks the spongy construction continued. Five box drains, strongly built of flat stones at a depth of five feet, led from it to a funnel-shaped sump set just above high water mark.

So well built and protected were the drains that on uncovering one of them it was found that no earth had sifted through to obstruct the water flowing along it. From the sump the water passed along a tunnel for a distance of 500 feet, sinking steadily until it reached the Money Pit somewhere below the 90-foot level.

The work involved in sinking the Money Pit was impressive, but the construction of the flood-tunnel system was unquestionably the work of an engineering genius. As the tide rose in the bay, water was soaked up by the coconut fiber sponge and channeled through the drains and the tunnel into the pit. As long as the pit remained undisturbed, the pressure of earth in the shaft held the water back. As earth was removed, the pressure lessened. Then, when the treasure chests were almost reached, the water broke through from below and flooded the shaft.

These discoveries strengthened the conviction of the treasure seekers that the Money Pit must conceal an immese hoard. Why else go to such trouble to protect it? They began to construct a 150-foot long cofferdam along the center of Smith's Cove, intending to enclose the area that fed the flood tunnel. Before the structure was completed, it was destroyed by an unusually high tide.

Unwilling to begin another dam, the workmen tried to intercept the tunnel's course across the island. Their first attempt, near Smith's Cove, missed the tunnel. Instead of trying again in that area, where the tunnel was closest to the surface, for some reason they went back to the Money Pit and dug still another shaft—the fifth to that time. At 35 feet they struck a large boulder. When they tried to shift it, a rush of water poured into the shaft. They took this to mean that they had found the flood tunnel, although a moment's reflection should have suggested that it was at too high a level. Heavy timbers were driven down in the hope of blocking the tunnel, and a sixth shaft was sunk 50 feet away from the Money Pit.

At 118 feet the workmen started tunneling from this latest shaft toward the original shaft. The tunnel was large, measuring three feet by two feet. At some point during the tunneling— fortunately when most of the workmen were at lunch—the Money Pit collapsed into the tunnel. The searchers believed that the two chests they sought were dislodged in the general upheaval and fell deeper into the Money Pit, though the evidence for such a conclusion is unknown.

The Truro Syndicate had spent close to $20,000 by then, and

# The Flood System Discovered

# More Setbacks

were obliged to bring their operations to a halt until more money could be raised. They had found no treasure, but they had discovered the secret of the flooding.

In 1859, after another nine years had passed, they tried again. Several more shafts were sunk near the original one, all with the aim of draining the Money Pit or diverting the course of the flood tunnel. At one time 33 horses and a work force of 63 men were employed at the pumps. But still the water poured in. In 1861 steam pumps were erected, but the boiler burst almost immediately. One man was scalded to death, and operations were once more suspended.

As other prospectors tried their luck, the area around the Money Pit became a jumble. There were shafts sunk into the ground on all sides, some filled with water that rose and fell with the tides, others filled with debris. In 1866 operations were taken over by a group known as the Halifax syndicate. They also built a dam in Smith's Cove which was destroyed by the tide. But they managed to locate the point at which the flood tunnel entered the Money Pit. This occurred at 110 feet, 10 feet below the level on which the chests were thought to have rested originally. The mouth of the tunnel was about four feet high by $2\frac{1}{2}$ feet wide, lined with round beach stones. The skill of those who had built it was awe-inspiring.

With the realization of the unique system of protecting whatever might be placed in the Money Pit, people asked themselves the question: "How had those who buried the treasure intended to recover it?" Some thought they must have planned to make their way somehow through the flood tunnel. Others guessed that some system of floodgates, which could be closed when required, must have been introduced. No one doubted that the treasure must still be there somewhere. Isaac Blair, one of the members of the Halifax company told his nephew Frederick, "I saw enough to convince me that there was treasure buried there and enough to convince me that they will never get it"

Frederick Leander Blair later played a big role in the history of the Oak Island treasure hunt. Born in 1867 he was 24 years old when a new group of prospectors formed the Oak Island Treasure Company in 1891. He drew up the company prospectus, in which it was stated that they intended "to use the best modern appliances for cutting off the flow of water through the tunnel. . . . It believes that such an attempt will be completely successful, and if it is there can be no trouble in pumping out the Money Pit as dry as when the treasure was first placed there."

Alas, for such high hopes. Like all but one of the previous syndicates, the new company sank its intercepting shaft not at Smith's Cove but at the Money Pit end of the tunnel. Eventually, like all their predecessors, they returned to the Money Pit itself. Its position was now hard to identify, but the workmen managed to make their way into it through a side tunnel from one of the adjoining shafts. They dug upward till they came to a platform left by one of the previous operations. Money then ran out, and work was not resumed for eight years, the next time in 1897 at Smith's Cove. Blair drilled five holes across the mouth of the flood tunnel there.

Salt water was struck at the third drilling point, a charge of

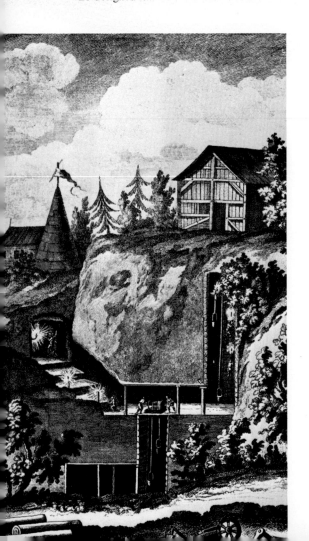

Below: this engraving, taken from Frenchman Denis Diderot's *Encyclopaedia*, published in the second half of the 18th century, shows the primitive mining methods at the time when the Money Pit was probably constructed. It demonstrates, if any such evidence were needed, the incredible ingenuity of the man or men who designed it.

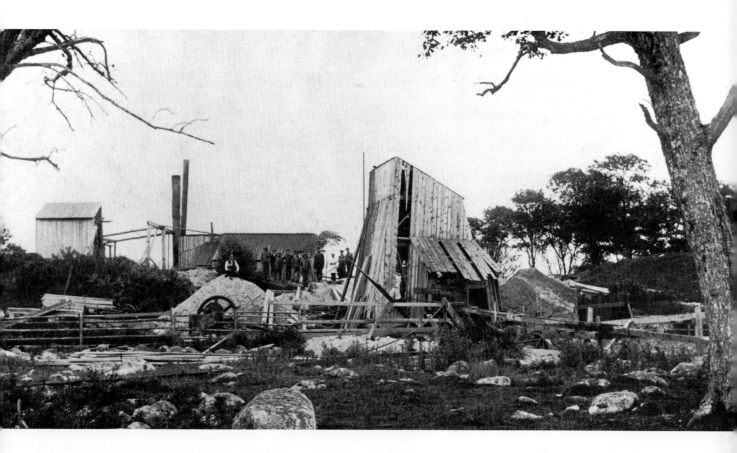

160 pounds of dynamite was lowered, and on being detonated produced great turbulence in the water of the Money Pit 450 feet away. Believing the flood tunnel to be blocked, Blair's team returned to the Money Pit, but pumping still failed to empty it. The team then proceeded to drill into its depths.

First they sent down a three-inch pipe inside of which their drill would operate more efficiently. This pipe was brought to a stop at 126 feet by an edge of iron, and all efforts to force the pipe past it failed. A 1½-inch drill was then put down inside the pipe. This passed the obstruction, went down to 151 feet, and struck a layer of soft stone afterward identified as cement. Twenty inches below the cement the drill bored through five inches of oak wood. The searchers believed that they were on the verge of learning what lay in the Money Pit at last. But then the drill began to behave oddly. It dropped two inches and rested on something that seemed to be large objects of metal which could be moved slightly from side to side. The movement of these objects hindered the descent of the drill but it finally got below them, only to come in contact with loose metal. This resisted the drill in a different way. At that time boring was done by raising and dropping the drill rods, and small pieces of metal fell into the space left each time the tool was drawn up. At one point a small piece of a substance identified as parchment was brought up, and this fragment still survives. On it the letters V.I. could be read. Finally the drill went past the layer of metal pieces into another layer of the large metal objects.

The nature of the metal is not indicated in the report written by William Chappell, one of the men present, but no one doubted

Above: this photograph of the head of the Money Pit was taken around 1896–7, during the period of activity by Blair's Truro Syndicate. The aim of this syndicate was to locate the flood tunnel, undermine it, and then to destroy it as an obstacle to reaching the treasure.

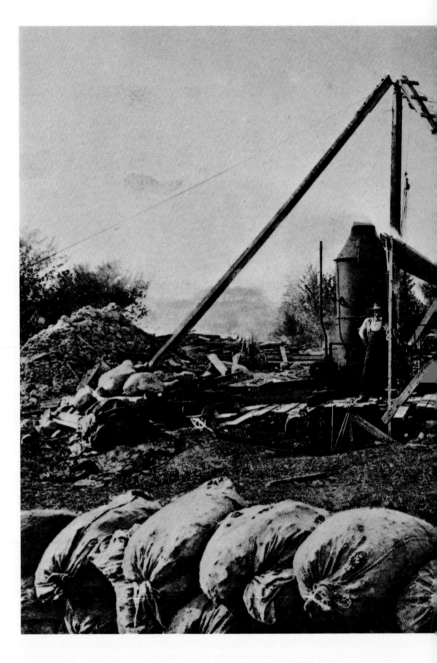

Right: this photograph was taken during the period of the Blair Company workings on Oak Island in about 1915. By November 1920, Blair was telling people that "the Pit caved in and more or less filled up . . . The ground surrounding the Pit has also caved in more or less and the spaces in and around the Pit are full of water." Nevertheless, Blair continued to act as a kind of consultant to other men digging for the treasure until his death in 1945, still convinced that the treasure would be found.

that they had located a chest containing small metal pieces that might well be coins, between two layers of metal bars. Edward Hopper, a syndicate member who was at the shaft that day, wrote to a friend in London: "Never in my life have I known the kind of excitement that gripped us at that moment. We felt we were about to uncover the most cunningly concealed secret on the face of the earth. The riches down below seemed but of lesser importance, it was the solution of the riddle that had us all agog."

The next act was to secure the drill by piping below 126 feet. Samples could then be obtained of the small pieces of metal. After the drill was withdrawn, a 1½-inch pipe was lowered inside the three-inch pipe; but at 126 feet it was deflected by the iron object and struck the hard wall of the pit. When the 1½-inch drill was reinserted, it followed the course of the deflected pipe. The hole down to the chest was lost! Other drills were immediately

# A Quagmire of Clay and Mud

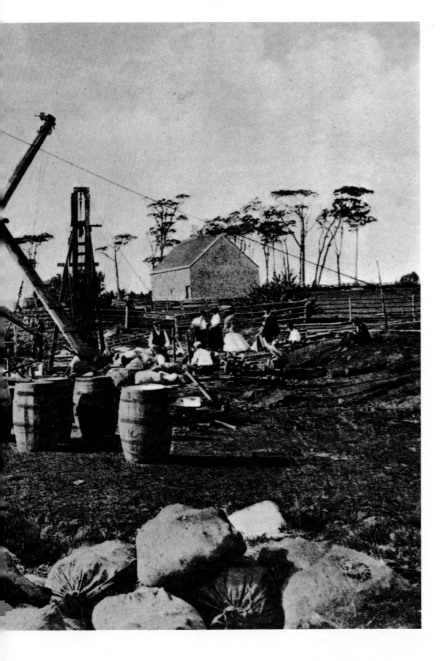

sent down, one of which appeared to strike the outer edge of the chest. Another one penetrated a channel of water that spouted up the pipe at the rate of 400 gallons a minute, drenching everything within range.

Blair concluded that there must be a second flood tunnel. To test for it he poured red dye into the pit—and sure enough a red coloration appeared at three separate places 600 feet from the pit, this time on the south shore. He sank no fewer than six shafts —the fourteenth to the nineteenth overall—between the Money Pit and the shore in an attempt to intercept the second flood tunnel. All of them had to be abandoned when water flooded in. The area soon became a quagmire of clay and mud, and the position of the Money Pit became more uncertain. Finally the syndicate, having spent $115,000, had to call a halt. Blair lacked the resources to continue on his own, but he managed to buy out

# Captain Kidd's Treasure Map?

the other shareholders and in 1905 acquired a long lease of the eastern end of the island. Until his death as a very old man in 1954 he never abandoned hope that the treasure would be found. One after another, optimistic prospectors appeared on the scene, sought his advice or enlisted his aid, poured their money into the bottomless Money Pit, and left empty-handed.

In 1909 came Captain Harry Bowdoin, a New York engineer with rich and powerful friends. Bowdoin cleared out the Money Pit to a depth of 113 feet and put down a core drill. At 149 feet they drilled through what appeared to be a layer of cement, and enthusiasm mounted when it was suggested that this could be the roof of a treasure chamber. But below this layer the drill brought up only yellow clay; an analysis of the cement showed it to be "natural limestone pitted by the action of water." In 1912 someone tried to freeze the watery mud at the bottom of the Money Pit, but this also came to nothing. Still other attempts were made about this time, and in the resulting criss-cross of shafts, the exact location of the Money Pit was once again lost.

In 1931 William Chappell, who had been in the 1897 syndicate with Blair, returned to Oak Island with $50,000 and sank a shaft where the Money Pit was believed to be. He uncovered a pick, a miner's seal-oil lamp, and an ax head thought to be 250 years old. Blair could not understand what had happened to the wood, the cement, and the metal pieces that had so tantalizingly eluded him and Chappell when they had brought up the circle of parchment so many years before. He came to believe that the treasure had dropped further into some natural cavity in the rock as a result of all the activity in the Money Pit. Greater understanding of the geological formation of the island was later to show that in fact the underlying limestone contained many cavities and sink-holes.

In 1933 came a British Columbian named Thomas M. Nixon, who believed that the Incas had deposited a treasure on Oak Island. He proposed to enclose the entire Money Pit area within a circle of interlocking steel pilings. If he had carried out this costly operation it might have solved many problems, but in-

Right: the second of two shafts sunk by wealthy New Jersey businessman Gilbert D. Hedden in 1936. Careful research had convinced Hedden that the Oak Island Treasure was that of the 17th-century pirate Captain William Kidd. Hedden's shafts went down 150 and 124½ feet, and numerous bores were made by his team which struck timbers at depths between 148 and 157 feet. Hedden then gave up, but he remained convinced that the treasure was there, between 160 and 170 feet below ground.

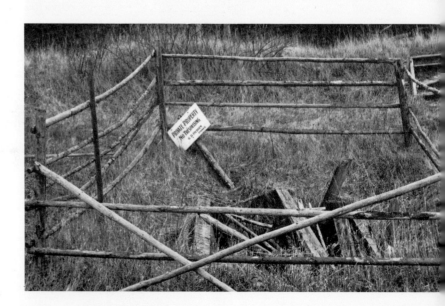

stead he did no more than sink some bore holes around the Money Pit and depart, like so many others before him, with nothing to show for his trouble.

Nixon was followed by Gilbert D. Hedden, a wealthy New Jersey businessman. In the course of two seasons of digging and drilling, he came to the conclusion that the chests that once held the treasure must have rotted away in the constantly waterlogged soil. He guessed that the treasure lay scattered through the clay. He also took the trouble to explore the island, and made a significant discovery in the tangled undergrowth on the edge of the south shore. A triangle of beach stones had been arranged on the ground with a curved line enclosing the base to give it the appearance of a rough sextant. The sides of the triangle were 10 feet long, and an arrow made of stones slanted across the base line to the apex. This arrow pointed due north, to the Money Pit.

Hedden did not stumble on this sign by chance. He was led to it by following directions in the book *Captain Kidd and his Skeleton Island*, written in 1935 by Harold Wilkins. This book included a chart of an island that resembled Oak Island in several particulars, and contained the following directions:

18 W and by 7 E on Rock

30 SW 14 N Tree

7 by 8 by 4.

Below: the map in British writer Harold Wilkins' book *Captain Kidd and his Skeleton Island*, first published in 1935. Hedden was struck by several similarities between the island on the map and Oak Island, and went to England to meet Wilkins. He then convinced Wilkins that the map, drawn from memory after seeing briefly some charts believed to have belonged to Captain Kidd himself, was of Oak Island. Further examination of the charts, however, showed them to date from 1669, when Kidd was only 20 years old and had probably not yet accumulated enough treasure to bury elaborately on any island.

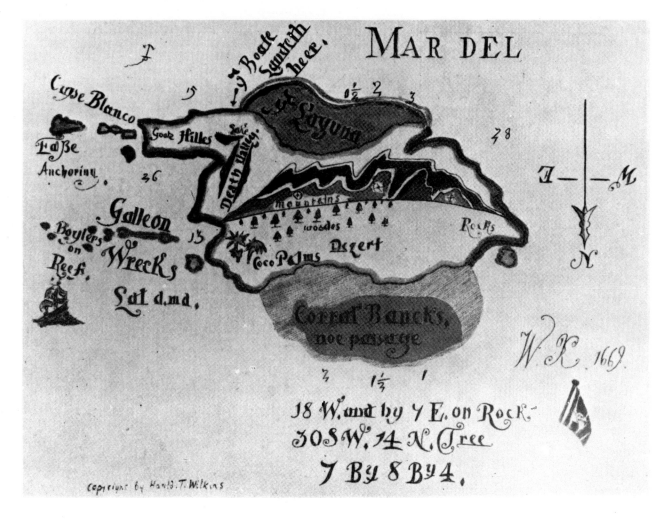

Right: Captain Kidd supervising the burial of treasure in a cave, while one of his men takes notes of the exact spot. After seeing the map on the previous page, both Hedden and Blair were certain that it was Captain Kidd's treasure that lay buried on Oak Island.

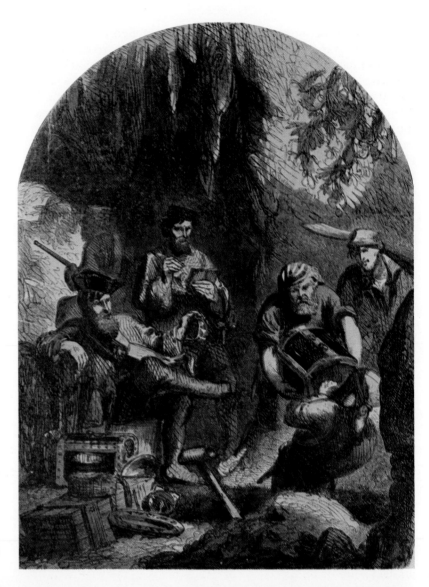

Below: Captain Kidd (far right) at the bar of the British House of Commons in March 1701. He was questioned by the House about his piracy, for which at that time he was being tried, because it was not clear whether he was acting on his own behalf or on the orders of certain English peers whose ship the *Adventure* he had captained. Whatever the truth, Kidd was found guilty of murder and piracy and hanged in London in May of the same year.

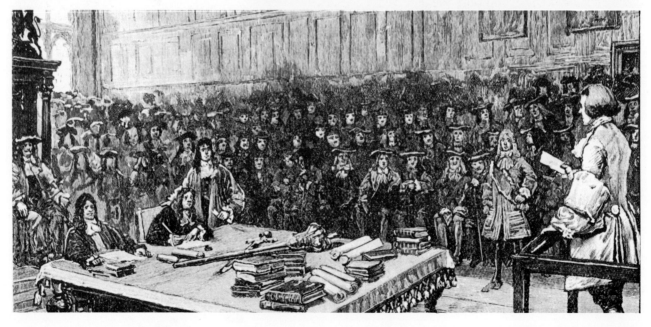

Carrying Wilkins' book in his hands, Hedden searched the ground around the Money Pit and discovered a large granite stone due north of it in which a hole had been drilled. This reminded Blair, who was still the unofficial advisor for all search operations, of a similar drilled stone he had discovered at Smith's Cove 40 years before. They rediscovered the second boulder and found that the distance between them was just over 25 rods, a rod being an ancient unit of measure equivalent to $16\frac{1}{2}$ feet. Hedden and Blair called in two land surveyors who calculated a position 18 rods from the drilled stone on the west and 7 rods from the drilled stone on the east. Thirty rods southwest of this brought them to the tangle of undergrowth where lay the arrow pointing north to the Money Pit. The tree that had once grown above it had long since vanished, and in any case it was somewhat more than 14 rods north. What the final line of directions signified Hedden and Blair could not tell, but the first two lines were enough to convince them that the treasure in the Money Pit was Captain Kidd's.

Hedden went to England to consult Wilkins, who was incredulous when told of the Oak Island mystery pit. He denied all knowledge of Oak Island and explained that he had drawn the map in his book from memory after being allowed a glimpse of some apparently authentic Kidd charts in the possession of Hubert Palmer, a collector of antiques. As for the directions, he insisted that they had come out of his head. However, Wilkins was so impressed by the use Hedden had put them to on Oak Island that he later came to believe he himself was a reincarnation of Captain Kidd!

The Kidd-Palmer charts, as they are called, are four in number. They were found secreted in three sea chests and an old oak bureau that had been acquired by Palmer between 1929 and 1934. All had apparently at one time belonged to Captain William Kidd. One is said to have been handed down in the family of his jailer at Newgate prison where he was hanged in 1701 for acts of piracy in the Indian Ocean. All the charts depicted the same curving island and several bore the date 1669. The charts, which are now in Canada, are considered to be genuine 17th-century charts, and their existence adds another mystery to the Oak Island enigma. The reference to the China Sea in one of them has been held to be a deliberate attempt to mislead, while at the same time making a punning reference to Oak Island by playing on the French for oak, *chene*. Against this theory is the fact that in 1669 Kidd was only in his 20s, and though his movements at that time are obscure, it is doubtful that he could have amassed a sizeable treasure so early in his career.

After Hedden came Edwin H. Hamilton, a machine engineer. He drilled down to 180 feet, deeper than anyone before him, located the original Money Pit, and made two important discoveries. He found that the second flood tunnel entered the Money Pit at 150 feet and from the same side as the first one, which had been constructed at 110 feet. Both tunnels therefore came from Smith's Cove, one above the other. He also explained why Blair's red dye had appeared on the south shore: at 180 feet a natural stream flowed across the base of the pit from north to south in direction.

# The Story of Captain Kidd

Below: the body of Captain Kidd hanging in a gibbet at Tilbury point, in the Thames Estuary. After their execution by hanging, the remains of pirates were often chained up in this gruesome manner and the gibbet placed at some point from which it could be clearly seen from passing ships as a warning to their captains and crew of the cruel penalty for piracy on the high seas.

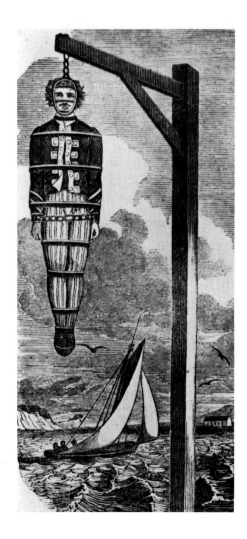

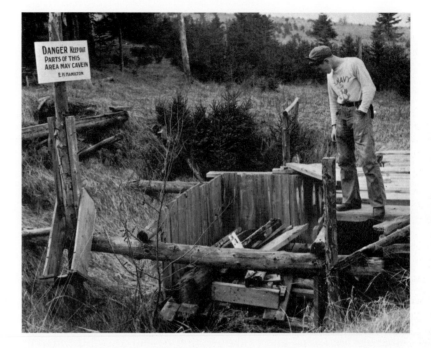

Right: a photograph taken in 1949 of the pit shaft dug by Edwin H. Hamilton. This shaft went down 180 feet, deeper than any earlier attempt, but apart from locating the second floor tunnel at 150 feet and a natural stream at 180 feet, he was no more fortunate than Blair or Hedden.

Dauntless prospectors continued to turn up. One man appeared equipped with only a pick and shovel. In 1955 a Texas oil drilling syndicate worked on the site for four weeks. Tragedy struck in 1963. Robert Restall, a former circus stunt rider, had worked on the pit for five years. On August 17, 1963 he was overcome by the exhaust fumes falling into the shaft from his pump. His 22-year-old son John and two other men died in a fruitless attempt to rescue him.

Excavations on a mammoth scale were carried out in 1965 by Robert Dunfield, an American petroleum geologist. He built a causeway from the mainland to bring a 70-foot clam digger to the island, and in six weeks he had excavated a vast hole 80 feet wide and 130 feet deep where the Money Pit had once been. Another deep crater obliterated the site of the stone triangle and a third, 80 feet wide and 100 feet deep, was dug near Smith's Cove. At the end of the year Dunfield had spent $120,000. He said, "I'm running out of nerve but I'm damned if I'll quit. I'm going on till I succeed or bust, and I intend to succeed." He didn't.

Rupert Furneaux, whose book *The Money Pit Mystery* (1972) is an authoritative guide to the checkered history of Oak Island, visited the island after Dunfield's assaults and found the eastern end "devastated." As he walked around the island he remembered the old saying that it would only give up its secret when the last oak had gone. He knew that for some years black ants had been causing extensive damage among the oak trees. In his wanderings he found only two oaks, both dead and toppling into the spruces that were taking their place. That was in 1967. Will Oak Island soon give up its secret?

Meantime, Furneaux has concentrated on trying to solve the mystery of who constructed the pit. He dismisses the pirate theory completely on the grounds that the task required special engineering skills. Besides, the construction of the two flood

# A Tragic Accident

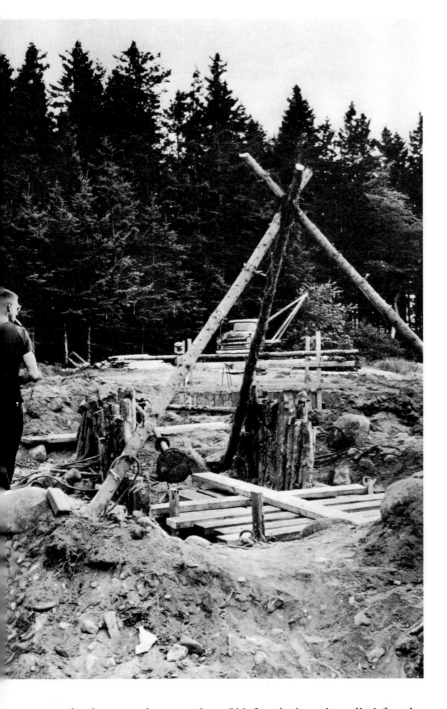

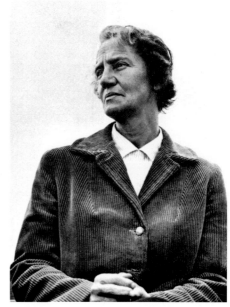

Left: the sealed shaft dug by Robert Restall. "Anyone can reach the gold who has enough backing and the proper equipment," he predicted. But in August 1963, after five years' work, he was overcome by pump fumes while working in the shaft. His son John and two other men were also killed.

Above: Restall's widow, Mrs. Mildred Restall, at the shaft where her husband and son were killed the previous day. Before his death, Restall had found a stone with the date 1704 on it. This convinced him that treasure had been buried that year.

tunnels alone, each more than 500 feet in length, called for the concerted effort of a disciplined body of men for a matter of weeks, if not months. A pirate crew, always eager for the next adventure and more booty, would hardly take such time and make such effort.

Furneaux decided that the pit must have been constructed by well-drilled workers under the direction of an able engineer. Putting himself in the position of his mystery engineer, Furneaux realized that his greatest problem must have been to keep the tunnelers working on a straight line from Smith's Cove to the Money Pit. The line of this tunnel is 14° south of the true east-west line. Workmen digging in the dim light of a tunnel would

# A Puzzle Solved?

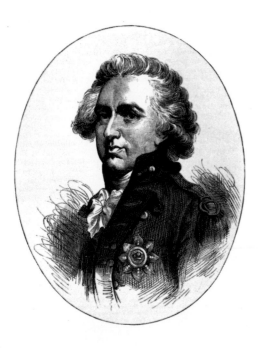

Above: Sir Henry Clinton, British commander-in-chief during the American Revolutionary War. One theory about the Money Pit suggests it was designed and dug on his orders, possibly by his extremely able military engineer John Montresor, as a safe place to conceal the large sums of money in his keeping in the event of defeat or withdrawal. It certainly seems that only a highly trained engineer could have devised the flooding system.

Right: the treasure hunt continues. As recently as 1970 a group of businessmen formed the Triton Alliance Company. By November 1971 they announced that they had drilled over 200 feet down, lowered a submarine camera television, and had glimpsed the faint outline of a number of chests or boxes. But divers who went down the same shaft to an unspecified depth did not find anything.

find it easiest to follow the direction indicated by one of the bold cardinal points of the compass, in this case west. This could only have been possible in a year when the magnetic variation from true north, and true west, was 14°.

Such a variation had occurred twice in recent centuries: in 1611, which was clearly too early, and in 1780. Bearing in mind the description by the boys who discovered the pit in 1795 that the clearing had been recently worked and new wood was springing up, the year 1780 looked a likely answer.

It is Furneaux's belief that British engineers dug the pit on Oak Island, possibly on direct instructions from Sir Henry Clinton, British Commander-in-Chief against the Americans in the Revolutionary War. He was stationed in New York from 1778 to 1782, but he had orders to fall back on Halifax if necessary. Furneaux deduces that Clinton may have felt it wise to prepare a safe place for concealing the large sums of money sent to him from England for the conduct of the war, if he had to fall back on Halifax. In some years these sums exceeded £1 million. Oak Island may have been suggested to Clinton by his close friend John Montresor, principal engineer in the British Army and the man who had surveyed Mahone Bay some years earlier. The soldiers who carried out the work presumably came from Halifax 40 miles up the coast, and their lights while working on the island may have given rise to the legend of its haunting. The names of the British military engineer officers serving in America at that time are

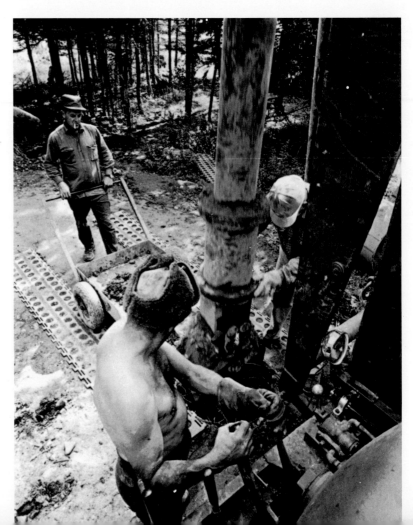

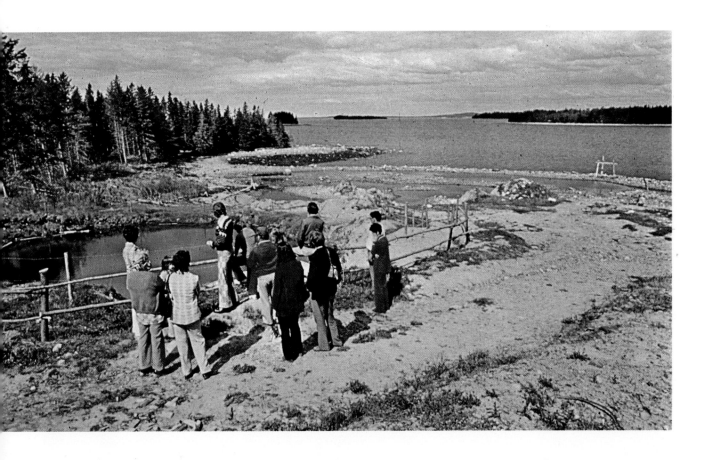

known, but which of them was in charge of the work on Oak Island, if Furneaux's supposition is true, has yet to be discovered.

How did the British hope to recover the money from the pit, protected as it was with flood tunnels? Furneaux's answer is that the money was never intended to be buried deep. After the pit had been dug, but before the flood tunnels had been connected, the officer in charge—possibly accompanied by a few trusted workmen—tunneled into the sides of the pit at a much higher level, outward and then upward. These high chambers were designed to be the repositories of the money. Recovery might even have been possible from the surface without digging into the pit at all. Anyone not knowing this would expect the treasure to lie at the bottom of the pit and would dig down, eventually to be overwhelmed by the inrush of the tide—which is just what occurred. They would continue to think the treasure lay at the bottom of the pit—as also occurred. Furneaux adds that if the money was actually buried on Oak Island, it must have been recovered shortly afterward or there would have been a big discrepancy in the British Army's accounts.

This solution, attractive though it is in many respects, still leaves some questions unanswered. What were the objects encountered by the pod-auger in 1849 and by the drill operated by Blair and Chappell in 1897? What happened to those objects? How did a fragment of parchment get so deep in the ground? Many believe a treasure still lies somewhere in the mysterious Money Pit, now a mass of puddled clay and mud on Oak Island. But the attempts to prove it over the past nearly 200 years have cost five lives and a fortune in money.

Above: tourists looking at the muddy mess that almost incessant excavation has made of the Money Pit today. Will anything ever be found to justify the five lives and a fortune in money that this extraordinary riddle has already cost?

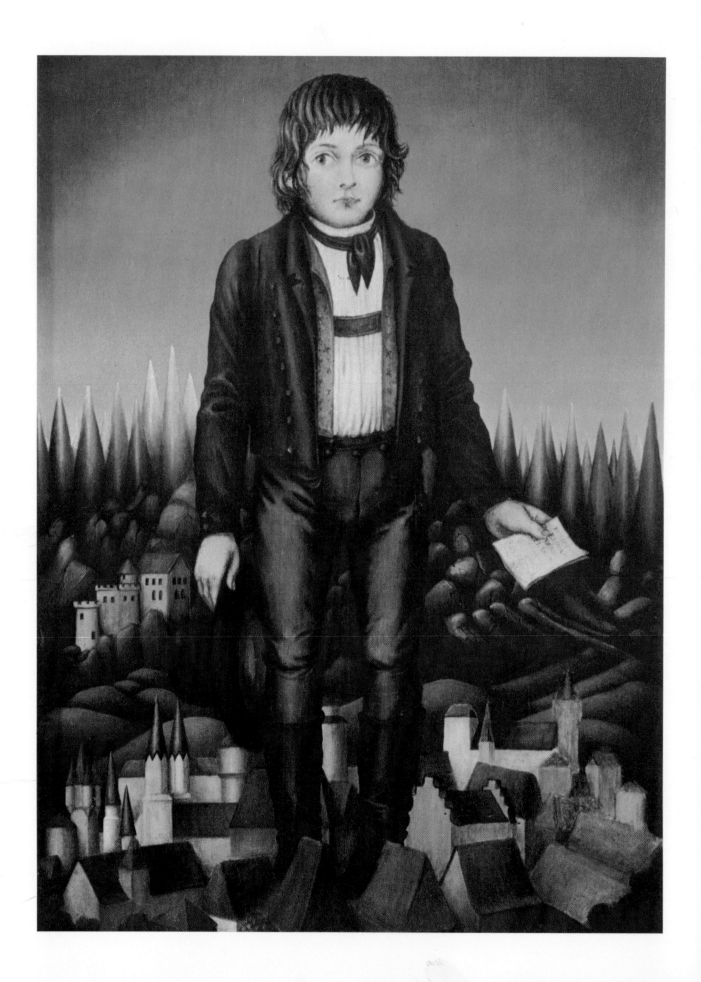

# Chapter 5
# People Without a Past

People who seem to appear out of nowhere are just as fascinating
and mysterious as those who seem to disappear into nowhere.
Scandalous rumors are the usual response. Was Caspar Hauser,
the 17-year-old who simply turned up in Nuremberg in 1828, the
rightful heir to the Grand Duke of Baden? Could the Man in the
Iron Mask have been a disreputable stepbrother of King Louis XIV?
Is Anna Anderson the Grand Duchess of the last Russian imperial
family, as she has claimed for more than 50 years? People without
a past: will their riddles ever be solved?

On Whitmonday in the year 1828 Georg Weichmann, a shoemaker of Nuremberg, Germany, noticed an oddly dressed youth
of about 16 wandering aimlessly in the square near his home. The
youth, a total stranger, looked like he might be drunk by the way
he moved so uncertainly. Weichmann approached him.

The youngster handed Weichmann a letter addressed to the
captain of the 6th Cavalry Regiment, then stationed in the
Bavarian city. The shoemaker took the time to find out where the
captain was housed, led the boy there, and left him after ringing
the bell.

When the door was opened by a servant, the youth handed
over his letter and said in a broken dialect, "I want to be a soldier
like my father was." The captain was away, but his wife ordered
food and drink to be brought to the young stranger, who looked
worn out and could walk only with difficulty. He rejected what
was offered, but when plain black bread and water were put before him, ate as though he were starved. When asked who he was
and where he came from, he seemed not to understand what was
being said to him. To all queries he either repeated, "I want to be
a soldier like my father was," or grunted a few disconnected
words such as "horse," "home," "my father"—all of which he
seemed to have learned by heart. He frequently pointed to his
feet and wept, as though in pain.

When the captain returned, he could get no further with the
boy. The envelope addressed to him turned out to have two letters

Opposite: a contemporary picture of Caspar
Hauser, the mysterious youth, as he first
appeared wandering in the streets of
Nuremberg, Germany in May 1828.

# The Arrival of Caspar Hauser

within, both of which added to the mystery rather than clearing it. The introductory letter said that the writer, who did not identify himself, had had the child left with him on October 7, 1812, and had never let him go out of the house. It added: "If his parents had lived, he might have been well educated; for if you show him anything, he can do it right off." The second letter, written to give the impression that it was from the youth's mother to the writer of the first letter, was dated 1812, 16 years before. It said that the youngster's name was Caspar, and it asked that he be taken to Nuremberg at the age of 17 because his dead father had belonged to the 6th Cavalry Regiment. Since the 6th Cavalry had been stationed in Nuremberg for only a short time, the letter could hardly have been written so long before. Both letters were believed to be forgeries.

The captain decided that the matter was one for civil authorities, and turned the youth over to the police. At the police station the same situation occurred. The youth made no sensible answers to questions, seeming to have no comprehension of what was going on around him. Sometimes he repeated his few stock of words or pointed, weeping, to his feet. When a kindly soldier gave him a small coin he was delighted and called out, "horse, horse," making signs that he wanted to hang the bright object around a horse's neck. His manner was that of a three-year-old child, but no one could decide whether he was a born idiot or someone who had lost his wits. A few even suspected that he might be an imposter. When provided with paper, pen, and ink he immediately wrote the name Caspar Hauser in a firm legible hand. He could write nothing else, and no more information could be obtained from him since his replies were irrelevant. He ignored threats of punishment, showing neither fear nor defiance. Finally he was taken to a nearby prison for vagabonds and suspicious persons; there he fell asleep instantly on a hard straw bed.

Apart from the two letters, Caspar's only possessions were some pious tracts and the clothes he stood up in—worn shoes, a red leather hat lined with yellow silk, a black silk kerchief around his throat, and a gray suit that looked as if it had been made from the cast-offs of a gentleman. In his pocket he had a white handkerchief with a red border and the initials *C.H.* worked in red.

When Caspar wept his face became ugly, like the puckered face of a crying baby, but when he smiled his face lit up so attractively that people said it was the face of an innocent child. The soles of his feet were as soft as a baby's, as though he had never before worn shoes and never walked. In fact, he moved like a child learning how to walk, often losing his balance and falling.

The jailer became deeply interested in Caspar and put him in a room in his own apartment where he could watch him unobserved through a secret opening in the door. After careful observation the jailer decided that his charge was neither an idiot nor a madman nor an imposter. In his opinion Caspar was a child in experience and behavior—if not in age—and he believed some great mystery lay beneath this unnatural state.

One day a friendly soldier gave Caspar a white wooden toy horse, which utterly delighted him. When other toy horses were given to him, he was content to play with them all day. He offered each one a tiny portion of his bread and water, and apologized to

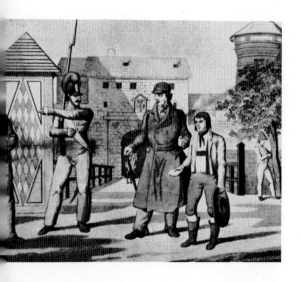

Below: Caspar Hauser is here shown being presented to the soldiers in Nuremberg in accordance with the instructions in a letter he carried.

them if he knocked them over. When he fell off a rocking horse one day and hurt his finger on the floor, he complained that the horse had bitten him. Such behavior is characteristic of the very young.

At first all communication with the strange boy called Caspar Hauser had to be carried on by signs, except for the few words he knew and kept repeating. But under the jailer's careful guidance he began to learn rapidly, showing an eagerness to acquire knowledge on all subjects. About six weeks after his arrival in Nuremberg, the Burgomaster drew out of him a halting account of his previous life.

For as long as he could remember, Caspar said, he had been kept in a cell about six-feet long, four-feet wide, and five-feet high. This tiny room had two shutters that were kept permanently closed. His feet were bare, and he sat and slept on a mat of straw. His food consisted of black bread and water which was placed in his cell while he was asleep. Sometimes the water had a bitter taste and he fell asleep directly after drinking it; when he woke again his clothes had been changed and his nails trimmed. He had two wooden horses and a wooden dog to play with. A man looked after him, but Caspar had never seen his face. Shortly before his departure from the cell this man showed him how to write the words "Caspar Hauser." His impressions of the journey to Nuremberg were confused, as well they might

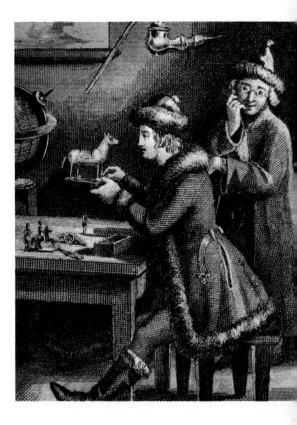

Above: Caspar playing with a white wooden horse that one of the soldiers gave him. He later described how he had grown up in a tiny room with two wooden horses and a wooden dog to play with, but no human contacts whatsoever. The man who had looked after him had never shown his face. Also in the picture is Professor Daumer who took Caspar in and looked after him.

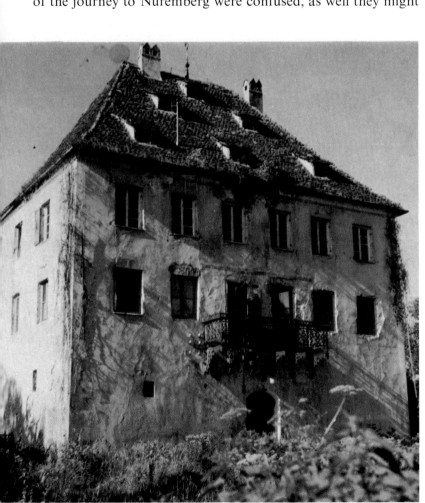

Left: Castle Pilsach. It has been suggested that it was in a windowless small room in this remote castle the young Caspar grew up, looked after by its caretaker, Franz Richter. In 1828 Richter's wife died and he found the boy too much of a responsibility. He therefore sent him alone to the city of Nuremberg, where he was later found.

Right: Louise von Hochberg and Charles Frederick, Grand Duke of Baden. Louise was the Grand Duke's second wife, and was only 19 when she married the 60-year-old Charles Frederick. One theory explaining the appearance of Caspar in Nuremberg in 1828 is that he was one of the Grand Duke's great grandchildren by his first wife, and therefore a claimant to the title. Louise, who is believed to have been the mistress of Charles Frederick's son Ludwig, is also believed to have smuggled the true heir out of the way to ensure that one of her own sons inherited the title.

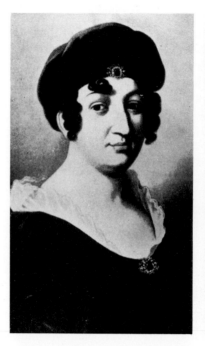 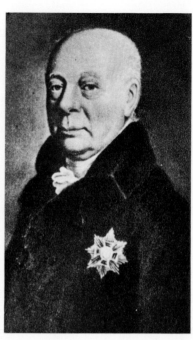

be. On coming into the open air for the first time he fainted, and walking in shoes was a torture to him.

The Burgomaster appealed to anyone who had known Caspar Hauser to come forward, but no one did. The city of Nuremberg then adopted him and entrusted him to a Professor Daumer with whose family Caspar went to live. His good nature and open-heartedness impressed everyone, and one observer described him as "a being such as we may imagine in Paradise before the Fall."

The appearance of this mysterious youth from out of nowhere created great excitement throughout Europe. Rumors abounded. Some said that Caspar had been kept in isolation to hide his noble birth. This idea gained more and more credence—and accusing fingers pointed finally at the Grand Duke of Baden.

The ruling family of Baden was renowned for the extravagance and immorality of its princes and the violence that ended so many of their lives. Karlsruhe, the capital of Baden, had been founded in the early 18th century by the Margrave Charles William who kept a harem of 160 beautiful girls. He was succeeded in 1738 by his grandson Charles Frederick who ruled for 73 years. Three sons were born to Charles Frederick by his first wife, and after her death in 1783 the 60-year-old Margrave married a 19-year-old lady-in-waiting at the court. Unknown to him, she was already the mistress of his third son Ludwig. On the day of her marriage she was created Baroness and later Countess Hochberg, but because she was not of royal birth, her children stood little chance of succeeding her elderly husband. Within six years she gave birth to four boys and a girl—popularly believed to be Ludwig's children.

The margrave's eldest son Charles Ludwig died in 1801 after his carriage overturned, although no one else was injured. It was said that the prince had received a blow on his head. Even at the time the death was considered suspicious, and in later years it

Below: Ludwig, Grand Duke of Baden, the third son of Grand Duke Charles Frederick by his first wife. Louise von Hochberg was apparently his mistress and bore him four sons and a daughter while married to his ageing father.

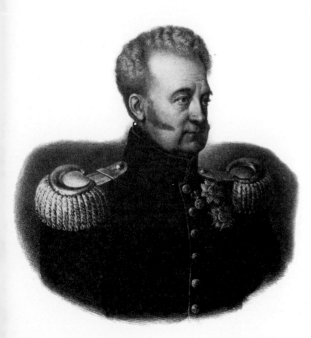

was regarded as the first unholy fruit of an alliance between Ludwig and the Countess to ensure the succession of their children.

In 1806 Napoleon created the aged margrave a grand duke and arranged a marriage between his stepdaughter, Stephanie de Beauharnais, and the Grand Duke's 20-year-old grandson and heir, Charles. This was a setback for the conspirators, but they met it by encouraging Charles to ignore his young wife by a life of dissipation. For four years he lived apart from her, but then her beauty and intelligence won through and he settled down to married life. In 1811 she bore a daughter, and in that same year the aged Grand Duke died and young Charles became the new ruler. In 1812 Stephanie bore a son. Was this baby switched with another to do him out of his succession? Did he appear 16 years later as Caspar Hauser?

Those who believed that Caspar was the Grand Duke's rightful heir said he had been smuggled out of the palace like this. The Countess Hochberg took a recently born and sickly baby from one of her peasants. She then dressed herself up as "the White Lady," a ghost traditionally said to make its appearance just before a death in the royal family, and concealed the ailing baby

# Caspar–Victim of a Conspiracy?

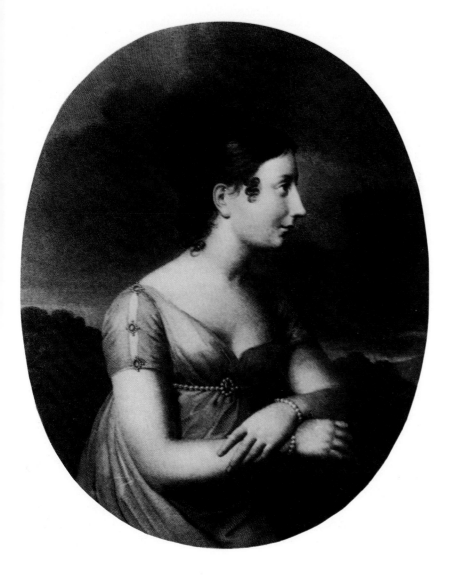

Left: Stephanie de Beauharnais, wife of Charles Frederick's grandson and heir, Charles. It is suggested that Caspar Hauser was her son, the rightful heir to the Grand Duchy, and was removed by the ambitious Louise to prevent him inheriting the title. Stephanie did indeed give birth to a son in 1812, who would have been 16 in the year 1828, when Caspar was first found. The baby died mysteriously shortly after birth.

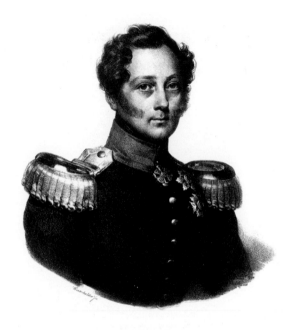

Above: Charles, Grand Duke of Baden. Caspar, it has been suggested, was his son, but was switched for the sickly baby that soon died. A second son also died under mysterious circumstances, and Charles himself died in 1818 after a lingering illness which suggested poison.

Right: two gentlemen looking at a portrait of "the White Lady," the Baden family ghost. The conspiracy theory proposes that Louise dressed up as the ghost in order to smuggle the baby Caspar out of the palace.

under her veil. Making her way to the newborn prince's bed-chamber along secret passages which had a secret door in a tapestry, she could give a ghostly impression of appearing and disappearing. A lackey who caught sight of her fell to the ground in a faint. A watchman saw her vanish through the wall.

The royal baby's two nurses had been drugged, it was said, and the wet nurse was allowed out of the palace for the night. The substitution was easily and swiftly made, and the infant prince removed to a castle outside the city. When the wet nurse returned to the nursery she was refused entry on the grounds that the baby was very ill. She tried to get to Grand Duchess Stephanie but was told that she also was ill and too weak to be disturbed. When the wet nurse finally managed to reach the Grand Duchess she found the royal mother frantic with anxiety because she too was being denied sight of the child. Later that night the Grand Duchess was told that her baby was dead, having been in the care of Margrave Ludwig's physician. She never saw his dead body, nor did the wet nurse. The body was examined by doctors who had never seen the baby alive. The verdict of death was cerebral meningitis, which could mean that the skull had been opened in an effort at treatment. At all events, the body was unrecognizable when the Grand Duke saw it. This substitution theory requires a large number of confederates, especially among the palace servants, but it need not be rejected on that count.

In 1815 the Grand Duke, who was only 29, was struck by a lingering illness that he came to believe was caused by the steady

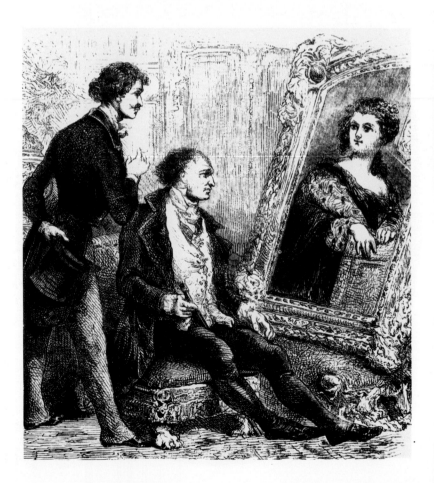

administration of poison. The following year a second son was
born. For a year he was closely guarded by trusted attendants,
but a week after his first birthday he developed a fever. The
Grand Duchess' physician did not want Margrave Ludwig's
physician to attend the child, as had been the case with the first
boy, but he was overruled. The child died the next day. Grand
Duke Charles followed him to the grave a year later and Margrave Ludwig at last took power. One of his first acts was to
recognize the Hochberg children as his heirs. Ludwig was still
ruling when Caspar Hauser turned up in Nuremberg.

By then, in 1828, the Countess was dead and Grand Duke Ludwig had become a prey to morbid melancholy. Ludwig's chief
aide was a certain Major Hennenhofer, who had been instrumen-
tal in the successful plot to abduct the royal heir in 1812. He is
said to have wanted the stolen prince killed at the beginning, but

# A Tangled Tale

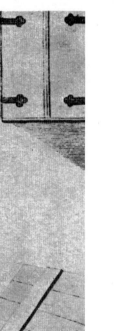

Left: the first attempt on Caspar's life. He
claimed he was attacked by a man in dark
clothing wearing leather gloves and a silk
mask. The attacker struck the mysterious
youth and fled, leaving him unconscious in
the cellar of the Daumers' house.

was overruled by the Countess who felt that the survival of the
prince was her only hold over Ludwig to prevent him from
marrying and producing other children that would supplant hers.
If Caspar were the prince, he was still a threat to Ludwig, so why
was he allowed to go free? The substitution theorists say that the
plotters thought he would disappear into the Bavarian army.
Since that plan had miscarried, and Caspar was protected by the
city of Nuremberg, Hennenhofer reverted to his original plan of
assassination. In October 1829 Caspar was discovered unconscious from a stab wound in the cellar of Professor Daumer's
house. On recovering, he said he had been attacked by a man
wearing a black mask. Caspar's critics, who say he was never
anything but a cunning imposter, say he must have stabbed himself in order to regain the limelight. Whatever the truth, he was
removed from the Daumer household to the care of a Nuremberg

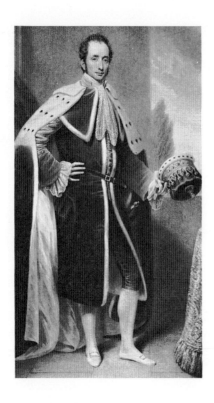

Above: Lord Stanhope, the eccentric
English nobleman who took a great interest
in Caspar and visited him frequently. In
1831 Stanhope removed him to Ansbach,
a town near to the city of Baden, and
employed a teacher and a bodyguard to
look after the mysterious boy.
Below: Queen Caroline of Bavaria. A sister
of Charles, Grand Duke of Baden, she said
that she saw a family likeness when she met
Caspar on his return to Nuremberg in 1833.

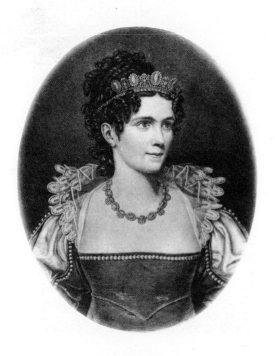

businessman. At this point in the mystery, Philip, 4th Earl Stanhope, enters.

Lord Stanhope belonged to an English family noted for its eccentricity and wild behavior. Was it only a whim that made him interested in the case? Whatever it was that drew him, he made several visits to Baden. He called on both the Grand Duke and Hennenhofer and ingratiated himself with Grand Duchess Stephanie, who was greatly agitated on learning that her first-born son might still be alive. From this time on, the erratic English noble was never without funds, though he had previously been chronically short of money.

In May 1831 Stanhope arrived in Nuremberg and proceeded to charm himself into Caspar's affections. He showered him with clothes and money, walked arm in arm with him through the streets, and soon began talking of his wish to adopt him. This proposal met with opposition, but Stanhope overcame it all. In November he took Caspar from Nuremberg to Ansbach, a town 20 miles closer to Baden, lodged him with a Protestant pastor named Meyer, and employed Police Lieutenant Hickel to act as his bodyguard. An unhappy period in Caspar's life began.

Meyer was short-tempered and suspicious of Caspar; Hickel actually believed he was an imposter. In spite of escaping outright cruelty because of the wide interest in him, Caspar underwent petty persecution at his guardians' hands. Fortunately for the youth, he formed many friendships in Ansbach, and was eventually apprenticed to a bookbinder. As for Stanhope, no sooner had he inveigled the youth away from Nuremberg than he ceased to spend much time with him. After a while he declared that Caspar was an imposter and left Ansbach. Soon his letters stopped and Caspar was left completely in the care of Meyer and Hickel, whom he came to mistrust. In September 1833 he made a return visit to Nuremberg, where he renewed contacts with old friends and was introduced to the King of Bavaria. The King's mother, Queen Caroline, was an aunt of the heir said to have died in 1812, having been a princess of Baden. She recognized a family likeness in Caspar and became a firm believer that he must be her nephew.

A few weeks after this royal recognition Stanhope wrote that he was returning to Ansbach. On his way he visited Baden, apparently leaving at the end of November in the company of Hennenhofer.

On December 11, 1833 the 21-year-old Caspar Hauser returned from a walk in the park with a mortal wound in his side. He told Meyer that a man had asked him his name and, after hearing it, had stabbed him in the ribs. Meyer refused to believe Caspar and charged the young man with having once again inflicted a self-injury to gain attention. Doctors were summoned, but the police were not informed. Three days later it was clear that Caspar was dying. Calm and conscious to the last, he resisted all efforts by Meyer to get him to confess that he was an imposter, and he maintained to the end that the story of the attack on him was true.

Who killed him is unknown. Queen Caroline of Bavaria accused Lord Stanhope to his face of the murder, though no record exists to show that he arrived in Ansbach until after Cas-

# Who Killed Caspar?

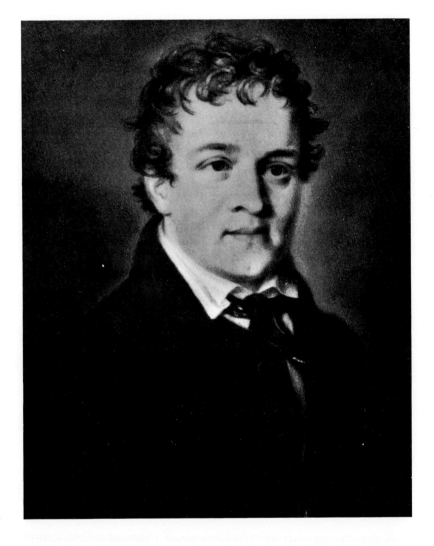

Left: Caspar Hauser in 1830, two years after he first appeared in Nuremberg. By this time he spoke fluently, had learned to read and write, and could handle everyday utensils as well as any other adult.

Below: Caspar's tombstone in the town of Ansbach where in December 1833 he was stabbed to death by an attacker who first asked him his name. The tombstone inscription reads: "Here lies Caspar Hauser, Enigma."

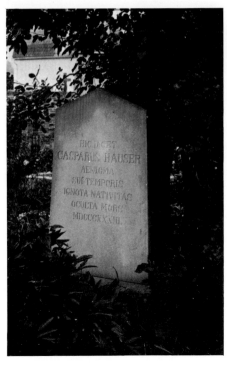

par's death. Whether Caspar Hauser was in truth the missing prince of Baden was never decided and probably never will be. There seems no reason to doubt that for many years of his life before arriving in Nuremberg he was kept closely confined in the manner he described. But all the evidence relating to the ducal family of Baden is largely circumstantial, if persuasive, and is unlikely to be proved.

On his tombstone in Ansbach cemetery are carved the following words: "Here lies Caspar Hauser, Enigma." He remains an enigma to this day.

The unfortunate Caspar Hauser was ignorant of his past through no wish of his own. Very different are those who deliberately obscure their origins so as to advance in a career where public knowledge of their lowly birth would be a hindrance. Such imposters flourished in Europe in the 18th century, a period in which high birth and rank were held to be the true mark of a man's worth. It was also a time when documentation was scanty and false statements of birth hard to disprove.

The most celebrated and attractive of these adventurers is the man known as Count Alessandro di Cagliostro. Something of a genius as a confidence man, he first emerged from obscurity in the summer of 1776 in London, where he had become famous for

# Two Charlatans From Nowhere!

his skill in predicting winning lottery numbers. He was then a man in his early 30s and, as an enemy was later to put it at the opening of a scurrilous poem: "Born, God knows where; supported, God knows how; From whom descended—difficult to know."

Cagliostro had arrived in London from Portugal, but his titled name was Sicilian. As for his birthplace, he maintained that he did not know it. He claimed to remember passing some years of his youth in Arabia, then a remote and inaccessible country, where he studied the secrets of the occult with an alchemist named Althotas. Althotas really existed, so perhaps Cagliostro was speaking the truth, or simply adding a little imagination to the basis of truth.

He is known to have visited Egypt and Turkey selling drugs

Right: Count Allesandro di Cagliostro and his wife Seraphina. Their real names were apparently Joseph Balsamo and Lorenza Feliciani. They first appeared on the European scene in the 1760s, when they began a grand career of fraud and mystification.

Below: Cagliostro predicting winning lottery numbers for some of his clients. He certainly seems to have established a reputation for this kind of clairvoyance and was besieged by people wishing to profit from his apparent system.

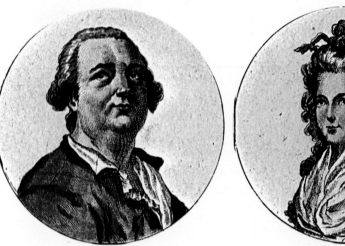

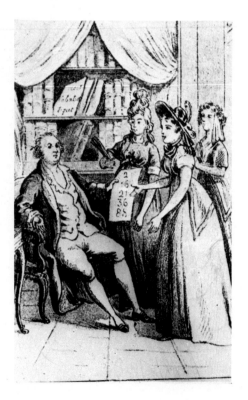

and amulets. In Italy in 1769 he married a remarkably beautiful 15-year-old whose name he changed to Seraphina. He seems to have had a genuine, if sporadic, gift for clairvoyance, and in London some seven years later managed to predict at least one winning lottery number. At once he was besieged by people eager to learn his system. Partly to escape them, partly because like most dissemblers he was a compulsive traveler, he hurried away to Germany and then to Poland. There he made a reputation for success in curing the sick, and founded a local Order of Egyptian Masonry, a mystical society not unlike later occult societies. He also sold bottles of the "elixir of life," ably assisted by Seraphina. Young, slim, and beautiful, she would casually refer in company to her son's recent promotion to the rank of captain in the Dutch army. Those who heard her expressed amazement that someone who looked so young could have a son old enough to be in the army. She replied simply, "He is 28." No further effort was needed to sell the elixir.

The miraculous potion was probably nothing more than an aphrodisiac, but by means of it and the count's genuine achievements as a faith healer, the Cagliostros reached the pinnacle of their success. That was in Paris in the years before the French Revolution. It pleased the count to keep his origins a secret and to conceal the source of his considerable wealth. Some of it no doubt came from the fees of Parisians who flocked to elaborate seances in his house, there to talk with the mighty dead such as Julius Caesar and Alexander the Great. His rooms were filled with Egyptian statuettes, and two lackeys dressed as Egyptian slaves were in attendance in the public rooms. Cagliostro's costume for these seances was a black silk robe embroidered with red hieroglyphics. It became the popular idea of a magician's robe for all time.

That he possessed real psychic powers is undeniable, but he stretched them with exotic tricks that weakened his standing. With success he grew arrogant and made enemies. Dragged into a scandal involving the theft of Queen Marie-Antoinette's diamond necklace, his reputation as a wonder worker crumbled. He wandered around Europe for a few more years, unwisely ending

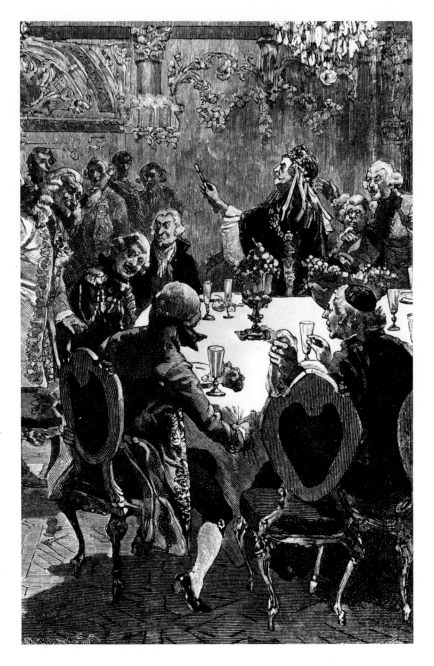

Left: Cagliostro at the peak of his powers gave a dinner in Paris at which he asked his guests to name six dead people whom he then proceeded to conjure up. On this occasion two of the "spirits" were the philosopher Voltaire and the great encyclopedist Diderot.

Below: King Louis XVI and his Queen Marie Antoinette question Cardinal de Rohan on the subject of the theft of the queen's diamond necklace. The cardinal was imprisoned in the Bastille, and Cagliostro was also sent to prison for a while. His apparent involvement in the affair was the beginning of his downfall.

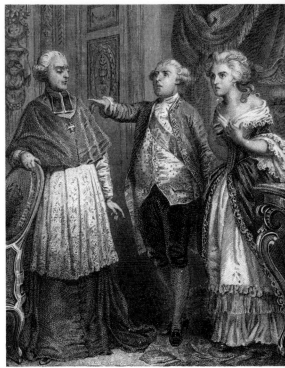

# The Mystery of Saint-Germain

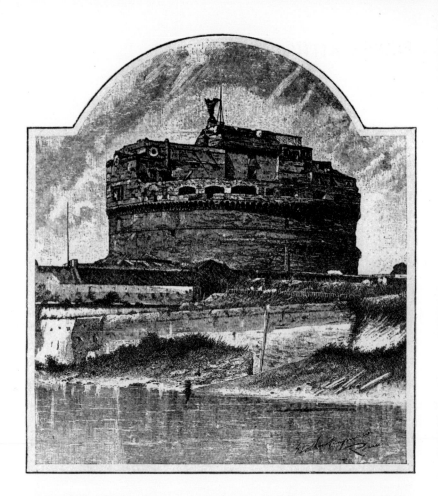

Right: the castle of St. Angelo in Rome. After the scandal of the queen's necklace, Cagliostro was forced to leave France and travel Europe. Finally he went to Rome where he was arrested by the Inquisition on charges of practicing the black arts and thrown into this prison during his trial.

up in Rome where he was arrested by the Inquisition and tried for heresy. In the city of the Pope the count's influential Freemason friends were unable to help him. Found guilty, he was imprisoned in an underground cell hewn from the rock in the mountain fortress of San Leone near Montefeltro. There, some time around 1795, he died. Some say he hanged himself in despair.

The Inquisition records show that he confessed to having been born in Palermo as Giuseppe Balsamo, son of a tradesman, and that he had spent his childhood in petty thievery. Not all his biographers accept this as fact inasmuch as it was probably extracted under torture. Some favor an Arabian or Levantine origin. No one knows the truth about this cunning but generous-hearted charlatan.

In the 18th century, Paris was the social capital of Europe, the big magnet for adventurers. A generation before Cagliostro, another strange count made his appearance there. He was the mysterious Count de Saint-Germain. No one has ever been able to discover the true name, family, or nationality of this extraordinary individual. His early life is totally wrapped in obscurity. Some said he was related to the Spanish royal family, others that his mother was an Arabian princess.

Like Cagliostro he began his career as a seller of elixirs of immortality, and he allowed it to be believed that he himself had been alive for many hundreds of years. He was a man of wit, taste, and profound learning. In Paris he captivated Louis XV and, still more important, the king's mistress Madame de Pompadour. Astonishingly wealthy, he always wore diamonds of the finest quality, frequently giving them away as presents.

In the company of the credulous he would talk of Henry VIII and other bygone kings as though he had known them intimately, providing so much detail that his listeners felt compelled to believe him. He had a servant who supported him loyally and could be as drily witty as his master. On one occasion at dinner the count was telling the party of a conversation he had enjoyed with King Richard I during the crusades. There was a murmur of disbelief around the table. Turning to his servant standing behind his chair, the count asked him if he had not spoken the truth.

"I really cannot say," replied the man without moving a muscle. "You forget, sir, I have only been 500 years in your service."

"Ah, true," said Saint-Germain, "it was a little before your time."

With people whom he could not dupe he confessed that a moderate diet and sensible exercise would achieve more than any elixir. He once admitted that he had read innumerable memoirs of life in former times, and that it was his excellent memory of their content which enabled him to sound like a man who had knowledge of life hundreds of years ago. The source of his great riches is as unknown today as to his contemporaries. He may have been a spy in the pay of the English or the Prussians, or both. He may have repaired flawed diamonds which he sold at many times their worth. He may have been born wealthy. Whatever the truth, he revealed nothing and was never discredited.

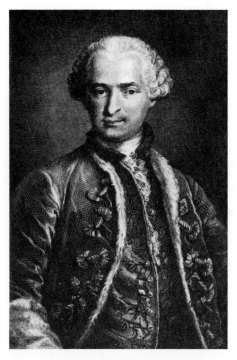

Above: the mysterious Count de Saint-Germain. Despite the numerous legends that surround the life of this elusive figure, little is actually known about him. He achieved a position of some influence at the French court of King Louis XV, and is said to have appeared in Paris after his death foretelling the French Revolution.

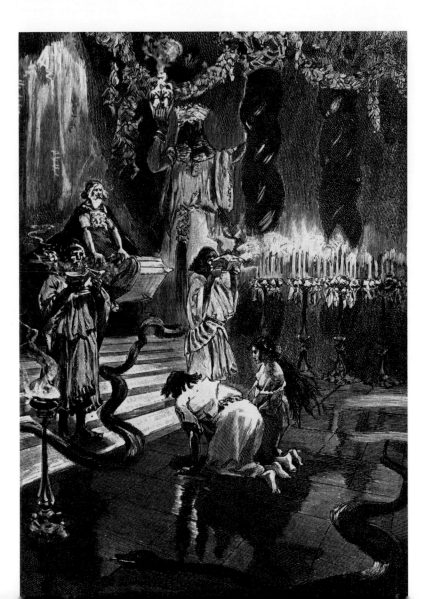

Left: an artist's impression of a meeting which never took place, between Saint-Germain and Cagliostro. Both men practiced pseudo-magic and organized cabalistic ceremonies, but while Saint-Germain was simply a shabby charlatan, Cagliostro does appear to have had genuine psychic gifts.

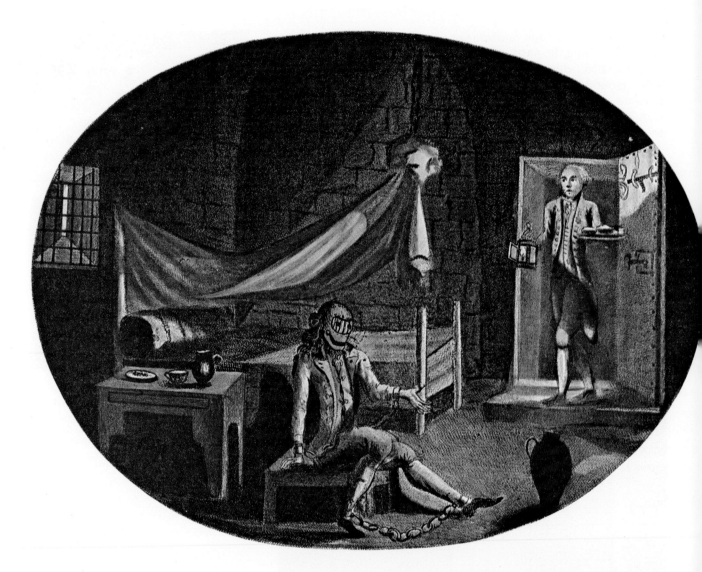

Above: the Man in the Iron Mask is
probably the most extraordinary mystery
of all time. Who the man was has only
recently been established with any
certainty, but the nature of his crime, and
the real reason for his 34-year incarceration,
still remain a baffling, intriguing riddle.

He ended his days quietly, living in the palace of his friend the
Prince of Hesse-Kassel. There in 1784 he died, taking all his
secrets with him to the grave.

Most mysterious of all those whose past is unknown is the
Man in the Iron Mask. The secrets of this enigmatic figure, who
was held in strictest confinement for over 30 years in a succession
of France's top security prisons, have never been unearthed
despite the efforts of historians, government officials, and other
interested investigators. Only recently has his name even been
established. His crime is still a deep mystery.

Whatever this crime was, it apparently did not warrant the
death sentence. Nevertheless it constituted so grave a threat to
the state and to the king—which in the reign of Louis XIV meant
the same thing—that the most remarkable precautions were
taken to prevent his identity from becoming known. He was forbidden contact with any other prisoner. His name did not appear
in the prison records and was never used, either in direct address
or correspondence. His jailer had strict orders to kill him instantly if he ever tried to talk of his life prior to his arrest. The
most chilling arrangement of all, and the one that has captured
the imagination of successive generations, was that his face was

never to be seen. He was obliged to wear a mask in front of every-one save the governor of the prison.

Rumors about a mysterious prisoner began to circulate within a few years of his death in the Bastille in 1703. Fifty years later these speculations were given a base of firm evidence with the chance discovery of a private journal kept by Etienne du Jonca, the King's Lieutenant in the Bastille during the relevant period. The first journal entry relating to the prisoner records his arrival at the Bastille in 1698 when he had already spent 29 years in prison, always in the custody of the same governor. It says: "Thursday, September 18 at three o'clock in the afternoon M. de Saint-Mars, Governor of the Chateau of the Bastille, made his first appearance, coming from the command of the Iles Sainte-Marguerite-Honorat, bringing with him, in his litter, a prisoner he had formerly at Pignerol, whom he caused always to be masked, whose name is not mentioned."

Five years later du Jonca records the death and burial, under the false name of *Marchioly*, of "the unknown prisoner, always

# The Enigmatic Man in the Mask

Left: Louis XIV of France giving orders to M. de Saint-Mars, governor of the Bastille, about the detention of the mysterious prisoner. One theory suggests that Louis XIV was in fact an illegitimate son, and the prisoner the true king.

# The Prisoner of Noble Birth

masked with a mask of black velvet." Different versions describe the mask as made of iron, or reinforced with steel, or fitted with a chin piece of steel springs to allow the prisoner to eat while wearing the mask. But according to du Jonca—the only eye-witness—it was made of black velvet.

The only other physical description of the masked prisoner comes from a doctor who in his youth helped attend the prisoners of the Bastille. He said he had often been required to treat the "unknown prisoner." He never saw his face but he examined his tongue and the rest of his body. "He was admirably made," said the doctor, "his skin was dark, his voice interesting." The medical man also pointed out that the mystery man "never complained of his lot or gave any indication of who he was."

The puzzling aspects of the case made rumor flourish. One tale had it that the prisoner was an illegitimate offspring of the Queen Mother and her Chief Minister Cardinal Mazarin, and therefore an elder stepbrother to King Louis XIV. Because he resembled the king so much, he could not be allowed his liberty without causing a scandal. According to another story, he was the king's twin brother, smuggled out of the palace at birth to avoid future rivalry and strife in the realm. He was kept in prison as an adult, and masked in iron so that he would never be seen in public, but he was given special and courteous treatment as a royal person-

Right: this 18th-century illustration shows the Marquis de Louvois visiting the "unknown prisoner" on the Ile Sainte-Marguerite before he was taken to the Bastille by Saint-Mars. The respect that the Marquis showed to the prisoner added to the legend that he was a man of noble birth, or even of royal blood.

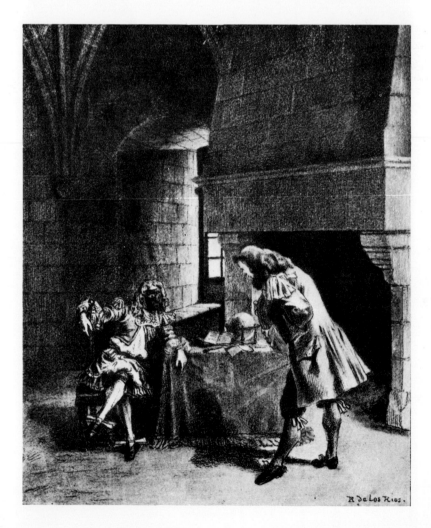

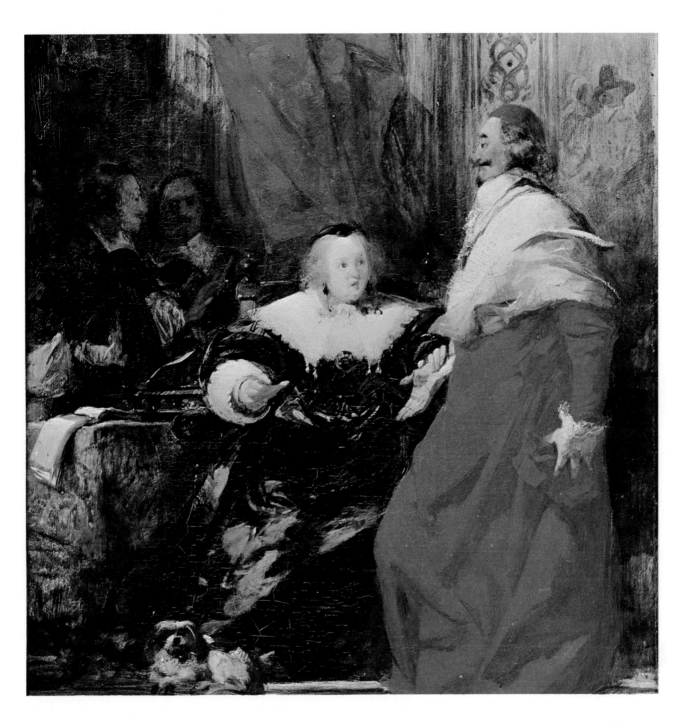

age. This is the version fictionalized by the great French novelist Alexandre Dumas, and it became so popular that the prisoner, like the title of Dumas' novel, is thought of only as *The Man in the Iron Mask*.

Yet another theory suggests that Louis XIV was the illegitimate child, and the prisoner the true king. It was said that the rightful heir had been imprisoned on the Ile Sainte-Marguerite, an island fortress in the Bay of Cannes, where eventually a son was born to him by the daughter of one of his jailers. This child was smuggled to Corsica and named "Buona-Parte," meaning "good stock" in Italian. His direct descendant was Napoleon Bonaparte, who was therefore the true heir to the throne. Other

Above: Anne of Austria, widow of King Louis XIII, and her Chief Minister, Cardinal Mazarin. One of the numerous theories about the "unknown prisoner" was—and is —that he was the offspring of an affair between the queen and her minister, and that his facial likeness to Louis XIV was the reason for the mask. The mask, however, was not iron, but of velvet with metal reinforcement, according to the only eyewitness whose evidence has been recorded.

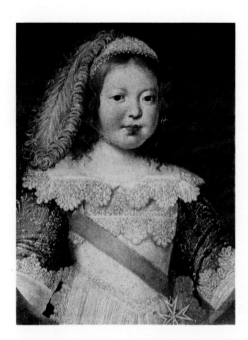

Above: a painting of Louis XIV as a child.
A second theory about the "unknown
prisoner" is that he was Louis' twin brother.
That would also explain the mask and the
eagerness of the king to keep him out of
sight of the people of France.

Right: this old map of the Bay of Cannes
shows the two islands clearly. It was on
the Ile Sainte-Marguerite, the larger of
the two, that the Man in the Iron Mask was
imprisoned.

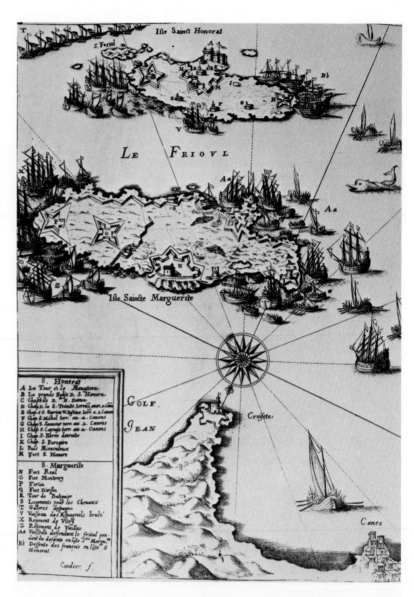

more unexpected identifications of the prisoner named him as an
Englishman, either an illegitimate son of King Charles II or a
son of Oliver Cromwell. Extravagant theories but, people
reasoned, no more extravagant than the efforts taken to conceal
the prisoner's identity. After his death, all the furniture and
equipment he had used was burned or melted down, and his
linen, bedclothes, and cushions destroyed. The walls of his room
were scraped and whitewashed in case he had concealed a message or made some mark that would reveal his name. All the floor
tiles were taken up and replaced. Whatever the secret about the
man, it was clearly one that the authorities were determined to
keep hidden.

Louis XIV's great-grandson and successor, Louis XV, is said to
have been told the truth, whereupon he remarked, "If he were
still alive I would give him his freedom." Louis XVI ordered a
search of the Royal Archives to satisfy the curiosity of his wife,
Marie-Antoinette, but few of the relevant papers could be found.
Documents discovered during the French Revolution estab-

listed that the prisoner cannot have been a member of the royal family, and he was tentatively identified as an Italian, Ercole Mattioli. Marchioly, the name under which the masked prisoner was buried, closely resembles this, and Mattioli had certainly offended the king. He had been the intermediary between Louis and the Duke of Mantua in a delicate scheme whereby the king hoped to acquire an important citadel on the Italian frontier. Mattioli double-crossed Louis who angrily ordered him to be abducted from Italian territory and imprisoned for life. The offender was incarcerated in Pignerol in the same tower as the masked prisoner—but there was never any doubt as to who he was. Indeed, the whole point of abducting and imprisoning him was to show the world that a man could not cheat the king of France and get away with it. The resemblance between his name and the name Marchioly in the prison death register was seen as yet another attempt to cover up the masked man's identity.

The archives of the Ministry of War eventually proved to be the source of further knowledge of the "unknown prisoner." Over 100 letters were discovered that related to the conditions of

## A Threat to King Louis XIV?

Below: this forbidding building is the monastery of Les Lerins on the Ile Sainte-Marguerite. This is one of the places on the island in which the mysterious prisoner was kept. One ingenious theory has it that he seduced the daughter of one of his jailers, and that their son was smuggled to Corsica, where his direct descendant was Napoleon Bonaparte. If therefore the real reason for his incarceration was that he was the true heir to the throne of France, this theory makes excellent Bonapartist propaganda.

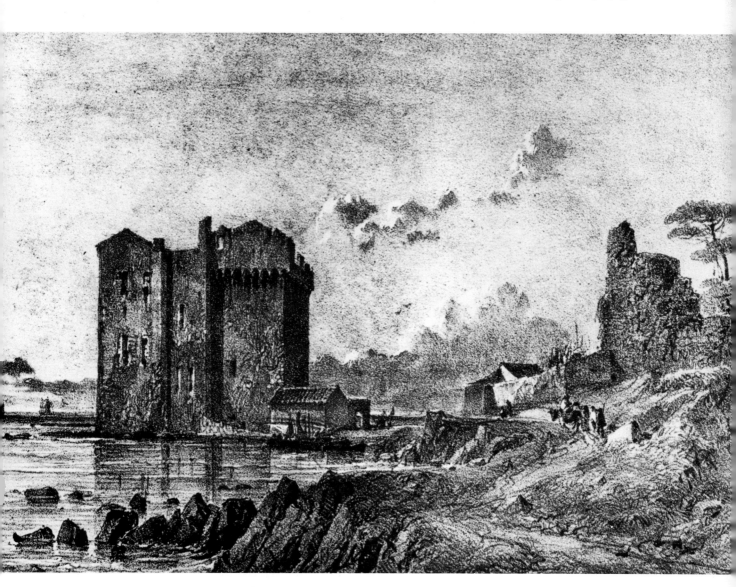

# A Death in the Bastille, 1703

his captivity, letters regularly passing between the prison governor Saint-Mars and the king's ministers. From these it became clear that the chief duty of Saint-Mars throughout his long service to the crown as governor of four successive prisons was to look after the masked man. Other eminent prisoners came into his custody from time to time. Their identities are known, and any letters refer to them by name. But his most important charge is always referred to as "the new prisoner" or "the prisoner you sent me." With the passage of time he became "the prisoner in the lower tower," and finally "the ancient prisoner."

It is now known that the mystery prisoner was arrested in Dunkirk in 1669, presumably either attempting to flee the country or having been lured back to it. He was taken across the whole of France to Pignerol on the Italian frontier, and remained there for 12 years until accompanying Saint-Mars on his transfer to the nearby Fortress of Exiles. Apart from his lack of liberty, his confinement seems to have been relatively civilized, certainly a

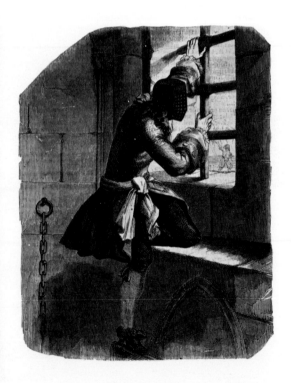

Above: a 19th-century illustration of an attempt by the Man in the Iron Mask to escape. According to one legend, he threw out of the window a plate on which he had written his name, but any who found out his name apparently came to regret the knowledge, for the penalties were swift and severe. Ironically, his name seems to be the one thing we know about him.

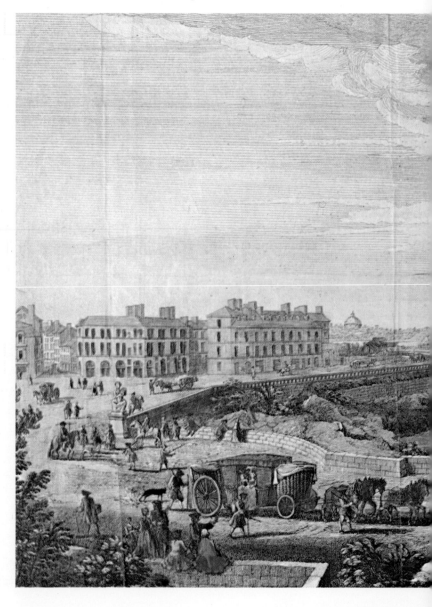

far cry from the dank dungeon in which Cagliostro ended his days. He was allowed books to read, although each page was carefully examined for secret writing. He was given musical instruments to play, and was kept supplied with good clothes. Strangely enough, he never complained. Saint-Mars reports of him that "he lives contentedly, like a man completely resigned to the will of God and the king." There is never any indication that he believed his imprisonment to be unjust.

In 1687 Saint-Mars was appointed governor of the island fortress of Sainte-Marguerite, and a special cell was built on the edge of a cliff to accommodate "the ancient prisoner." It is still pointed out to visitors as the Prison of the Mask. The unknown man was conveyed there in a chair covered with waxed cloth intended to prevent anyone from seeing or speaking to him during the journey. The cloth was so effectively sealed that he almost suffocated beneath it. After 11 more years in his island prison, he was once more conveyed across France to the Bastille in Paris,

Below: the Bastille in the 18th century. After 12 years in the fortress of Pignerol on the Italian frontier and a further 20 years on the Ile Sainte-Marguerite, the Man in the Iron Mask was moved to the Bastille in September 1698. It was here, in November 1703, that he died suddenly and was buried in an unnamed grave in a nearby churchyard. After his death all his possessions, linen, clothes, bedding, even the doors of his cell and the furniture in it, were destroyed. Even the flagstones of his cell were prised up in case he had left a message of some kind underneath them.

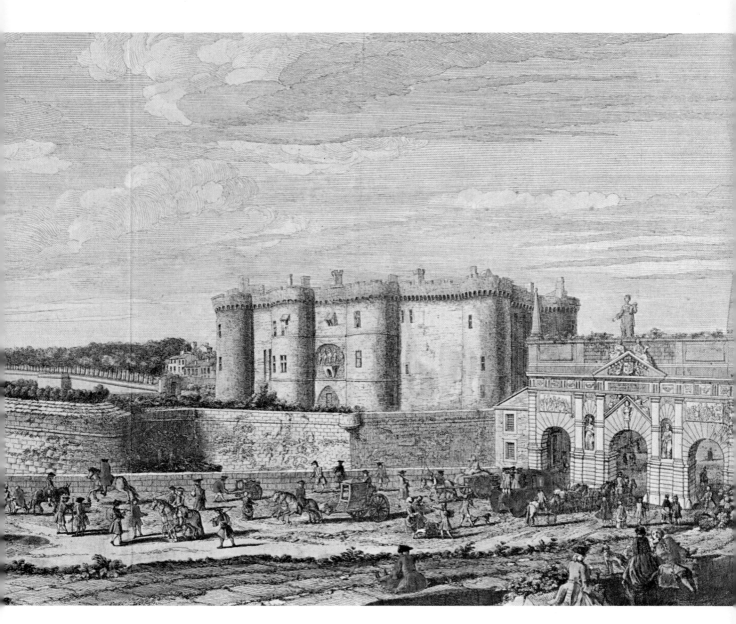

# His Name Revealed

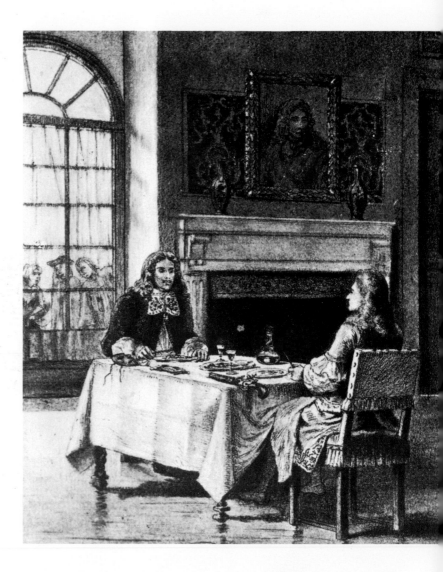

Right: on the journey from Cannes to Paris in 1698, Saint-Mars and his prisoner spent a night at Saint-Mars' own chateau in Palteau. Here the local people noticed that the prisoner sat with his back to the window, so they never knew whether he took off his mask, while Sainte-Mars sat opposite him with two pistols on the table.

this time in a litter. The cortege had to make several overnight stops on the way, one of them being at Governor Saint-Mars' own chateau in Palteau—a place his duties can seldom have allowed him the opportunity to enjoy. Long afterward the peasants on the estate recalled that Saint-Mars and the prisoner ate together. The prisoner's back had been turned to the window, and they had not been able to see his face, masked or unmasked. But they had seen clearly that Saint-Mars, sitting opposite his prisoner, had two pistols beside his plate.

Who was the masked prisoner, and why did his identity have to be kept such an absolute secret? By a fortunate error on the part of those who compiled the Ministry of Wars archives, a letter to Saint-Mars from the king himself has survived. It is dated July 1669. All subsequent attempts to conceal the masked man's name behind such evasions as "the prisoner in the lower tower" are rendered useless by the survival of this royal letter. It reads: "I am sending to my citadel of Pignerol, in the charge of Captain de Vauroy, sergeant-major of my city and citadel of Dunkirk, the man named Eustache Dauger. You are to hold him in good and safe custody, preventing him from communicating with anyone at all by word of mouth or writ of hand."

For a long time no trace of an Eustache Dauger could be found. At last someone noticed that a lieutenant in the King's Guards had borne the name Eustache d'Auger. He had been overlooked because his family was more commonly called de Cavoye after the name of a property they owned in Picardy. But when attention was focussed on Eustache d'Auger de Cavoye, a signature was discovered in which he spelled his name "Dauger." A record of his birth in 1637 exists, but not of his death, and references to him disappear after 1668, the year before the name appeared in the king's letter. Knowing the name of the masked prisoner does not by any means solve the mystery. Finding the reason for

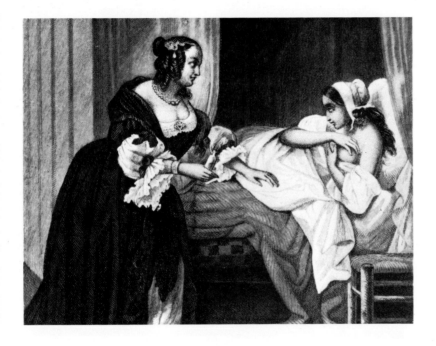

Left: the notorious Marquise de Brinvilliers began her career as a poisoner by trying out her potions on patients in the Hôtel Dieu, a Paris hospital. She later went on to poison her father and her two brothers, but failed in her attempt to poison her sister-in-law, the last obstacle to her inheriting the family estate. The Marquise, realizing she was suspected, fled to Germany, where she entered a convent. French agents tricked her into being returned to France, where she was tried and found guilty on her own confession when threatened with torture. If the Man in the Iron Mask was, as seems likely, Eustache Dauger, it is possible that his incarceration was to make him a scapegoat for other highly placed people, including the king's mistress, Madame de Montespan, who were apparently involved in the Poisons Trial. Below: the Marquise de Brinvilliers on her way to execution. Her head was cut off, her body burned, and her ashes scattered.

his imprisonment has proved altogether more difficult. Could the story go something like this?

Eustache Dauger was one of six soldier brothers, four of whom were killed in battle. His fifth brother, Louis, became a close friend of the king and was eventually created a Marquis, but his own career was questionable. At the age of 21 he and some other young members of the nobility celebrated an unholy Black Mass, and he escaped punishment only through the influence of his mother. Seven years later in 1665 he was obliged to resign his commission after a drunken quarrel in which a page was killed. In the same year his mother disinherited him, tired of having to settle his debts. Short of money and without an occupation, Eustache seems to have drifted toward the intriguers of the court. In the 1670s the sensational Poison Trials implicated many leading members of the court and French society in a sordid web of trafficking in poisons and practicing Devil worship and the Black Mass. The affair was hushed up when it was seen to involve no less a person than the king's mistress, Madame de Montespan. Since she is known to have taken part in Black Masses as early as 1667, Eustache, a friend of her family, may well have been one of her associates. Early talk of her misbehavior may have led to

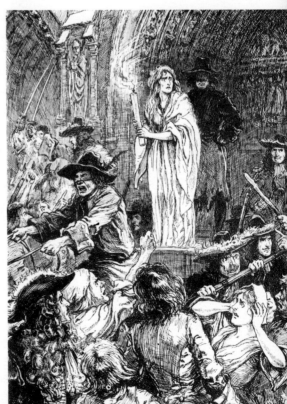

# Grand Duchess–
# or Great Fraud?

Below: the Grand Duchess Anastasia, the
youngest of the four daughters of Czar
Nicholas II of Russia. Is it true that she
alone escaped the murder of her family in
Ekaterinberg (now Sverdlovsk) on the night
of July 16, 1918?

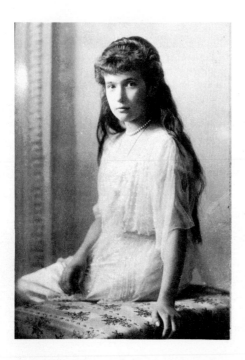

Right: the Czar and his family in the years
before the revolution and their imprisonment. The Grand Duchess Anastasia is on
the far right.

Opposite: an artist's impression of the
scene on the night of July 16, 1918, when
the imperial family and their household
staff were awakened, told to dress, and
taken to the cellar of the house in which
they were imprisoned. Most died at once
from shots fired at point blank range, but
according to the records Anastasia and one
of the maids survived the first volley and
were then finished off with bayonet thrusts.
The bodies were then stripped, dismembered,
and burned.

his removal to a place where he could not verify the rumor.

While this speculation could provide a reason for Eustache
Dauger's imprisonment and the secrecy with which he was surrounded, it does not explain why he had to wear a mask. Even 29
years after his arrest, the circumstances of his arrival at the
Bastille show that it was still imperative that he not be recognized.
The suspicion that he resembled somebody eminent and powerful is a very tempting one, and it may be significant that his
brother Louis, the Marquis de Cavoye, is said to have resembled
the king, a likeness borne out by a study of the Marquis' portrait.
Perhaps Eustache's likeness to the king was still more striking
than his brother's—but whether this was by chance or an indication of some hidden relationship is a matter of guesswork. Maybe
a likeness to his respectable brother was considered enough to
disclose his identity.

Though we now know who the secret prisoner was, and can
make a guess as to the sort of offense for which he was imprisoned, the full facts of the case—especially his masking—will
probably never be discovered. King Louis XIV, Prison Governor
Saint-Mars, and the few others who were in on the secret kept
what they knew to the death.

Royal families have shrunk in size and importance in the 20th
century, so pretenders to the throne and court scandals do not
capture public attention in the way they used to. But one claimant to royal lineage has kept in the public interest for the last 50
years. She is the woman who today still claims to be the Grand
Duchess Anastasia, youngest of the four daughters of Czar
Nicholas II of Russia. She insists that she escaped death when
the victorious revolutionaries executed her imperial father,
mother, three sisters, and young brother in 1918.

It is unlikely, but just possible, that one of the victims of that
bloody affair did escape. After the 1917 revolution broke out, the

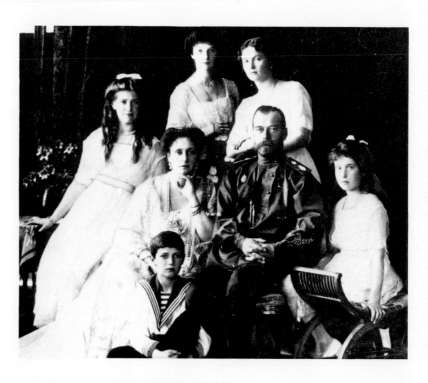

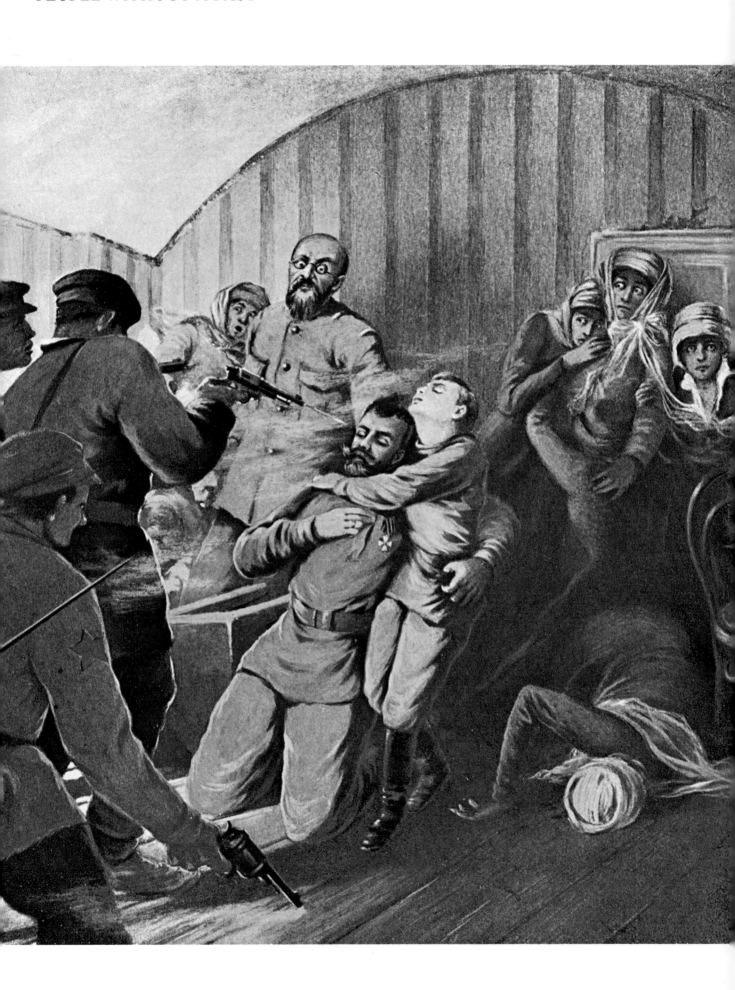

Right: the Mommsen Sanatorium, Berlin. It was to this hospital that a young woman of about 20, with no papers or other form of identification, was taken in February 1920 after a police sergeant had saved her from drowning in a canal in the city.

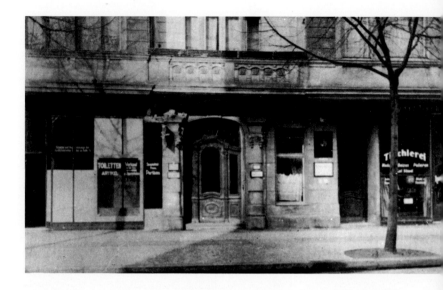

Below: is this woman really the Grand Duchess Anastasia? Photographed in Berlin in 1922, she does indeed bear a resemblance to the Romanov princess. But opponents of her claim point out that when she was first discovered in Berlin she could not speak a word of Russian.

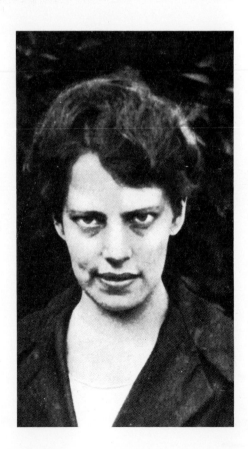

czar and his family were kept in a succession of prisons, in conditions of increasing severity. They ended up in a merchant's villa at Ekaterinburg (now Sverdlovsk), where their Bolshevik guards took delight in humiliating the former rulers. By July 1918 counterrevolutionary armies were approaching, and the order was given to execute the imperial family. According to accepted reports, they were awakened in the middle of the night and told to dress and go to the cellar of the villa. They were shot at point blank range, and most died at once; but Anastasia and a maid had to be finished off with bayonet thrusts. Since the eye-witness reports admit that Anastasia did not die by the bullet, it is conceivable that she also escaped death by the bayonet. After the execution, the bodies were taken to a disused mineshaft in some woods, stripped, dismembered, and burned with fire and acid. Since the victims included the maid, a valet, a cook, and the czar's physician in addition to the imperial family, it is again just possible that one of the bodies was overlooked in the darkness.

The woman now known as Anna Anderson claims that she had only been wounded in the cellar, and that upon regaining consciousness she was in a farm cart being driven by the man who had saved her, a Red Guard named Alexander Tchaikovsky. The two of them made their escape from Russia into Rumania, where she married him. Soon afterward he was killed, and she made her way to Germany with her brother-in-law in the hope of getting help from the wife of Prince Henry of Prussia, whom she called her aunt. Deserted by her companion soon after reaching Berlin in February 1920, she threw herself into a canal in a fit of despair.

Up to this point the story of her life has only her word for it. From the moment a police sergeant dragged her from the canal, however, the events of her life are chronicled. During her stay in a hospital her claim to be the Grand Duchess Anastasia attracted attention. Many influential people were convinced by her manner, others as vigorously disputed her claim. There were many members of the Romanov family outside Russia, and they naturally were drawn into the controversy. This was partly out of self-interest because as heirs to the former czar, they would

# Did She Survive?

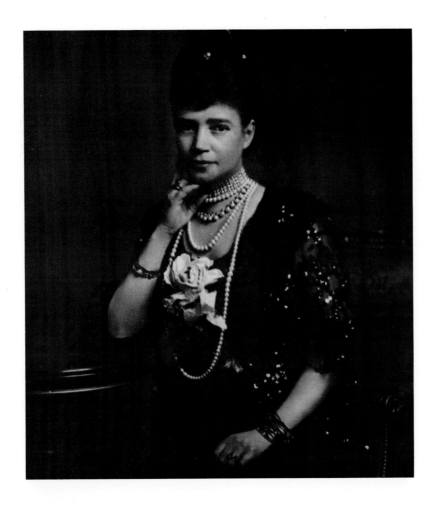

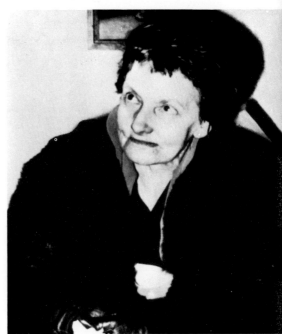

Above left: Anastasia's grandmother, the Dowager Empress Marie, who would surely have been able to establish the truth or otherwise of Anna Anderson's claim. Unfortunately they did not meet, and the Empress Dowager died in 1928.

Above: Anna Anderson as she is today. Most of her life has been spent in Germany, but she did go to the United States for 2½ years. It was in America that she was first called Anna Anderson. It was not a happy period, because her stay with her "second cousin," Princess Xenia of Russia, was not a success, and for about a year the mysterious woman was confined to a mental home. Members of the Romanov family living in Europe and the United States are divided in their opinion about her, but Anna Anderson has never wavered in her claim.

share the inheritance of his property in Germany. Some of the Romanovs said that they recognized Anastasia in Anna Anderson, others declared that she was an imposter, still others could not make up their minds. For nearly 50 years the case has been taken through a number of German courts without reaching a conclusion.

Opponents point out that when Anna Anderson was discovered in Berlin, she could not or would not speak a word of Russian. They claim that she is Franziska Schankowska, the daughter of a Polish landworker, and that the scars she says remain from the wounds received in the cellar at Ekaterinburg are in fact the result of an accident in a bottle factory where Franziska worked. Supporters argue that Anna Anderson bears a striking resemblance to the young Anastasia, and has an intimate familiarity with uncommon details of Russian court life.

Plays and films based on the Anastasia story have her traveling to Denmark to meet the Dowager Empress Marie, who would be the grandmother of the grand duchess. Unfortunately, this meeting never occurred. If it had, the matter might have been settled long ago. Nonetheless, Anna Anderson's determination and force of character have won her many devoted friends over the years. Is she the Grand Duchess Anastasia, supposed to have died in 1918 at the age of 17? No certain judgment has yet been made. As in the case of Caspar Hauser, the Man in the Iron Mask, and so many others, the mystery remains.

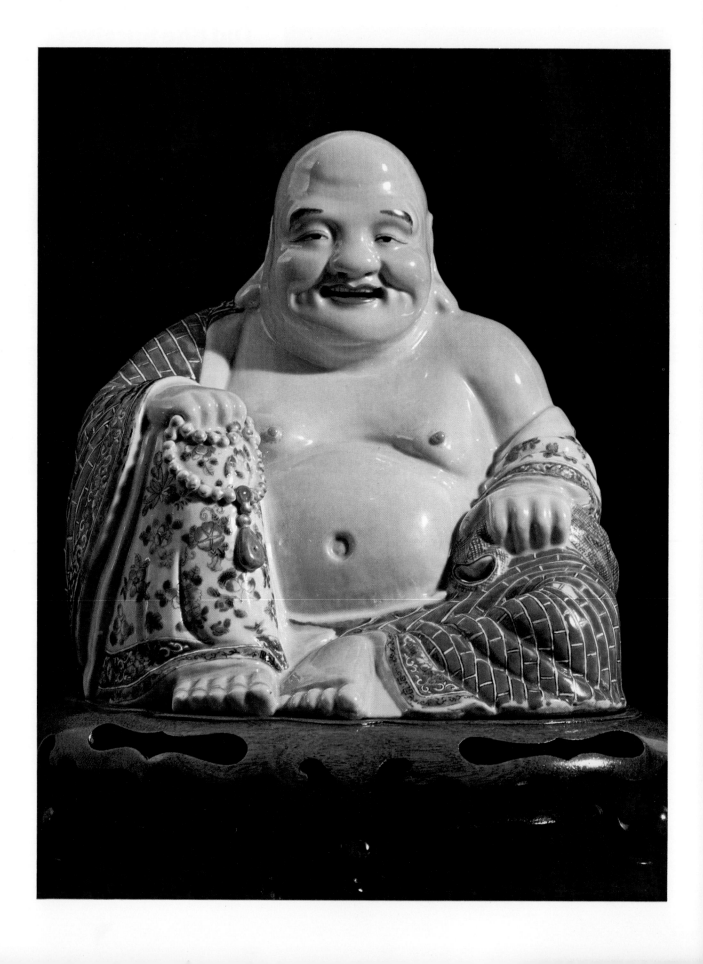

# Chapter 6
# Jinxes and Curses

Why do some objects seem to bring misfortune on the people who come into contact with them? What makes them jinxed? How does a jinx or a curse work? Why should an ivory statuette cause toothache or an unknown force fling coffins around in a family vault? Here are the stories of some of the ships, gems, cars, and houses that have been associated with a run of bad luck—and of men and women who, wittingly or not, make things go wrong through the curse of the "evil eye."

The year was 1928. The city, Kobe, Japan. A middle-aged English couple, the C. J. Lamberts, stood in front of a junk shop window. "That's what I'd like," said Marie Lambert, pointing to a tiny statuette of a half-naked fat man seated on a cushion. She recognized the laughing man as Ho-tei, the Japanese god of Good Luck. "Let's find out what he costs," said her husband, as they walked into the shop. They were pleasantly surprised to find that the figurine was cheap, even though it was made of ivory. It seemed almost too good to be true. Back on their cruise ship the Lamberts examined their purchase closely. The statuette had the creamy color of old ivory and was beautifully carved. As far as they could see, its only minor imperfection was a small hole underneath, plugged neatly with an ivory peg. If the carver had used the base of an elephant's tusk for the statue, which was possible, the tiny hole would be natural as the point where the nerve of the animal's tooth had ended. Altogether, the statue seemed to be one of those rare bargains that tourists dream about. The Lamberts hoped the presence of the "Laughing Buddha," as Ho-tei is sometimes called, would insure good luck for the remainder of their voyage.

Ho-tei was originally a 6th-century Buddhist monk who devoted his life to helping the poor, taking special care of children. Statuettes of Ho-tei, who later became a god, show him holding in his right hand a string of beads or a fan, and in his left hand a sack. Sometimes a small child is hanging onto his back or

Opposite: Ho-tei, originally a 6th-century Buddhist monk who devoted his life to helping the poor, is today the Japanese god of Good Luck. But a small Ho-tei figure brought nothing but bad luck to one English couple.

# God of Good Luck?

Right: this is the Ho-tei that caused the Lamberts so much trouble that they were happy to get rid of it. What was it about this particular Ho-tei that was jinxed?

Below: the Lamberts were a widely traveled couple. Here they are photographed landing by chair-lift from their ship in a small Peruvian port called Mollendo, an experience C. J. Lambert describes as "a thrilling method of landing" in his book *Together We Wandered.*

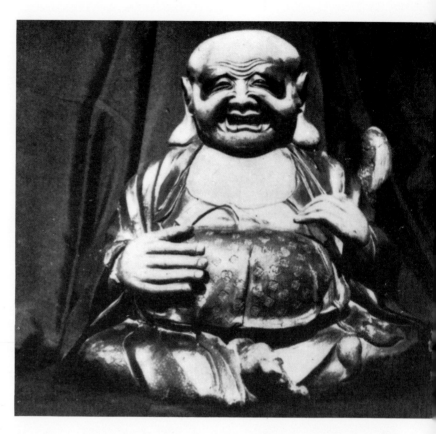

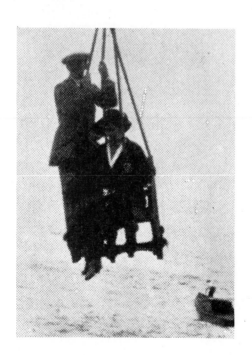

Opposite: this terracotta Ho-tei doll from Japan expresses very well the joyful, merry quality of the little god the Lamberts were pleased to have bought so cheaply.

sitting on his shoulder, illustrating a legend that he once carried a child to safety across a dangerously flooded river. The legend of St. Christopher, who features on many good luck charms in the West as the protector of travelers, is believed to be a Christianized version of the legend of Ho-tei.

Marie Lambert packed the statuette in one of her suitcases. On the second day out, on route to Manila, the next scheduled stop, Mrs. Lambert began to suffer from a toothache. The ship's doctor prescribed painkillers, but they did little good. Once in Manila, both Lamberts contracted an unpleasant fever whose chief symptom was pain in all the joints, and Marie Lambert had to delay her visit to a dentist. When she finally got to one, his drill slipped during treatment and drove through the nerve of her tooth, increasing her pain instead of curing it.

On the next lap of the voyage, which took the ship to Australia, Mr. Lambert in turn was prostrated with an agonizing toothache. While in Cairns he went to a doctor, who told him there was nothing wrong with his teeth. In fact, the ache had stopped while he was at the dentist's. It started again as soon as he returned to his cabin. Two days later he consulted another dentist, and the same thing happened. Finally, in Brisbane he desperately ordered a dentist to start pulling out his teeth and to keep on pulling until the pain stopped. When the first tooth came out, the pain went away. However, it started again as soon as Lambert returned to the ship. He had not noticed that the Ho-tei figurine was in his suitcase at the time his toothache started.

In Sydney the Lamberts left their luggage checked, and the toothache ceased. On the voyage to New Zealand the luggage

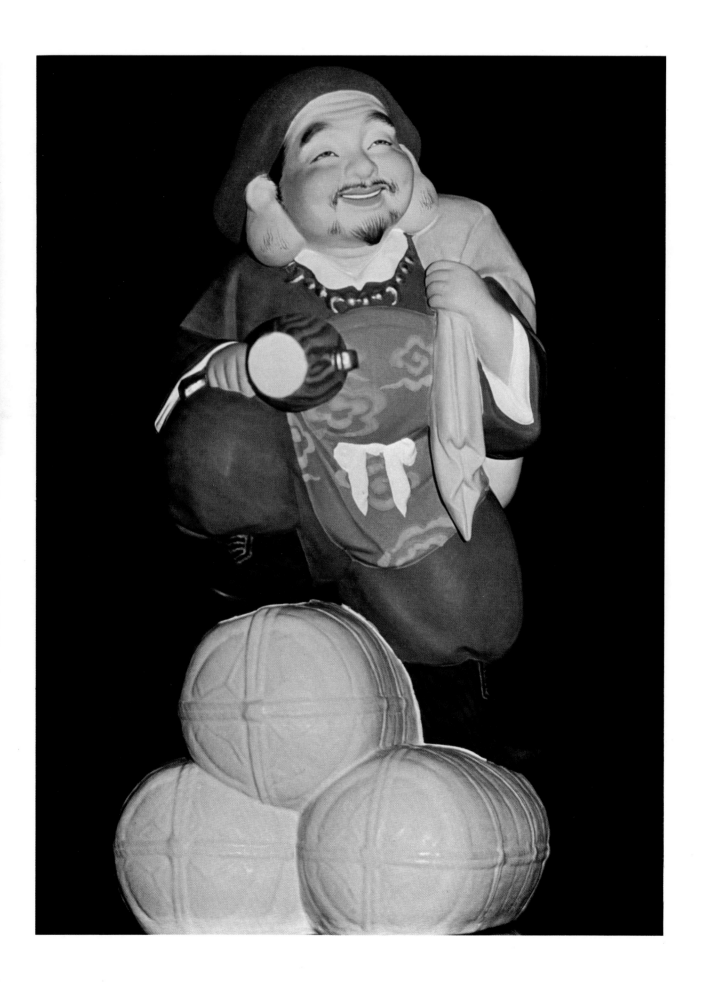

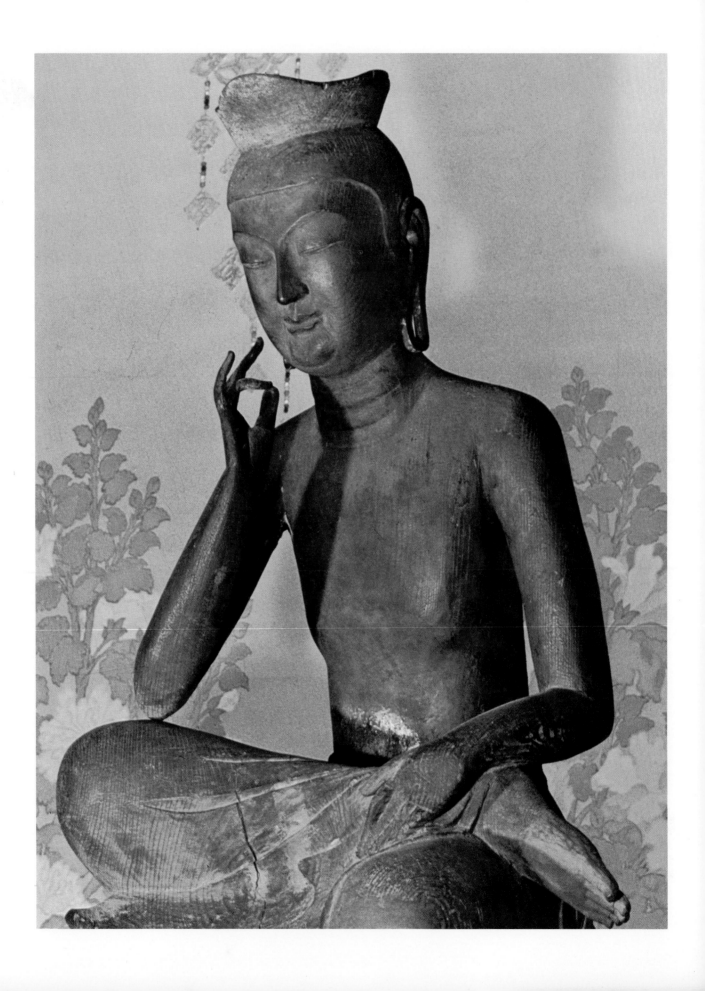

was in their cabin only once, when they repacked; Lambert's toothache started again. When the luggage went into the hold, the pain stopped. While on shore in New Zealand he had no toothache, and there was only one bout of toothache on the continuation trip to Chile—when the Lamberts repacked their luggage in the cabin.

In the United States the couple visited Lambert's mother, who was so delighted with Ho-tei that they made her a present of the little god. When her excellent teeth started aching a few hours later, she handed back the gift saying that she felt it was "bad medicine." In spite of this hint about the statuette's ill effects on its owners, the Lamberts did not connect Ho-tei with their own toothaches till they were on their way across the Atlantic to Britain. A fellow passenger who was interested in ivory borrowed the figurine overnight to show her husband. In the morning she mentioned that she and her husband had both had toothaches. The Lamberts then thought about their toothaches, and realized that they had always occurred when Ho-tei was in their cabin. Marie Lambert wanted to throw the statuette overboard at once, but her husband was afraid that the god might retaliate by rotting every tooth in their heads. So they brought Ho-tei back to London with them.

Lambert took the figure to an oriental art shop and showed it to the Japanese manager, who immediately offered to buy it. Lambert explained that he could not take money for it, and described the troubles it seemed to have caused. The manager sent for an old kimono-clad Japanese, and the two men examined the statuette carefully. From what they then told him, Lambert gathered that his Ho-tei had been a temple god. In the East the statues of such gods are sometimes given "souls" in the form of small medallions hidden inside them. That probably explained the ivory plug in the base of the figure. The old man placed Ho-tei in a shrine at the end of the shop and lit joss sticks in front of it. Then with an expression of awe, he bowed Lambert out of the shop.

Colin Wilson, who tells this story in *Enigmas and Mysteries*, adds that C. J. Lambert derived some profit from his uncomfortable adventure. He recounted it in a travel book that sold well. Lambert could never bring himself to revisit the shop in which he had left Ho-tei, however.

Lambert's understandable assumption was that a god had been taking revenge on unbelievers who had removed him from his temple. But is it possible for a god, or a priest following that god, to fix the power to cause harm into an inert substance? Skeptics take the view that all runs of misfortune are caused by the victims, who unconsciously bring disaster upon themselves. We have all known people who seem to attract bad luck—we call them "accident prone." They usually appear to be suffering from plain undeserved misfortune. Yet we still have the feeling that there is some connection between their personality and their lack of good fortune. There may be something about the attitude of such people—a certain expectation that the worst will happen— that triggers off the accident. The subconscious attitude may of itself be capable of causing the accident to occur. On the other hand, the subconscious attitude could affect the quality of atten-

# The Luck of The Lamberts

Opposite: the Lamberts noticed that there was a small hole underneath the figure which had been neatly plugged with an ivory peg. Many Japanese statues, such as the one shown here, have cavities for relics. Was the Ho-tei the Lamberts bought holding some kind of relic which meant "bad medicine" for them?

# The Jinxed Battleship

tion the accident prone person brings to day-to-day behavior, and so could allow mishaps to occur more frequently. Even with our limited knowledge of the power of the mind, this possibility cannot be ruled out. However, many people—in civilized countries as well as among primitive tribes—would go as far as to call the consistently accident prone "accursed."

The idea of being accursed does not extend only to people. The famous ship *Mary Celeste*, found drifting in the mid-Atlantic with all aboard mysteriously missing, had been dogged by bad luck from the moment of its launching. Few sailors doubt that there are such things as jinxed ships, unlucky from the day they were launched or before.

The 26,000-ton battleship *Scharnhorst* was such a ship. Launched in October 1936 as the pride of Nazi Germany, it should have had a long and successful career ahead; but from the beginning there were clear signs that all was not going well. Before the ship was half built it rolled over on the side, crushing 60 workmen to death and injuring over 100 others. It took three months to raise it back into position. Workmen had to be drafted to complete the battleship because the rumor had spread that it was jinxed. Later events seemed to substantiate the rumor.

When the time came for the important launching, Hitler, Goering, Himmler, and many other top Nazis were present. Unfortunately, the *Scharnhorst* was not, having launched itself the night before. In the process, it ground up two barges as it hit the channel.

The exceptionally powerful long-range guns of the *Scharnhorst* were first used in the bombardment of Danzig in 1939, with unfortunate results. During the attack one of the guns exploded, killing nine men, and the air supply to one of the gun turrets broke down, suffocating 12 gunners. A year later, during the bombardment of Oslo, the *Scharnhorst* was hit by more shells than all the rest of the German fleet combined. Fires broke out in over 30 places, and the ship had to be towed out of reach of the shore batteries. In making its way home for repairs, the battleship had to lie hidden from British bombers by day and move by

Right: the *Scharnhorst*, shown at its launching ceremony. The ship seemed unlucky from the very start. When only half built, the ship rolled over on its side, killing 60 ship workers. When Hitler and Goering arrived for the grand launching in 1936, they discovered that the *Scharnhorst* had somehow launched itself the previous night, destroying several barges.

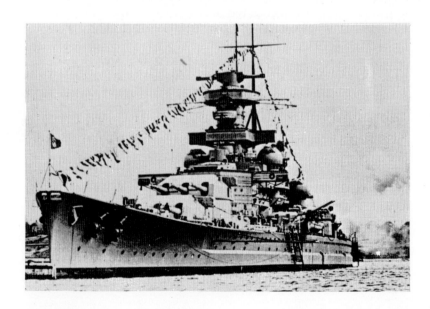

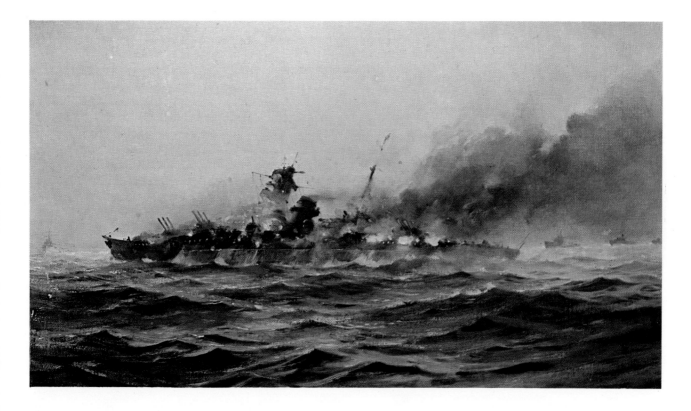

night. At last it reached the safe haven of the Elbe river, but immediately ran into trouble again. Unknown to the *Scharnhorst*, the *SS Bremen* lay ahead. The ocean liner was one of the world's largest, and the glory of Germany. Too late the watch sounded an alarm, and seconds later the battleship rammed the prize liner. The *Bremen* sank and settled into the mud, where British planes bombed it to pieces.

After being repaired, the *Scharnhorst* was sent north in 1943 to cruise the coast of Norway and intercept convoys on their way to the Soviet Union. On the way there it passed and failed to notice a British patrol boat lying in the water with a disabled engine. When the battleship was safely over the horizon, the patrol boat radioed a warning. Several British warships steamed to the area and located the German battleship, but the *Scharnhorst* managed to escape the slower pursuers after a short exchange of fire. One of the pursuers caught a glimpse of the *Scharnhorst* from about 16,000 yards away, and the commander decided to fire a last shot. Knowing that the *Scharnhorst* would try to get out of the line of fire, he made a guess as to which direction to aim and gave the order to fire.

Living up to its jinx, the *Scharnhorst* turned directly into the path of the broadside from the British battleship. Flames shot up from the decks, and within minutes the German ship had plunged to the bottom of the icy sea with most of the crew. Only 36 survived out of a total of 1900. Years later it was discovered that two of the crew had succeeded in reaching a small rocky island where they made a windbreak from their raft. But the *Scharnhorst* jinx pursued them even there, for evidence showed that they were killed when their emergency oil heater exploded.

The jinx on the Lockheed Constellation airliner AHEM-4

Above: *The Sinking of the Scharnhorst*, a painting by C. E. Turner. The ship was destroyed on December 26, 1943 with only 36 survivors out of a total crew of 1900.

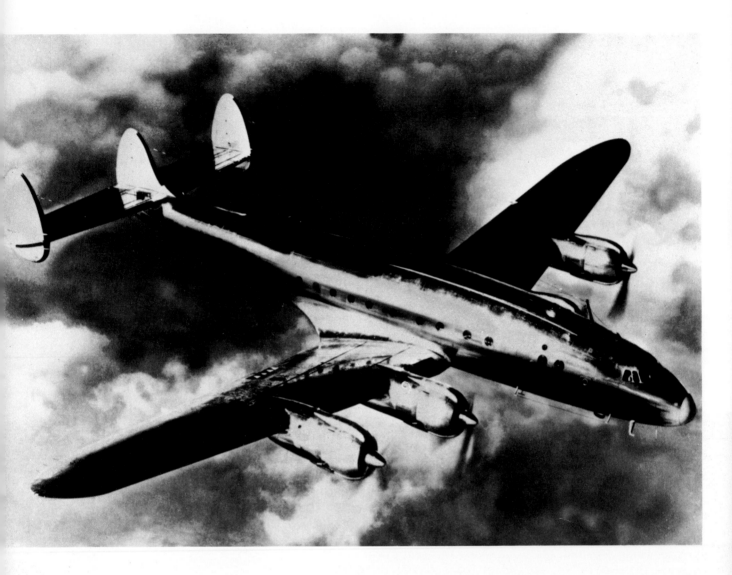

Above: a Lockheed Constellation airplane, like the Constellation AHEM-4 that was pursued by misfortune from 1945 to 1949. The chain of mishaps began with the death of a mechanic who walked into one of the plane's propellers, and ended with the death of everyone on board in a crash near Chicago.

began the day in July 1945 when a mechanic walked into one of the plane's propellers and was killed. Precisely one year later, on July 9, 1946, Captain Arthur Lewis died at the controls while the plane was over the Atlantic ocean. Precisely one more year later, on July 9, 1947, a newly installed engine burst into flame shortly after takeoff. The captain, Robert Norman, succeeded in putting out the flames with a fire extinguisher, but then found that the plane lacked enough power to climb above the roof of an apartment building directly in their path. Norman switched on the takeoff power and just managed to climb out of danger, but when he tried to ease the power off again, the controls remained jammed. He and his copilot finally wrestled the controls back by sheer force, and landed without further mishap.

July 1948 passed uneventfully. But on July 10, 1949, the airliner crashed near Chicago, killing everyone on board including Captain Robert Norman. The AHEM-4's jinx was his bad luck.

Besides ships and planes, there are records of cars and houses that seem to have brought disaster to their owners. One example is the car in which the Archduke Franz Ferdinand, heir to the dual monarchy of Austria-Hungary, and his wife were assassinated at Sarajevo in July 1914—a murder that precipitated the outbreak of World War I. Shortly after the start of the war, General Potiorek of the Austrian army came into possession of the car. A few weeks later he suffered a catastrophic defeat against the Serbians at Valjevo, and was sent back to Vienna in disgrace. He could not endure the shame of this and died insane.

The next owner of the car was an Austrian captain who had been on Potiorek's staff. Only nine days after taking over the car, he struck and killed two peasants, then swerved into a tree and broke his neck.

At the end of the war, the Governor of Yugoslavia became the owner of the car. After four accidents in four months—one of which caused him to lose an arm—he had had enough, and sold the car to a doctor. Six months later the car was found upside down in a ditch. The doctor had been crushed to death inside it. The car was next sold to a wealthy jeweler who committed suicide only a year later. After a brief spell in the hands of another doctor, who seems to have been all too anxious to get rid of it, the car was sold to a Swiss racing driver. He was killed in a race in the Italian Alps when the car threw him over a wall. The next owner was a Serbian farmer. Having stalled the car one morning, he persuaded a passing motorist to give him a tow—and became the car's tenth victim in a bizarre accident. Because he forgot to

# Planes and Cars

Below: in the back seat of a car that seemed to be jinxed is the Austro-Hungarian Archduke Franz Ferdinand and his wife, seen here on the actual day of their deaths by assassination in Sarajevo in August 1914. General Potiorek, who was later to be affected by the car's bad luck, is sitting directly in front of the duchess.

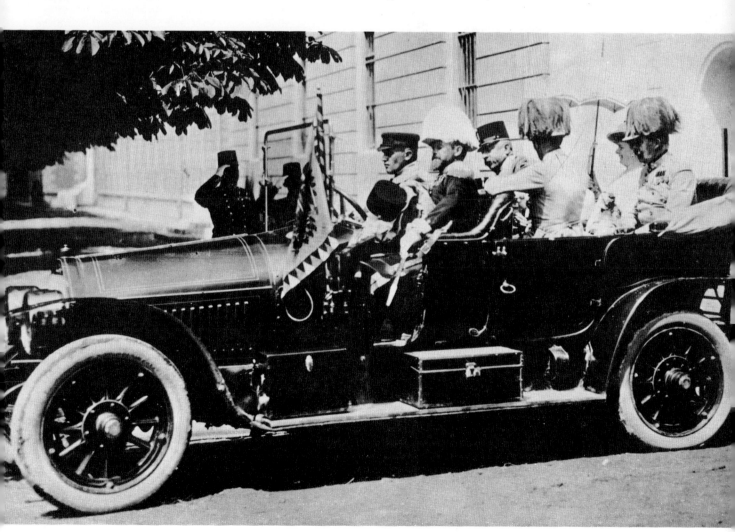

# Castle of Fate?

turn off the ignition, the car started up, smashed the horse and cart, and overturned on a bend. The car's final owner was Tibor Hirshfeld, a garage owner. Returning from a wedding with six friends one day, Hirshfeld tried to overtake another car at high speed. He crashed and was killed along with four of his companions. The car was then taken to a Vienna museum, where it has been ever since.

Would anyone dream of a fairytale castle as being jinxed? Probably not, but the beautiful castle of Miramar near Trieste seems to have brought bad luck to those who lived in it. Miramar castle was built in the mid-19th century by the Archduke Maximilian, a younger brother of the Emperor Franz Josef of

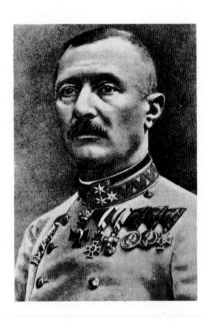

Above: General Potiorek, who escaped harm at Sarajevo, became the next owner of the car. Within a few weeks he suffered utter defeat in battle and was sent back to Vienna in disgrace.

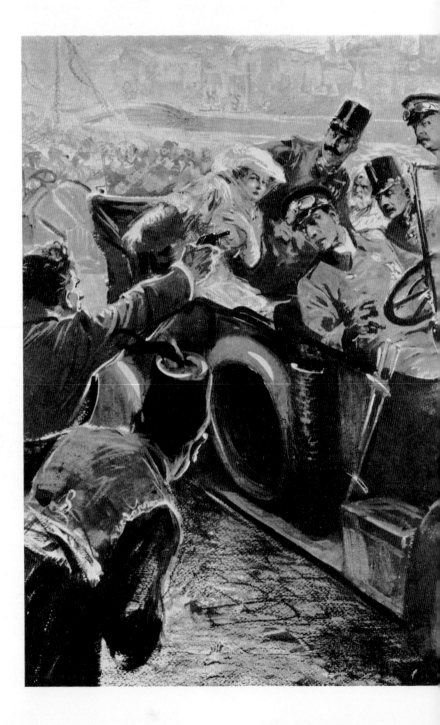

Right: the assassination. Within six weeks of the double murder half the civilized world was at war, and the terrible blood-letting known as World War I had begun.

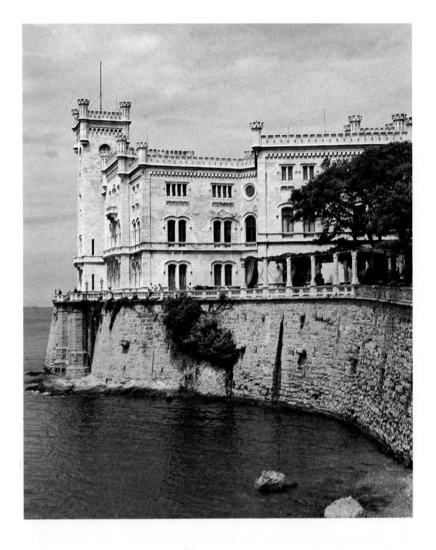

Left: the beautiful castle of Miramar, near Trieste, which brought disaster to those who were closely connected with it.

Below: Archduke Maximilian. It was the archduke who built the white palace with delicate white towers called Miramar, and it was at Miramar that he made the fateful decision to become the Emperor of Mexico.

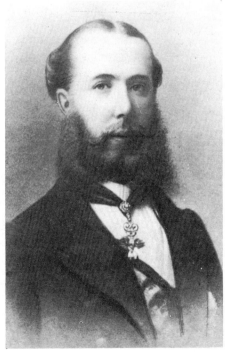

Austria-Hungary. Maximilian had once been blown ashore near Trieste while sailing in a small boat, and some fishermen gave him shelter. Inspired by the beauty of the place, he decided that day to make his home there. Later he built a white palace with delicate towers, terraces of granite, and flights of marble steps leading down to a landing stage guarded by sphinxes. The garden was planted with firs and flowering trees, and visitors described it as one of the most beautiful places on earth. The first owner started the catalog of misfortunes connected with Miramar. It was there that Maximilian accepted the fatal offer of the imperial crown of Mexico, which resulted in his death in front of a Mexican firing squad three years later. His wife Carlotta, who was only 26, went insane.

The Empress Elisabeth, wife of Franz Josef, was the next resident of Miramar, living there with her son Rudolf. Rudolf came to a tragic end in 1889 by committing suicide with his beloved, and the Empress was assassinated in 1898 by an Italian anarchist who believed in Italian liberation from Austria. The next to live at Miramar was Archduke Franz Ferdinand, Rudolf's cousin and heir to the imperial throne. He and his wife were assassinated in Sarajevo, starting the jinx of the car as well. At the end of World War I, when Trieste passed from Austrian

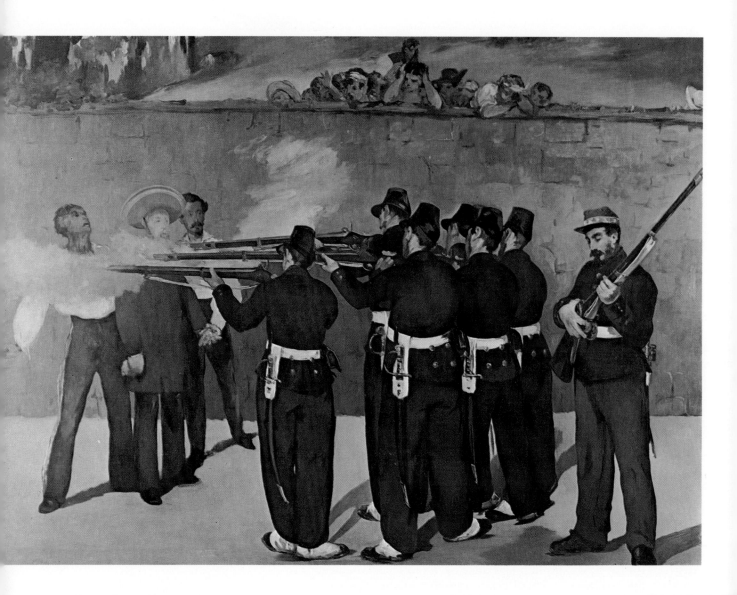

Above: the execution of Maximilian, the
unsuccessful Emperor of Mexico. His wife
who had ruled with him lost her sanity in
the equally unsuccessful struggle to
rally support for him in Europe when his
situation in Mexico became desperate.

to Italian hands, the Duke of Aosta, a cousin of the King of
Italy, moved into Miramar. He died in a prison camp in Kenya
during World War II. After that, two British Major Generals
became residents of the castle of Miramar. Both died of heart
attacks.

Skeptics maintain that misfortunes such as these occur either
by chance, in the case of the *Scharnhorst*, or as the result of fears
and tensions. For example, the crew of the airliner AHEM-4
knew that a mechanic had walked into the propeller and been
cut to pieces. The subsequent owner of Franz Ferdinand's car
knew that the Archduke and his wife had met violent death in it.
The rationalist view is that the belief in jinxes developed as early
peoples felt the need to discover a pattern in the misfortunes that
befell them. Cattle sickened, children died unexpectedly, storms
destroyed crops. For a society that believed the human being
was the center of creation, and that everything which happened
did so for a humanly comprehensible reason, two explanations
presented themselves. Either some object associated with the
victim contained within itself the power to bring harm, or some
god or person of evil intent was willing harm on someone. The

idea of the jinx and the curse was born—the jinx connected with objects, the curse with spirits or humans.

The destructive power of a curse is real and undisputed. People who believe they are under a curse to die will often obediently proceed to die. Those most likely to react in this way are primitive peoples whose lives are rigorously ordered by ritual and taboo. Such were the Maoris of New Zealand, and such still are many Amazon Indians of South America. In earlier times a Maori chief was a sacred figure, and it was taboo to touch him or objects that had belonged to him. It was accepted that any transgression would be punished by the angered ancestral spirits of the tribe. Sir James Frazer in *The Golden Bough* tells of a Maori warrior who unwittingly ate the unfinished dinner of his chief. When he learned what he had done, he was immediately seized by violent stomach cramps and convulsions. He died of the seizures at sundown the same day. Knowing he was fated to die, his body and mind combined to bring his death about.

A modern story of a curse that was connected with a strange death is that of the so-called "curse of the Pharaoh." It struck after the opening of Tutankhamun's tomb in Egypt in 1923. The first of several men to die was Lord Carnarvon, who had financed the dig. Three months after the archaeological discovery he was bitten by a mosquito, and the bite became infected. At five minutes to two on the morning of April 5, 1923 he died. At this precise moment two unusual incidents occurred: all the lights in Cairo went out and remained out for some time, and back in England, Lord Carnarvon's dog howled and died. No satisfactory explanation has ever been forthcoming for either of these coincidental events.

The famous blue diamond known as the Hope Diamond brought bad fortune to most of its owners over a long period of time. Gemologists believe that the Hope Diamond, a product of the great Golconda mines of southern India, must have been cut

# The "Curse of the Pharaoh"

Left: first of many victims of the so-called "curse of the Pharaoh" was Lord Carnarvon, seen here at Tutenkhamen's tomb (center, wearing a bow tie). Only months after this magnificent archaeological discovery, he died from an infected mosquito bite. At the moment of his death, all the lights in Cairo went out and his dog, back in England, howled once and died.

# Diamond of Doom

Below: the priceless Hope Diamond is today safely installed in the Smithsonian Institute in Washington. But this magnificent gem has a 300-year history of blood and passion in which kings and poor men, thieves and courtesans have looked upon its beauty and been driven mad.

from a larger blue diamond that was acquired by Louis XIV and disappeared during the French Revolution nearly 75 years later with the rest of the French royal treasure. It made its first appearance in its present form in 1830, and was bought by the British banker and gem collector Henry Thomas Hope. He escaped any evil consequences but the cousin to whom he bequeathed it, Lord Francis Hope, was plagued by problems. His wife, a noted actress, blamed all their marital troubles on the blue stone, and prophesied evil for all its owners. Her curse may have added to the unluckiness of the exquisite gem.

In the early 1900s the diamond was sold by Lord Francis Hope, who was said to be suffering grave financial trouble. Jacques Colot, a French broker, paid more than three times its original price for it, and sold it to a Russian noble, Prince Kanitovski. Colot went mad and committed suicide. The prince behaved as if he were mad. He lent the diamond to an actress at the Folies Bergères, and then shot her from a box in the theater the first

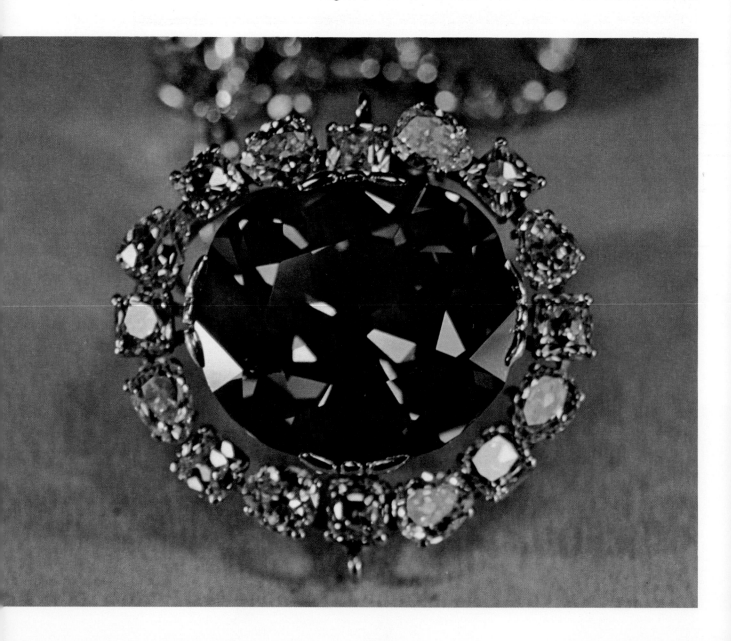

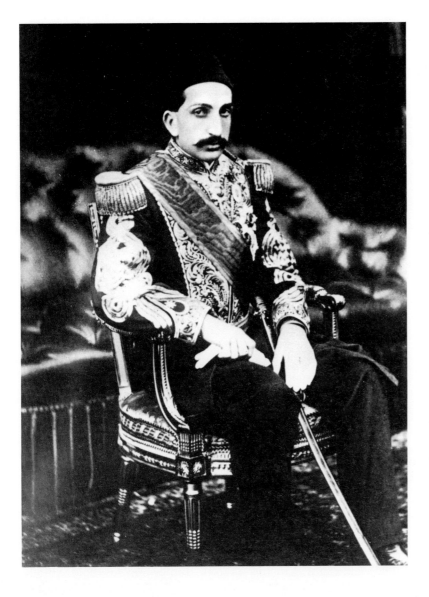

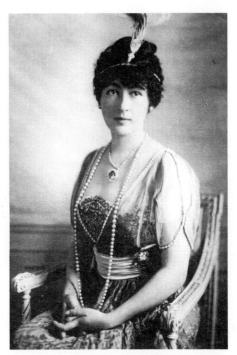

Left: Sultan Abdul Hamid II of Turkey. Known as "Abdul the Damned," he bought the blue Hope Diamond in 1908 and by April 1909 he had been deposed, the last true sultan of Turkey.

Above: Mrs. Evelyn Walsh McLean wearing the Hope Diamond. Her husband Edward Beale McLean bought it for her, but he was involved in the Teapot Dome scandal of the 1920s and afterward became an alcoholic, losing his mind as well. Although her life was marked by a series of tragedies, Mrs McLean refused to believe it was connected with the diamond, though she also refused to let her children touch it.

night she was wearing it. A few days later he was stabbed by revolutionaries. A Greek jeweler by the name of Simon Mantharides was the next to own the Hope Diamond. He is said to have been thrown over a precipice. In 1908 Abdul Hamid II, the sultan of Turkey known as "Abdul the Damned," bought the gem for tens of thousands of dollars. He was deposed in April 1909—the last of Turkey's sultans. Habib Bey acquired it next, putting it on exhibition in London in June 1909. In November he was drowned when the French liner *La Seyne* sank off Singapore.

In spite of this ominous record, the diamond was bought by Edward Beale McLean, proprietor of the *Washington Post*, as a gift for his wife. McLean was involved in the Teapot Dome scandal of President Harding's administration, and afterward became an alcoholic, losing his mind as well. The eldest of the four McLean children was killed by an automobile at the age of nine. The last owner, said to have paid in the millions for it, contributed the seemingly sinister Hope Diamond to the Smithsonian Institution, where it still rests.

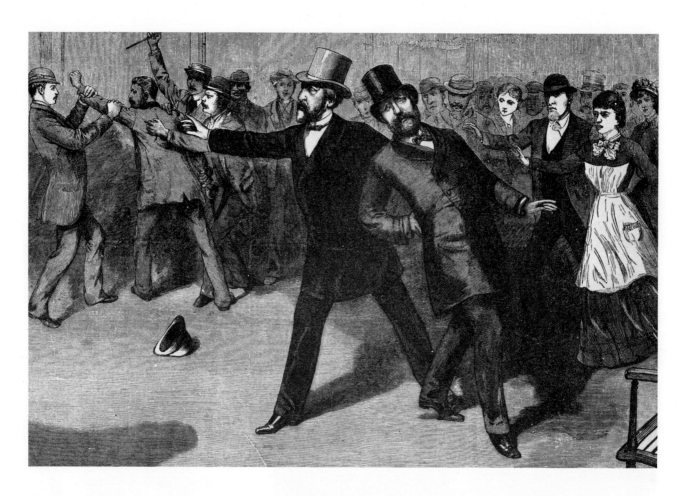

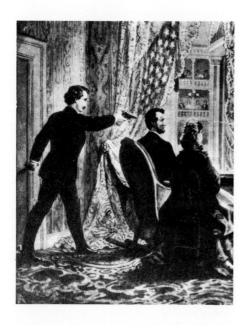

Above: the assassination of President Garfield in July 1881. Many writers have noted that since 1840 every American president elected in a year divisible by 20 has died in office. Four of these men were assassinated, Garfield, McKinley, and Lincoln, whose murder is shown below.

Is it a curse that decrees that every president of the United States elected in a year divisible by 20 will die in office? History shows that this has been the case since 1840. Three died naturally —William Henry Harrison, who was elected in 1840, Warren G. Harding (1920), and Franklin D. Roosevelt (1940). Assassins killed Abraham Lincoln (1860), James A. Garfield (1880), William McKinley (1900), and John F. Kennedy (1960). The pattern in itself is odd enough, but the fact that both assassinations and natural deaths fit into this pattern is odder still. When Roosevelt, first elected in 1932 and reelected in 1936 and 1940, survived to the end of his third term, it might have been thought that the jinx had been lifted. But it reasserted itself during his fourth term. Reelected in November 1944, he was dead the following spring.

No one can put a name to an apparent blight that strikes American presidents in given years. But in many countries the cause of a person's misfortunes is easily attributed—to the evil eye. The belief that certain individuals possess the power to bring disaster to another person simply by a look is still widespread today in the countries around the Mediterranean, particularly in Italy, and nowhere more so than in Naples and the south. In Florence and Tuscany this unlovely gift is known as *male d'occhio* (evil eye); in Rome it is called *fascina* (fascination). In the south it is *jettatura*, meaning a spell cast by touch, word, or look. Of the three, the look is the most penetrating and potent.

To ward off the dreaded power of the evil eye, most people

# The Curse of the Presidents?

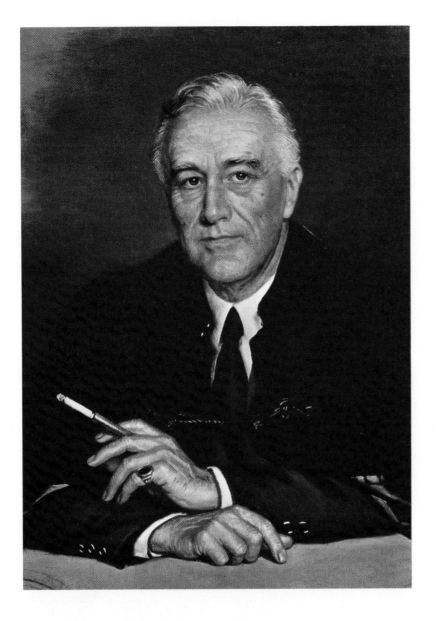

Left: President Franklin D. Roosevelt.
First elected in 1932, reelected in 1936 and
1940 (a year divisible by 20), Roosevelt
seemed to have beaten the sinister pattern.
However, in 1944 he became the only
president to be elected for a fourth term of
office. He died, in office, on April 12, 1945.

wear amulets most of the time. Some of these charms are
grotesque or ridiculous in design, meant to attract the attention
of the evil eye and distract it from the person wearing it. Many
are indecent or obscene for the same reason, the commonest of
all being the phallus or objects suggested by it. Snakes, fish,
crescent moons, pieces of coral, closed hands with the thumb
protruding between the first and second fingers, and horns of all
sorts, shapes, and sizes. The horn is believed to have the greatest
power of defense. Even to mutter the word *corno* (horn) is
better than nothing.

When obliged to speak to someone having the evil eye,
Neapolitans will hold their hand in a gesture of protection,
extending the first and fourth fingers in the sign of the horned
hand. Out of courtesy they may keep the hand behind their back
or in their pocket, but they will not relax the position of the
fingers till they feel safe from danger.

Some people probably trade on their reputation as bringers of
bad luck, the jinxes of their community, but others are entirely

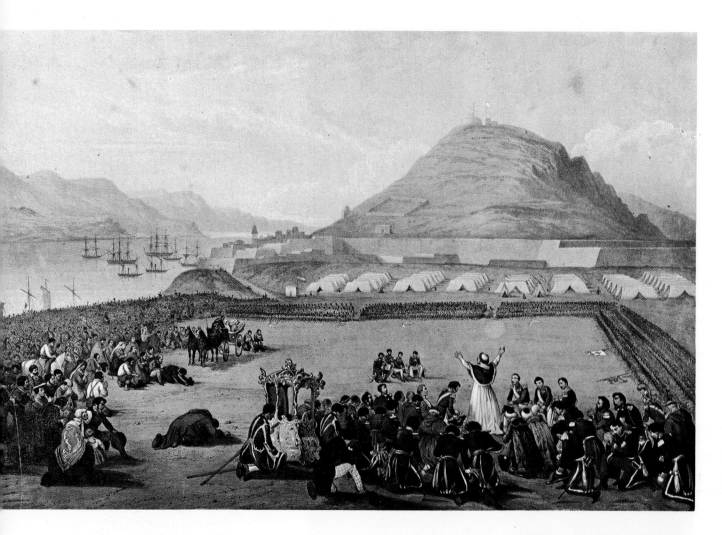

Above: Pope Pius IX blessing Italian troops
at Gaeta, south of Rome, during the war
against Austria in 1848. Pius IX was
believed to have, if not the power of the
*jettatura* or "evil eye," at least a way of
bringing disaster to any project he visited
or blessed. As one Italian wrote: "We all
did very well in the campaign against the
Austrians [in 1848] . . . suddenly he blessed
the cause and everything went bad at once."

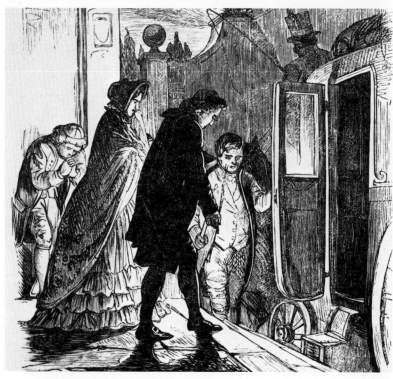

Right: Pius IX leaving Rome in November
1848. The pope had tried to follow a
middle course in the revolution and war
during that year, but a gradually deteriorat-
ing situation at last forced him to leave the
Holy City and seek refuge in the Kingdom
of Naples.

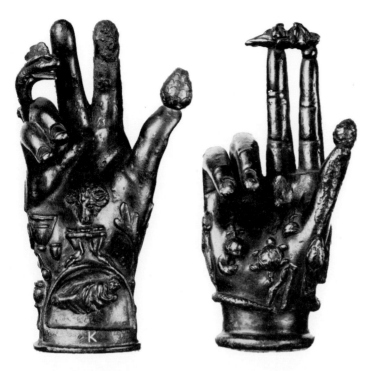

# The Evil Eye

Left: the sign of the hand with thumb and first two fingers raised was used as protective sign and symbol against the evil eye long before the Christian era, when it became a sign of blessing. These two amulets are Roman and date from the 1st century BC.

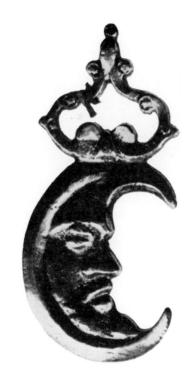

unwilling agents for the harm they cause and the terror they inspire. Apparently there is no way possessors of the evil eye can rid themselves of their fatal gift. It is as much a curse on them as on their victims—they are born with it and must live and die with it. Aristocrats and churchmen were frequently credited with having the evil eye. The most eminent churchman to have this reputation was Pope Pius IX. It is said that even devout Catholics, while asking for a blessing, would keep the horned hand pointed at him. F. T. Elworthy in *The Evil Eye* quotes this statement about whether the pope had the malevolent gift or not: "They said so, and it seems really to be true. If he had not the *jettatura*, it is very odd that everything he blessed made *fiasco*. We all did very well in the campaign against the Austrians in '48 [1848]. We were winning battle after battle, and all was gaiety and hope, when suddenly he blessed the cause, and everything went to the bad at once. Nothing succeeds with anybody or anything when he wishes well to them. When he went to S. Agnese to hold a great festival, down went the floor, and the people were all smashed together. Then he visited the column to the Madonna in the Piazza di Spagna, and blessed it and the workmen; of course one fell from the scaffold the same day and killed himself. . . . I do not wonder the workmen at the column in the Piazza di Spagna refused to work in raising it unless the Pope stayed away!"

The horned hand may or may not help against the evil eye. But there seems no way in which sailors can protect themselves if they sail in a jinxed ship. Many mariners are convinced that spirits of the dead are involved in jinxes, and point to the two most notorious jinx ships of the 19th century—the British vessels *Hinemoa* and *Great Eastern*.

On its maiden voyage in 1892 the 2000-ton steel bark *Hinemoa* carried a ballast load of rubble from an old London graveyard. During the voyage, four apprentice seamen died of typhoid. The first captain went insane, the second became a criminal, the third

Above: this charm in the shape of the crescent moon is from southern Italy, where belief in the evil eye is most strong. The crescent moon stood for many pre-Christian gods and goddesses, including the Egyptian Isis, the Greek Hera, and the Roman Demeter, so the use of this particular symbol is an extremely ancient defense against the evil eye.

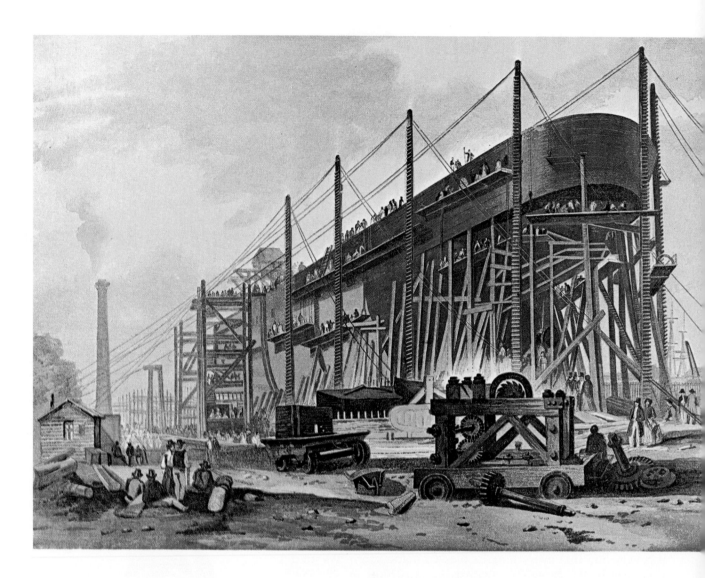

Above: the *Great Eastern* during its construction on the Thames in 1857. Three years' work had already gone into what was planned to be a steamship five times the size of the biggest vessel then afloat. The ship was designed to carry 4000 passengers, with power supplied by paddle wheels "larger than a circus ring." Designed by the British engineer Isambard Kingdom Brunel, it was to prove one of his few disastrous failures.

Opposite top: Isambard Kingdom Brunel. He had already designed two steamships, the *Great Western* in 1838 and the *Great Britain* in 1845, when he planned the *Great Eastern*, the "wonder of the seas," in 1854.

Opposite below: the *Great Eastern* afloat. It took a long and grueling series of launching attempts that lasted from November 1857 to January 1858 before the giant ship finally slid into the water.

was removed from his command on grounds of being an alcoholic, the fourth was found dead in his cabin, and the fifth shot himself. Under the sixth captain the *Hinemoa* capsized, and two sailors were swept overboard when it righted itself. The end came during a storm in 1908 when the bark drifted ashore on the west coast of Scotland, a total loss. Sailors say the vessel was jinxed right from the start by the presence of graveyard bones in the ballast on the maiden voyage.

The *Great Eastern* was built by the famous British engineer Isambard Kingdom Brunel starting in 1854, and was one of his few failures. In its day the passenger liner was the largest—and the unluckiest—ship in the world. The vessel was planned to be the wonder of the seas, a floating palace carrying 4000 passengers in luxury around the world. The six masts and five funnels were more than any other ship had ever carried. Marine jargon did not have enough names for so many masts, so they were referred to as Monday, Tuesday, Wednesday, Thursday, Friday, and Saturday. The colossal hull, 692 feet long, surpassed the dimensions of Noah's Ark. In fact, the *Great Eastern* had two hulls, one inside the other, three feet apart and heavily braced. Inside the hull there was an ingenious arrangement of longitudinal and transverse bulkheads, forming 16 watertight compartments. This was designed to make it virtually unsinkable—and it is true that while nearly every other calamity befell the ship, it never sank.

Hammering in the three million rivets, each one an inch thick and all driven in by hand, took 200 rivet gangs 1000 work days. Fatal accidents during construction were fewer than average—four workers and a spectator. But one riveter and his apprentice disappeared, and there was a rumor that they had been sealed up in a hull compartment and that their screams for help had been drowned in the din of the hammers.

The original backers ran out of money when the price of iron plate increased, and work stopped till Brunel had succeeded in raising more money. Launching the heaviest hull in history into the Thames river had to be performed sideways. It took an agonizing three months to get the vessel to move the 330 feet down to the water. Chains snapped, barges sank, innumerable hydraulic rams burst under the strain. Day after day Brunel worked to inch his giant structure a few feet closer to the water. The *Times* correspondent in London wrote: "There she lies on the very brink of the noble river which is to carry her to the ocean, but she will not wet her lips." When the launch was finally made on the last day of January 1858, it had cost £1000 a foot.

Total expenses had already reached over £1 million. The cost of completing the ship broke the next company, but once more Brunel managed to raise the money to carry on. The new board of directors set aside the original plan to take the *Great Eastern* on long voyages to India and Australia—for which the liner was uniquely suitable. Instead, they went after the quick profits of a North Atlantic run. Only the first class cabins were completed for the maiden voyage, the second and third class accommodation left for what turned out to be another nine years. The day

# The Great Eastern

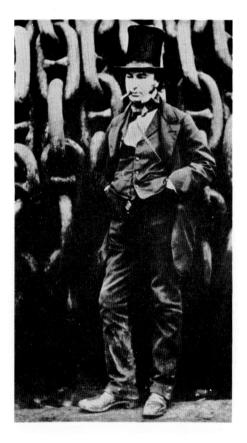

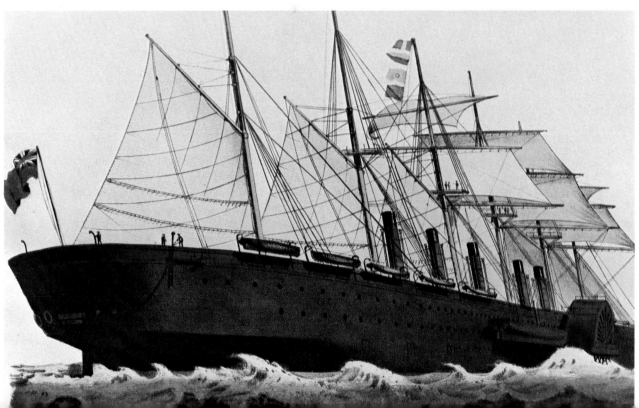

# "The Unluckiest Ship in the World"

Below: the *Great Eastern* in a hurricane in the Atlantic in September 1861. In a storm which would almost certainly have sunk any other ship, the *Great Eastern* lost both its huge paddle wheels, all its lifeboats, and the rudder broke and began smashing against the screw. But this was only the beginning of the *Great Eastern*'s misfortunes.

before the great ship was to sail, Brunel came down for an inspection. The famous engineer was prematurely aged at 53. Just after posing with colleagues for a photograph, he staggered and collapsed with a stroke. Brunel died a week later as news came through that one of the *Great Eastern*'s funnels had exploded as the liner steamed down the channel, because a steam valve had been left closed. Five men were scalded to death and another fell to his death in one of the great paddle wheels. The grand salon with its mirrored walls and sumptuous decoration was wrecked.

Repairs took longer than expected and the planned voyage to the United States was canceled. In order to get some return on their investment, the directors moved the by-then notorious ship to Holyhead, Wales and opened it to sightseers. Not long after, a howling gale tore it from its moorings and drove it out to sea. For 18 hours the vessel rode the storm while many nearby ships sank, proving how well it was designed. But the recently repaired salon was ruined again. Three months later the captain, the

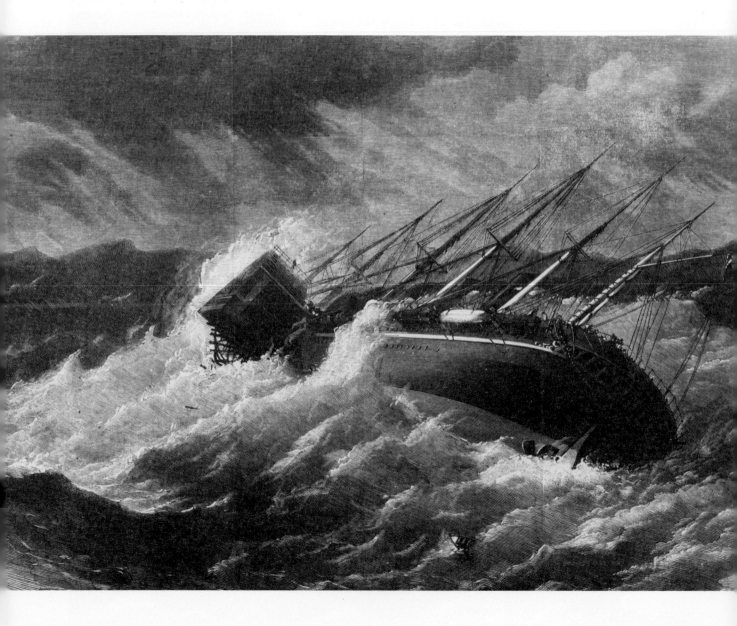

coxswain, and the nine-year-old son of the chief purser were drowned when a sudden squall upset their gig as they were going ashore.

Nothing casts a sharper blight over a ship's character than the death of the captain during or before a maiden voyage. When the news reached London the directors of the *Great Eastern*'s managing company resigned. The next board set a definite sailing date of June 9, 1860, but July 9 came and went. Most of the 300 ticketed passengers—all that the ship had beds for—tired of waiting and sailed on one of Sir Samuel Cunard's more reliable ships. When the *Great Eastern* finally left Southampton on June 16, only 35 paying passengers were aboard. The new captain, commanding a crew of 418, had never crossed the Atlantic before.

During the 12-day crossing the cheap coal that was being used as an economy measure damaged the funnel casings and made the main dining room so hot that passengers refused to sit there. Otherwise the voyage was uneventful, and the huge liner arrived

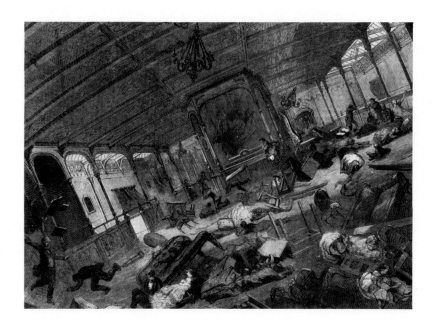

Left: the grand saloon of the *Great Eastern* during the hurricane of September 1861. One passenger, hearing frantic noises, untied himself from the stanchion to which he had lashed himself and staggered to it. "Tables and chairs were dancing to a hornpipe, the stove joined most heartedly in the fun, and the dancers seemed determined to break down all the nicely turned mahogany columns and banisters, which snapped like glass."

to a sensational welcome in New York. However, sightseers, incensed at the high $1 admission fee charged for visiting on board, tried to get their money's worth by pocketing souvenirs. Later, an announced two-day excursion turned into a nightmare. Two thousand people were faced with the problem of sleeping on only 300 beds. A pipe burst in the storage room and flooded the food supplies, leaving nothing available to eat except dessicated chicken, salted meat, and stone-hard biscuits. For this passengers were charged outrageous prices. Most of the passengers had to spend the night on the deck, where they had the unpleasant experience of being covered by cinders raining down from the five funnels. In the morning there was no water to wash off the grit. The passengers thought they could at least look forward to a speedy landing, but by some error of navigation the *Great Eastern* had gone off course during the night and was 100 miles

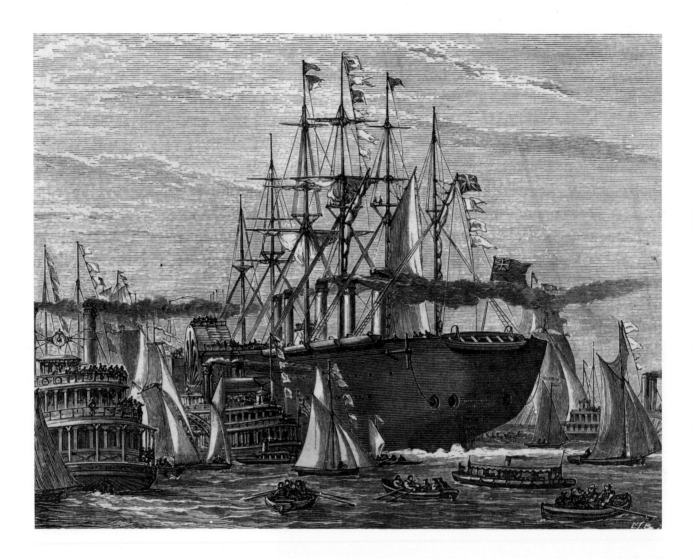

Above: the *Great Eastern* in New York
harbor after its first voyage across the
Atlantic in June 1860. Accidents, many of
them fatal, a disastrous attempt to earn
money by exhibiting the ship, and the 1861
hurricane marred the *Great Eastern*'s stay
in New York.

out to sea. There was no food left for breakfast or lunch. When
land was at last reached, the hungry, grimy, weary passengers
fought to disembark.

A second excursion was announced, but not surprisingly, only
a handful of tickets were bought. New York was disenchanted
with the great ship. Almost unnoticed it left for England with 90
passengers on board. But the return trip was not to be without
incident either. In mid-Atlantic a screw shaft gave out. At Milford
Haven the vessel fouled the hawser of a small boat and drowned
two of its passengers. Then the huge liner crashed into the
frigate *Blenheim*.

The next captain, the third, never sailed, resigning rather than
sail short-handed when the directors fired one-third of the crew.
Under the fourth captain, the ship sailed with only 100 passengers, even though there were 300 emigrants willing to travel
steerage. In fact, the *Great Eastern* never carried any emigrants
across the Atlantic, although in this respect it could have beaten
all competition and made great profits. The owners single-
mindedly concentrated on first-class passengers during the nine
years before second and third class accommodation was
installed—and the ship never came near getting a full comple-
ment of such travelers. Profits were also hindered because the

vessel was too cold to cross the Atlantic in the winter.

In September 1861 the *Great Eastern* was struck by a hurricane that would probably have sunk any other vessel. Both the side paddles were ripped off. All lifeboats were torn away. The rudder broke and began crashing against the screw. Repairs cost £60,000. The following year in Long Island Sound the ship struck a tall needle of rock unmarked on the charts; it tore a rip 83 feet long and 9 feet wide in the outer hull. This time repairs cost £70,000.

In 1864 the unlucky ship was put up for auction and bought for £25,000 to begin a new career as a cable layer. Misfortune still hounded it. When 1186 miles out from Ireland on the way to Newfoundland, an accident caused the cable to slip and the severed end sank three miles to the ocean bed. All efforts to recover it failed, so the ship returned to England. Another try in 1866 was successful, and on July 27 the first messages by undersea cable passed between Europe and North America.

As a vessel for laying cable, the *Great Eastern* at last justified its existence. In 1869 it sailed for India—the only time it visited the latitudes it had been designed for—and laid a cable between Bombay and Aden.

In 1874 the launching of the first custom-built cable ships brought an end to the only profitable employment the *Great Eastern* ever enjoyed. A mere 15 years after being launched, the great ship was brought back to Milford Haven where it remained rusting and blocking the shipping lines for the next 12 years. By 1886 the barnacles on the hull were six inches thick. In that year the owners managed to sell the onetime liner for £20,000, and it was gingerly taken around the coast of Wales to Liverpool. There the *Great Eastern* damaged the tug *Wrestler*, the last boat it was to crash into. Then this former "Wonder of the Sea," this

# A Giant Disaster

Below: the *Great Eastern* during the only profitable period of its wretched career, laying telegraph cable in the Atlantic Ocean between 1869 and 1874.

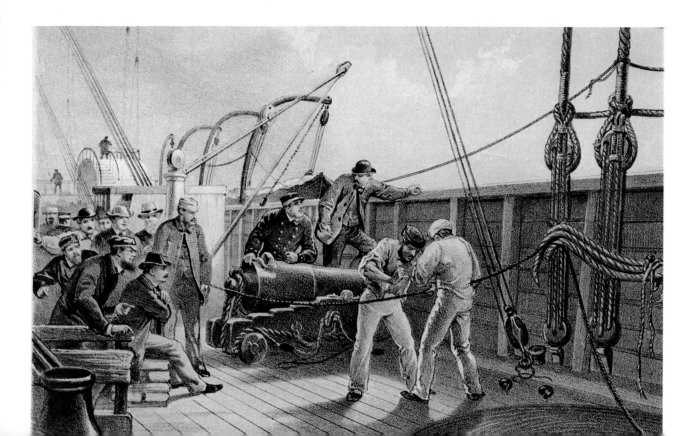

Right: only 30 years after its first journey through the English Channel, on which six men were killed when the funnel exploded, the vast hulk of this enormous ship was broken up for scrap near Liverpool, England. It was then that two skeletons were found inside the double hull. Were they the cause of bad luck?

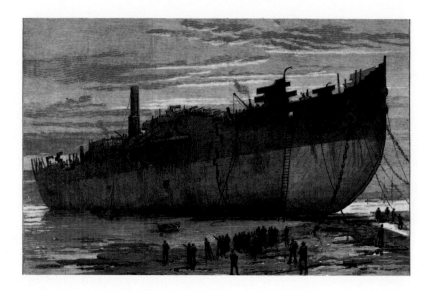

"Floating Palace," was painted with slogans advertising a Liverpool store. Later the vessel was taken to Dublin to advertise a brand of tea. Finally a firm of metal dealers bought the down-at-heel ship. It had been sold for the last time.

Breaking up the *Great Eastern* proved almost as difficult as building it. In fact, the wrecker's iron ball, suspended on a giant chain, had to be invented for the purpose in 1889. Inside the double hull, demolition experts discovered two skeletons—the riveter and his boy apprentice, who had vanished when the ship was being built. Few people doubted that they had discovered the cause of the ship's jinx.

Is there a more logical explanation? The sailors on board the *Hinemoa* knew that the ballast had been taken from a graveyard; the seamen on the *Great Eastern* during the maiden voyage knew that two workmen might have been sealed up in the hull. Couldn't it be said that they anticipated bad luck and went to meet it half way? Perhaps. But if that explanation satisfies some for jinxed ships, the same kind of reason can hardly account for the restless behavior of the coffins in the Chase Tomb.

In the churchyard of Christ Church, Barbados, on a headland overlooking Oistin's Bay, stands a small but strongly built stone tomb. It has been empty since 1820, and seems likely to remain so. Designed as a quiet resting place for the dead, it proved to be anything but.

The family vault, built of large blocks of local coral stone firmly cemented together, is recessed two feet deep into solid limestone rock. The floor space is 12 feet long by $6\frac{1}{2}$ feet wide; originally the entrance was closed by a heavy slab of blue Devon marble, which sealed the tomb between interments. It was built in 1724 by the widow of an English aristocrat, whose body does not seem to have been interred there unless his coffin was subsequently removed. The first recorded interment is that of Mrs. Thomasina Goddard on July 31, 1807.

In the following year the tomb came into the possession of the wealthy Chase family, whose head was Thomas Chase. On February 22, 1808 the small lead coffin of Mary Chase, his infant daughter, was interred in the vault. Four years passed and another Chase daughter, Dorcas, died—of uncertain age but apparently an adult. She was interred in the tomb on July 6, 1812. At that point there was nothing out of the ordinary in the state of the other two coffins.

Matters were very different when, on August 9 the same year, Thomas Chase himself was brought to the tomb. The coffins of both his daughters had been shifted—it looked as though by violence. That of the infant Mary had been thrown across the vault and lay head downward against the far wall.

The black laborers were alarmed at the sight, but the Chase family did not seem unduly upset. The coffins were returned to their original places beside the undisturbed one of Mrs. Goddard, and Thomas Chase's was placed alongside them. His was an exceedingly heavy lead coffin, requiring eight men to lift it. When the marble slab of the vault was put in position, great care was taken to seal it properly.

On the death of Samuel Brewster Ames, a baby who may have been a Chase relative, his coffin was brought to the tomb on September 25, 1816. All the coffins were in confusion, save that of Mrs. Goddard. Her coffin, which had been made of wood, had disintegrated but was in its place; the others had been flung about and upended. Thomas Chase's heavy lead coffin was lying on its side several feet to the left of its original spot. This time the Chase family was furious, assuming that the desecration was linked with the abortive slave rising that had been crushed with much bloodshed earlier in the year. But apart from the unlikeli-

# The Mystery of the Chase Tomb

Below: the empty Chase family vault on the island of Barbados as it is today. For many years the coffins inside were found in disarray every time the vault was reopened to receive another dead member of the important Chase family.

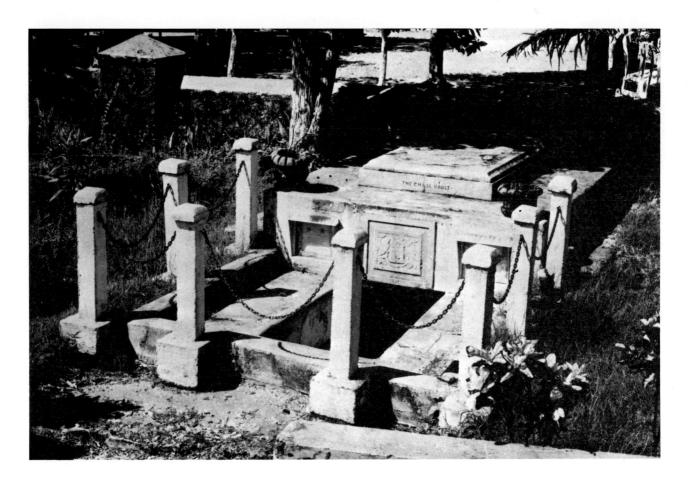

# A Family Curse?

hood that the superstitious blacks would be willing to enter a tomb, the sheer weight of Thomas Chase's coffin made it a well-nigh impossible task to have been accomplished unnoticed.

The coffins were rearranged, and the marble slab cemented into position. On November 17 of the same year, the tomb had to be opened again to receive Samuel Brewster, who had been murdered during the slave uprising and temporarily buried elsewhere. Once again the coffins were in the wildest disorder. Except for Mrs. Goddard's—undisturbed as always—they were leaning against the walls, crossing and overlapping each other. This time the minister of Christ Church, a magistrate, and two other men searched the vault thoroughly. They found no crack, no concealed entrance. A fairly big crowd had accompanied the funeral procession, and the findings confirmed their worst fears: the Chase Tomb was cursed. The black laborers had to be ordered sharply to enter the tomb and restore order. Mrs. Goddard's bones, which had fallen out of her disintegrating coffin, were wrapped up and placed against the wall. Once again the entrance was sealed.

Three years passed before the next, and last, coffin was brought to the Chase Tomb. The tomb's troubled history had created such sensational interest on Barbados that the governor, Lord

Right: these drawings by Nathan Lucas, an eyewitness, show how the coffins were originally arranged (left) and how they were discovered when the Chase tomb was opened in April 1820. It was after this that the tomb was abandoned.

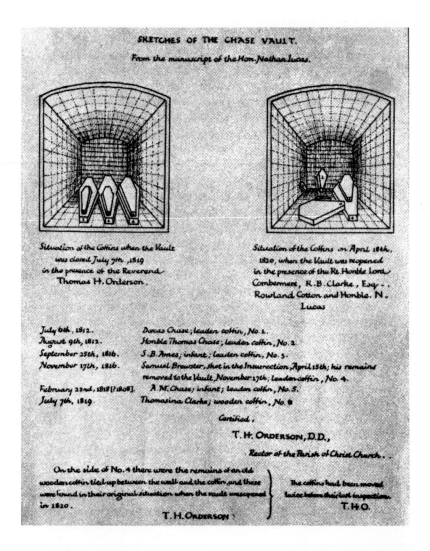

Combermere, the commander of the garrison, and many hundreds of spectators walked behind the coffin of Mrs. Thomasina Clarke on July 17, 1819. The vault was opened only with difficulty because Thomas Chase's heavy coffin was upended and resting against it, six feet from the place it should have been. The two children's coffins, which had rested on top of two larger ones, were on the floor. Only Mrs. Goddard's, the flimsiest of them all, was untouched.

Lord Combermere had been one of the Duke of Wellington's most successful cavalry commanders against Napoleon. It took a lot to frighten him. He personally supervised a meticulous examination of the interior of the vault. When nothing had been revealed by this search, he had the seven coffins put back into position, and ordered fine white beach sand to be sprinkled on the floor. This would show the footprints of anyone who entered the vault. The marble slab was put in place, and Lord Combermere and several others imprinted their personal seals in the wet cement sealing the slab.

Nine months later, on April 19, 1820, Lord Combermere was in the neighborhood of Christ Church again. He was due to return to England that year and was curious to know whether anything had happened inside the Chase Tomb. He found the seals on the slab unbroken. No footprints appeared on the sanded floor. The remains of Mrs. Goddard's coffin were against the wall where they had been left. But again the other coffins had been flung all over the place. One child's coffin was lying just inside the entrance. Thomas Chase's particularly heavy coffin and another one were upside down.

Experienced campaigner as he was, Lord Combermere knew when a situation was beyond his control. He ordered the coffins to be removed and buried elsewhere. Since then, the tomb has remained empty.

What power disturbed the coffins has never been discovered. Barbados suffers from earthquakes, but no quake would overturn a lead coffin and leave fragile wood unmoved. No moisture was ever detected in the vault, but even if water had somehow entered it and been able to shift the coffins, the wooden one would have been the first to move—and yet its position remained unaltered. Neither of these natural explanations—which seem to be the only two—are convincing. It also seems impossible that a human agency was involved. What about the supernatural?

Thomas Chase was the most hated man on the island. Both he and his daughter Dorcas were believed to have killed themselves—she, it was said, starved herself to death out of despair over her cruel father. The disorders began after her interment, as though the other corpses resented the presence of a suicide among them. Could some power associated with the corpse of Mrs. Goddard—whose coffin always remained undisturbed— have flung the coffins about the vault? Could the arrival of a second suicide and the corpses of three who did not die by their own hand have intensified the power? If the answer to these questions is "yes," the mystery still remains of what that power is, and why it manifested itself in this particular case. The curse on the Chase Tomb is as much a puzzle today as when it confronted the citizens of Barbados in the 19th century.

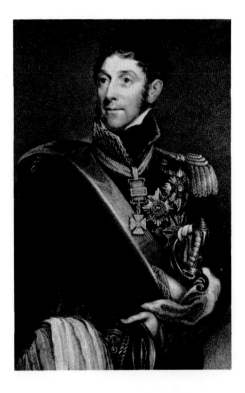

Above: Lord Combermere, the British governor of Barbados in 1820. It was he who finally decided that the Chase family mausoleum should be abandoned.

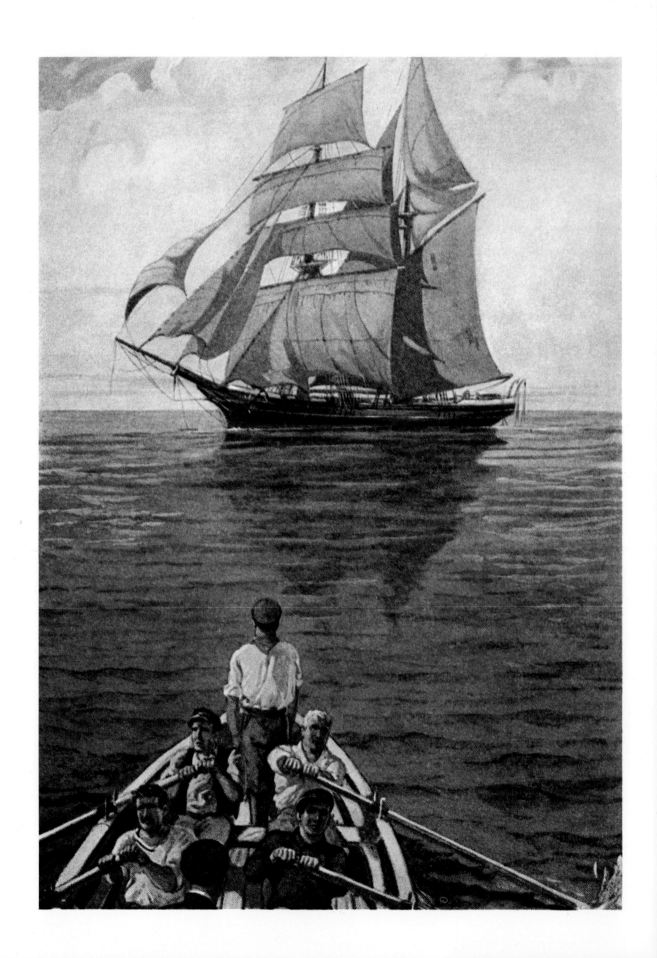

# Chapter 7
# Mysteries of the Sea

Who or what caused everyone on board the *Mary Celeste* to abandon the ship? Why was the seaworthy vessel, with cargo intact, left in apparent haste near dangerous rocks in the Atlantic Ocean? This mystery, unsolved and much discussed since 1872, is the most famous of the unexplained puzzles about crewless ships adrift, crews of corpses, and ships that seem to be capable of independent action of their own. No one has yet plumbed the depths of the mysterious seas to find the answers to such riddles.

The captain of the English brig *Dei Gratia* was the first to see the strange two-masted ship sailing an erratic course, with only the jib and the foretopmast staysail set. Though the vessel was on a starboard tack, the jib was set to port—a sure sign to a sailor that a ship was out of control, the crew either injured or dead. Captain Edward Morehouse decided to close in, but the sea was running high after recent squalls and two hours passed before he was near enough to read the name. It was the *Mary Celeste*.

Captain Morehouse knew the vessel well. He also knew Captain Benjamin Spooner Briggs, the man in command. Only a month ago their two ships had been loading cargo at neighboring piers in the East River in New York. The *Mary Celeste* had set sail for the Italian port of Genoa on November 5, 1872; 10 days later the *Dei Gratia* had followed across the Atlantic, bound for Gibraltar. Now Morehouse had caught up, only to find the ship drifting halfway between the Azores and the coast of Portugal. No one was at the wheel, no one on deck.

Morehouse sent Oliver Deveau, his first mate, to see what was amiss. Deveau was a large man of great physical strength, described as "absolutely fearless." He and two seamen rowed over to investigate the mystery. The ship seemed deserted. The first thing Deveau did on boarding her was to sound the pumps. He found that one of the pumps had been drawn to let the sounding rod down, so he used the other pump, leaving the first on the deck as he found it. There was a great deal of water between

Opposite: sailors leave their own ship to investigate an apparently deserted schooner, moving eerily under full sail across the ocean. A similar scene has been reenacted a number of times, for the tale of the *Mary Celeste* is only the best known of such riddles of the sea.

# A Deserted Ship

decks, probably as a result of recent storms, two sails that had been set had blown away, and the lower foretopsails were hanging by the corners. In spite of these problems, however, Deveau established that the *Mary Celeste* was in no danger of sinking.

Deveau and the second mate, John Wright, searched the vessel; they found no one aboard, alive or dead. They did find that the binnacle had been stoved in, destroying the compass, that two of the hatches were off, and that one cask of crude alcohol in the hold had sprung its lid. Otherwise the cargo seemed in good order and the ship's wheel, which had not been lashed, was undamaged. It looked as though the *Mary Celeste* had carried a yawl on deck, lashed to the main hatch. Two fenders were in position on the hatch, showing that a yawl could have been there, and two sets of rails had been removed apparently in order to launch it.

In the cabin Deveau and Wright discovered that the six starboard windows had been nailed up with planks, but there was no way of telling if they had been so fastened before the voyage

Below: the crew of the British ship *Dei Gratia* sighting the schooner *Mary Celeste* drifting about 600 miles west of the coast of Portugal on November 15, 1872.

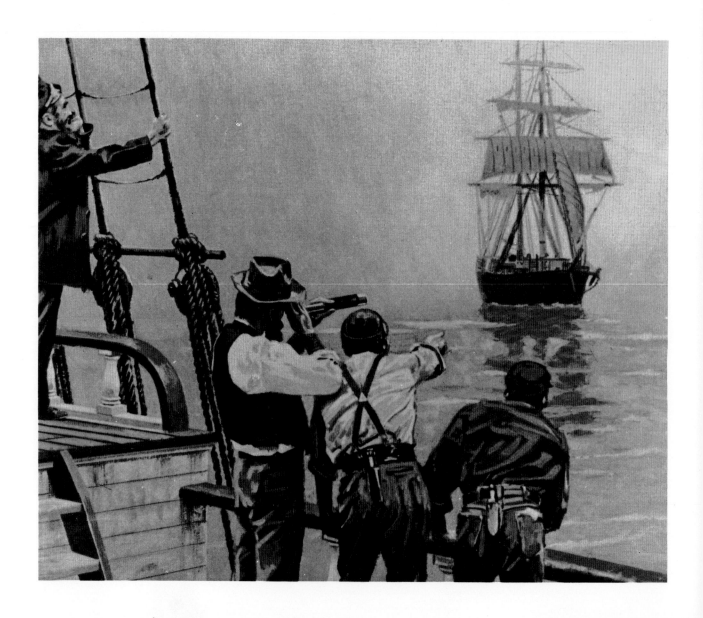

or during it. The port windows were shut but still let in some light. Much water had entered the cabin through the open door and through the skylight that was also open. The clock had been ruined by the water and much of the bedding and clothing was wet. Because the linen and clothes were difficult to dry out, Deveau concluded that they had been made wet by sea water. He later testified:

"The bed was as it had been left after being slept in—not made . . . I judged there had been a woman aboard. I saw female clothing . . . I noticed an impression in the bed, as of a child having laid there. There seemed to be everything left behind as if left in a great hurry, but everything in its place. There were boxes of clothing. There were also work bags with needles, threads, buttons, books, and a case of instruments, a writing desk. A harmonium or melodeon was in the cabin."

In those days it was not uncommon for a captain's wife to accompany him on a voyage, and Sarah Briggs had in fact done so. The couple had also brought their two-year-old daughter Sophia Matilda. They had left their other child, seven-year-old Arthur, with his grandparents in Marion, Massachusetts, to continue his schooling.

Almost as many legends have attached themselves to the *Mary Celeste* as there were barnacles on its hold. One of these is that a half-eaten meal was discovered on the cabin table, and that breakfast was still cooking in the galley. Deveau's sworn statement shows otherwise. Though the rack for stopping dishes from sliding off the table was in position, he reported, there were no eatables in the cabin, nor was any cooked food found in the galley. Pots and kettles had been washed up and stowed away. An open bottle of medicine was found, which suggested that whoever had taken it had left in too much of a hurry to put the cork back into the bottle. From the meager evidence, it was presumed that the ship had been abandoned some time in mid-morning—late enough for breakfast to have been cleared away, but not before Mrs. Briggs had made the bed. This presumption was partly based on the fact that no New England woman of Sarah Briggs' background would have allowed the beds to remain unmade till late in the morning, even at sea.

Less water had entered the seamen's quarters than the cabin. The seamen's chests were dry, and there were no traces of rust on the razors left behind. The crew had evidently gone in a great hurry, leaving behind as they did not only the contents of their chests—everything of value they possessed—but also their oil-skin boots and even their pipes, articles no sailor would abandon unless in a state of panic.

Looking for some explanation, Deveau studied the logbook in the mate's cabin. The last entry was dated November 24, and it gave the ship's position as 100 miles southwest of San Miguel Island in the Azores. There was some later information jotted on the log slate, found in the captain's cabin. It showed that the next day, November 25, at 8 a.m. the ship passed Santa Maria Island. Eleven days had passed since that final entry had been made. In that time the ship had continued for another 500 miles, apparently on course. For some undetermined period of that time, however, it had been unmanned. The date of the last entry

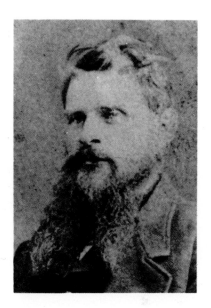

Above: Captain Morehouse of the *Dei Gratia.* In the investigation that followed the finding of the *Mary Celeste*, great play was made of the friendship between Morehouse and Captain Briggs of the *Mary Celeste.* The obvious theory was that the strange tale had been put together by the two of them to collect salvage money.

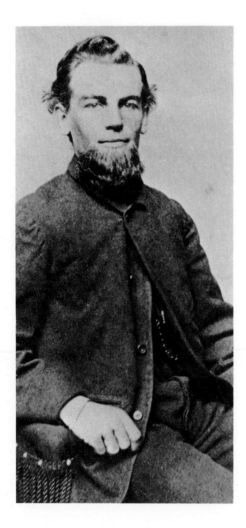

Above: Benjamin Spooner Briggs, captain and part owner of the *Mary Celeste*. Briggs came from a seafaring family and was a stern and able captain. His ship had apparently been abandoned in desperate haste, but to this day no one knows why.

on the log slate does not necessarily mean that the *Mary Celeste* was abandoned on the 25th. In small ships the log is not regarded as very important, and is seldom written up every day. For example, in the 18 days that the *Mary Celeste* had been at sea before sighting the Azores, only seven entries had been made in the log. There was no way of telling exactly when Captain Briggs took his wife, child, and crew of seven onto the yawl—if he actually did so. Neither was there any indication why they had left a sound and seaworthy vessel in an apparent hurry.

To some, the story of the *Mary Celeste* could be seen as a warning that the name of a ship should never be changed. Long John Silver of Stevenson's "Treasure Island" said: "I never knowed any luck as came of changing of a ship's name. Now what a ship was christened, so let her stay, I says." When the future *Mary Celeste* was built on Spencer's Island, Nova Scotia, in 1861, it was christened the *Amazon*. From the start the vessel was an unlucky one. The first captain died 48 hours after the *Amazon* was registered. On the maiden voyage, it ran into a fishing weir off the coast of Maine and damaged the hull. While being repaired, fire broke out amidships. In the Straits of Dover, it collided with another brig, which sank. By that time the ship had had three captains. Under the fourth, the *Amazon* ran aground on Cape Breton Island and was wrecked. It was salvaged, however, and then passed quickly through two or perhaps three other owners, one of whom renamed it the *Mary Celeste*. As such the vessel was bought by James H. Winchester, founder of an eminent shipping firm that still bears his name in New York. On discovering dry rot in the timbers, he rebuilt the bottom with a copper lining. He also extended the deck cabin and generally put the ship in excellent condition. The *Mary Celeste* had exchanged the red ensign of the British merchant navy for the stars and stripes.

Early in September 1872 the newly named vessel was tied up at Pier 44 in New York's East River being loaded with about 1700 red oak casks of commercial alcohol. In one of her last letters to relatives, Sarah Briggs described her reaction to this cargo, saying that she thought she had gone slightly daft with the "amount of thumping and bumping, of shaking and tossings to and fro of the cargo." She also mentioned "screechings and growlings," which could have been caused by sweating casks of a volatile liquid such as crude alcohol.

At a nearby pier the *Dei Gratia* was taking on a cargo of petroleum, and the two captains, Briggs and Morehouse, dined together the night before the *Mary Celeste* sailed. The curious coincidence that it was the *Dei Gratia* which later found the *Mary Celeste* abandoned was to sow suspicion in the minds of the members of the Board of Inquiry trying to decide what had happened.

Captain Briggs was master of the vessel and part owner, having purchased a few shares of the ship from Winchester. He was an experienced seaman of 37, robust, correct, and temperate. Having been brought up among New England puritans, he never allowed liquor aboard a vessel under his command.

In after years several grizzled sailors claimed to be survivors of the *Mary Celeste*, but the names of the crew of seven are all known. The first mate was Albert Richardson, who was married to Winchester's niece. Andrew Gilling, the second mate, and Edward Head, the steward-cook, were the other Americans of the crew. The four seamen were all German: Volkert and Boz Lorensen, brothers from Schleswig-Holstein; Arian Martens, and Gottlief Goodschaad (or Gondschatt). In one of her letters to her mother-in-law Sarah Briggs said that she was not sure how smart the crew would prove to be, but Captain Briggs was satisfied they were reliable.

When Deveau and White had completed their examination of the drifting ship, they returned to the *Dei Gratia* to report to Captain Morehouse. In spite of his friendship with Briggs, Morehouse apparently did not go aboard the *Mary Celeste* for a personal look. Either he or Deveau proposed taking the abandoned ship into Gibraltar to claim salvage. Deveau returned to the *Mary Celeste* later that afternoon with two seamen, taking their ship's small boat, a barometer, sextant, compass, watch, and some food prepared by their steward. In two days the *Mary Celeste* was ready to sail and the two ships set out, remaining in sight of each other till they reached the Straits of Gibraltar. At that point a storm separated them. The *Dei Gratia* reached Gibraltar on the evening of December 12, and the *Mary Celeste* arrived the following morning. Then, unexpectedly, the arguments began.

A claim for salvaging an abandoned ship on the high seas generally presents no problem because in the vast majority of cases the crewless vessel is dismasted, waterlogged, or otherwise in bad shape. But the case of the *Mary Celeste* was different. F. Solly Flood, the British Admiralty Proctor in Gibraltar, said in his report to London: "The account which they [the salvors]

# What Made Them All Abandon Ship?

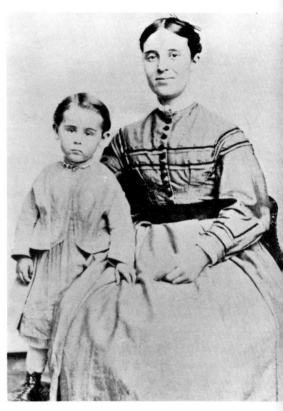

Above: Captain Briggs' wife Sarah and their five-year-old son Arthur. Mrs. Briggs and a two-year-old daughter, Sophia, accompanied Captain Briggs and a crew of seven on the *Mary Celeste*'s mysterious voyage from New York to the Italian port of Genoa with a cargo of commercial alcohol on board.

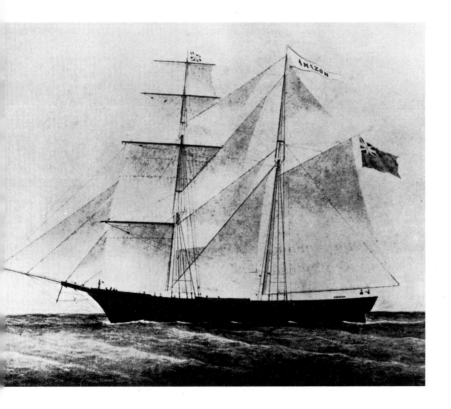

Left: the *Mary Celeste* in 1861 the year it was launched and when it was named the *Amazon*. In 1867 she was stranded off the coast of Nova Scotia, sold, renamed, again went aground on the same stormy coast, was finally seized for debt and bought by a ship's agent named J. H. Winchester and Co. Winchester gave her a copper-reinforced hull and put Briggs in charge as captain.

gave of the soundness and good condition of the derelict was so extraordinary that I found it necessary to apply for a survey."

The surveyors reported that the hull of the *Mary Celeste* was perfectly sound, and that the ship was not leaking and had not been in a collision. However, they remarked on two curious grooves which seemed to have been cut with a sharp instrument on each side of the bows, several feet back from the prow and a foot or two above the waterline. There was no damage within the ship, no trace of an explosion, no suggestion of a fire. The *Mary Celeste* was said to be in better shape than many of the small ships that did the Atlantic run. How could the captain, mate, and crew of the *Dei Gratia* swear that they had come upon this seaworthy and amply provisioned vessel drifting in mid-ocean? The British authorities in Gibraltar found such testimony hard to believe. In their view, it was far more likely to be a case of collusion between the crews of the two ships to claim the salvage money, the cargo alone being worth $30,000. Flood suspected even worse. He believed the case to be one of mutiny, piracy, and multiple murder. Described as a fussy and pompous man, Flood's good qualities were the counterpart of such faults: he was a painstaking investigator and he was dedicated to the rule of law. He was not going to let criminals, if so they proved, get away with their crimes.

Below: H.M.S. *Immortalité* finding the derelict ship *Margaret Pollock* in December 1872. Derelict and abandoned ships were a common hazard in the busy shipping lanes of the English Channel. H.M.S. *Immortalité* found two within four months, and after some speculation about the fate of the crews, sank them both to avoid collision with other ships.

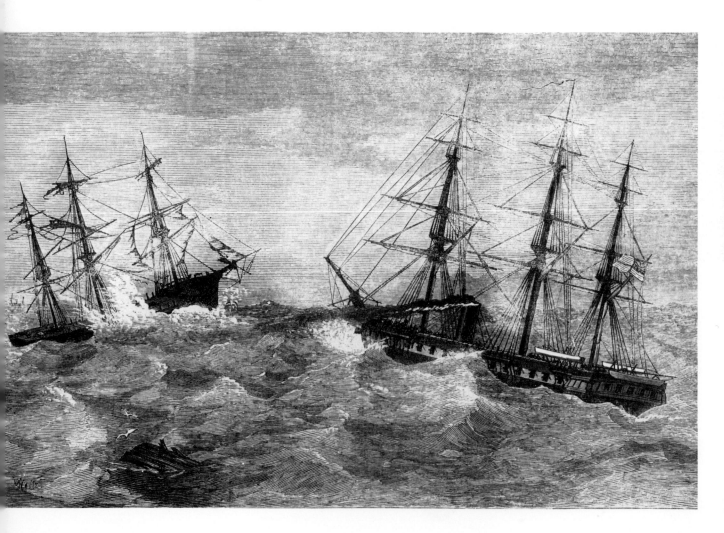

Flood suggested that the groove on the bows had been deliberately made to look as if the vessel had struck rocks. Horatio J. Sprague, the United States Consul in Gibraltar, hotly disputed this interpretation, and when the *USS Plymouth* put in at Gibraltar, he asked the captain to give his opinion of the grooves. Captain Schufeldt thought that the grooves were "splinters made in the bending of the planks which were afterward forced off by action of the sea without hurting the ship."

Meantime, Flood had found brown stains, which might have been blood, on the deck. More such stains were also found on the blade of an ornate Italian sword under the captain's berth. Deveau was closely questioned about these, but denied he had cleaned or scraped the decks to remove other similar stains. He maintained that his attention was fully occupied in running the ship, and he refused to accept that there was anything remarkable about the sword. It is a measure of the mistrust in which he and his companions were held that when samples of the brown stains were analyzed, the *Dei Gratia* crew was charged with the cost of analysis. Flood not only declined to reveal the report of the analysis, but also refused to give Sprague a copy. Even more surprising, he withheld the report from his own government! Could he have been hiding the fact that the results indicated no blood? Not until 1887, fourteen years later, was Sprague able to

# An Inquiry Begins

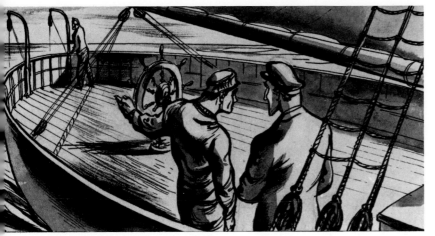

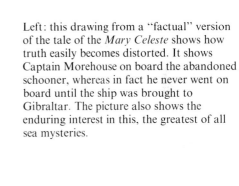

Left: this drawing from a "factual" version of the tale of the *Mary Celeste* shows how truth easily becomes distorted. It shows Captain Morehouse on board the abandoned schooner, whereas in fact he never went on board until the ship was brought to Gibraltar. The picture also shows the enduring interest in this, the greatest of all sea mysteries.

obtain a copy of the results of the analysis.

Flood also discovered irregularities in the log Deveau had kept while on board the *Mary Celeste*. At Captain Morehouse's instructions, he had written it up after arriving at Gibraltar. One entry stated that Morehouse had come on board the *Mary Celeste*, but Deveau insisted that he had made an error and that Captain Morehouse did not step foot on the ship till it had arrived in Gibraltar. Even more suspicious, in Flood's opinion, was the way the ship had continued on course for 11 days after November 25. He took this as an indication that the *Dei Gratia* crew must have boarded the *Mary Celeste* much earlier than they said they had.

Fortunately for the *Dei Gratia* crew, the members of the Board of Inquiry were experienced naval men. They knew that logs

# No Conclusion!

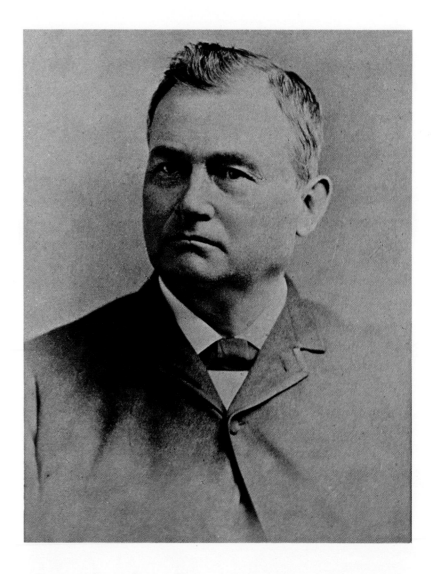

Right: James Winchester, American owner of the *Mary Celeste*. Winchester came to Gibraltar from New York to attend the inquiry into the *Mary Celeste* affair, but became angry when questioned closely about his ship, its crew, its captain, and even himself.

were not always kept without fail, and they could appreciate that Deveau, with only two men to help him sail the ship, had enough work on his hands without wanting to bother with paperwork. Unlike F. Solly Flood, they did not find anything untoward in the grooves on the bow or in the stains on the deck, and once all the available facts had been presented to them, they were quick to clear Morehouse and his men of any suspicion. In contrast, they spent a long time trying to work out what could have happened to Captain Briggs and his crew. When Winchester came over to Gibraltar from the United States in hopes of speeding the inquiry, he found himself subjected to such close questioning about his ship, the crew, the captain, the history, and himself that finally he got angered.

"I'm a Yankee with some English blood," he cried out, "but if I knew where it was, I'd open a vein and let the damned stuff out!"

When the court eventually handed down its judgment in March 1873, it confessed itself unable to decide why the *Mary Celeste* had been abandoned. This was the first time in its history it had failed to come to a conclusion. It awarded to the *Dei Gratia* a sum equivalent to about one-fifth of the combined value of the *Mary Celeste* and its cargo. The *Mary Celeste* was returned to Winchester, and under a new captain and a new crew, sailed to Genoa. There the cargo was unloaded—three-and-a-half months late, but otherwise intact. Winchester sold the ship as soon as it returned to New York, but its reputation as an unlucky vessel kept seamen from signing on as crew. The *Mary Celeste* changed hands rapidly, bringing little profit to any of its short-term owners.

In 1884 the ship was acquired by a disreputable captain named Gilman C. Parker, who deliberately ran it onto a reef in the West Indies for the sake of the insurance. Even this desperate measure brought no profit. The insurance companies became suspicious, asked awkward questions of the crew, and brought Captain Parker and his associates in the scheme to trial. Because the penalty for destroying a ship on the high seas was death by hanging, the jury, mindful of the ship's unlucky·history, was reluctant to convict. The defendants were freed on a technicality, but within eight months Parker was dead, one of his associates went mad, and another committed suicide. Their association with the *Mary Celeste* brought them nothing but grief.

As to what really happened to the *Mary Celeste* on that morning in late November 1872, somewhere between the Azores and Portugal, there have been many guesses. Surprisingly, interest in the subject was slow to develop, and for 11 years the mystery remained relatively unknown outside the seafaring community. Then an impecunious young doctor with an ambition to become an author wrote a story based on the affair. Entitled "J. Habakuk Jephson's Statement," the story appeared in *The Cornhill Magazine* in January 1884 with the ship's name changed to the *Marie Celeste*. In the story, the ship had been taken over as part of what would now be called a Black Power plot. According to the author's version of events, the lifeboat was still on board when the vessel was found.

When the identity of the writer became known, he was launched on the road to fame. The author was Arthur Conan Doyle, and his fictionalization of the *Mary Celeste* mystery started a flood of books and articles on the subject. Since then, so many books and articles have been devoted to the riddle that the Atlantic Mutual Insurance Company in New York has an entire room kept as a *Mary Celeste* Museum. One writer imagined that the *Mary Celeste* was attacked by a kraken or giant squid that picked off the crew one by one, sliding its tentacles through the portholes until it had consumed the last morsel of human flesh. Charles Fort suggested that the crew had been snatched away by a "selective force" which left the ship untouched. One of the more original theories had it that the crew built a platform under the bow in order to watch a swimming race around the ship between the captain and the mate. This explained the strange grooves. The platform collapsed and all were drowned. This explained the disappearance of everyone aboard. UFOs have also been held responsible.

What are some more logical ideas about the mystery?

One fact to be taken into account is that everyone left the ship in obvious great haste. Mrs. Briggs left her child's clothing behind, the seamen abandoned their pipes and oilskin boots. Clearly

Below: It was British writer Arthur Conan Doyle who did most to perpetuate the tale of the *Mary Celeste*. In 1884 a London magazine published a highly colored story by him based loosely on the facts and called "J. Habakuk Jephson's Statement." This illustration, which shows the captain's wife playing cribbage with two of the ship's passengers, accompanied the story.

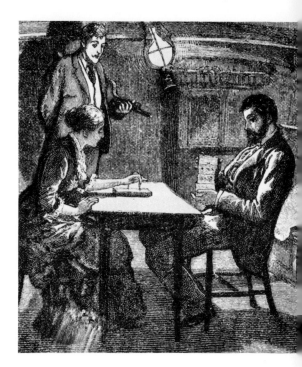

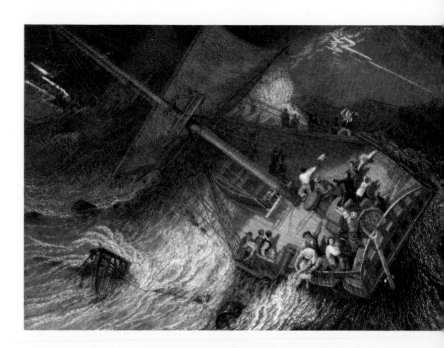

Right: a storm at sea. The ship has been blown almost completely over on her side by a giant wave that threatens to wash the crew from the deck within seconds. Was this possibly the fate of the crew of the *Mary Celeste*? But if so, why was everything in good order when she was found?

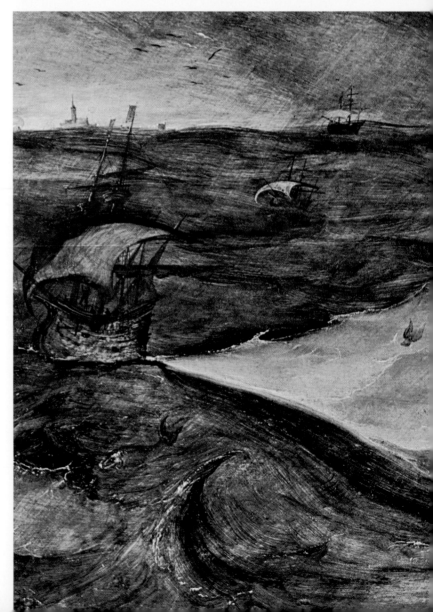

they left in panic, perhaps in deadly fear of something they believed was about to happen. They almost certainly left in the yawl, and they appear to have done so under the guidance of someone responsible—the captain or the first mate—because the chronometer, the sextant, and the ship's papers were not found on board and must therefore have been taken along.

There are three credible theories as to what caused the abandonment of the *Mary Celeste.*

The first was believed to be the likely explanation by Captain Morehouse and Captain James Briggs, brother of the mystery vessel's captain. Knowing that on the morning of the 25th the wind had dropped after a night of violent storm, they thought the ship may have been becalmed in the Azores and found itself drifting toward the dangerous rocks off Santa Maria Island. Everyone on board took to the yawl for safety, staying near the ship. But suddenly a wind got up and took the ship away, and though the men in the boat rowed frantically, the *Mary Celeste* drew farther from them. In the gales that again blew up in the afternoon, a single wave would have swamped the little boat.

# Swamped by a Sudden Squall?

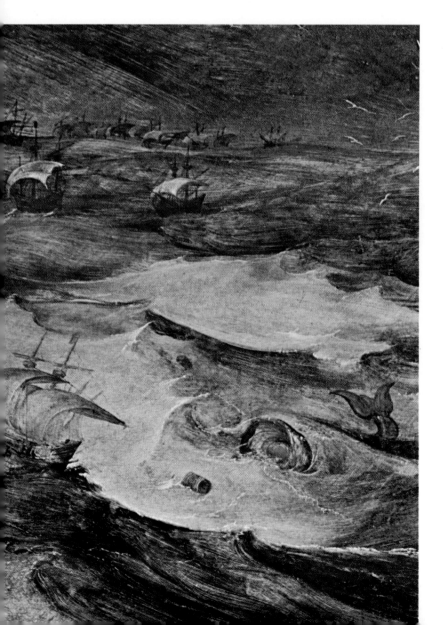

Left: another storm at sea, painted in about 1568. Here one of the ships is apparently being pursued by a huge whale, its jaws eagerly agape. Sailors are notoriously superstitious. Did one of the *Mary Celeste*'s crew spark off a panic by believing he saw more than was there?

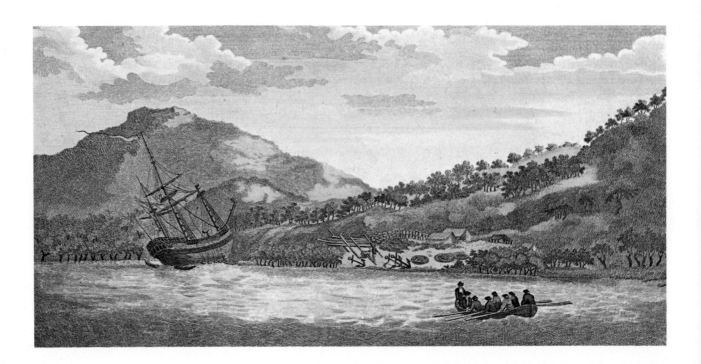

Above: Captain Cook's *Endeavour* aground on the Great Barrier Reef, the world's longest coral reef off eastern Australia, in 1768. The ship's carpenter, taking soundings, mistook the depth, panicked, and in the general hysteria that followed, the entire crew would have abandoned ship if Cook had not managed to restore calm. Is this what happened to the crew of the *Mary Celeste*?

Against this theory is the widely accepted surmise that the *Mary Celeste* kept to a steady course for several days after the 25th. This makes it more probable that the abandonment took place on a later date.

The second theory with a logical basis was proposed by Deveau and would explain why the pump plunger was found lying on the deck. He pointed out that the ship had been through heavy storms, and some of the water between decks had found its way into the holds. This may have given the impression that the ship was leaking, so the pump plunger was drawn and the pump sounded—by someone who misread the depth. He at once spread the alarm that the ship was on the point of going down. Panic followed.

This would be neither the first nor the last time a crew had panicked on grounds that later proved unjustified. For example, when Captain Cook's famous *Endeavour* was in difficulties off the East Australian coast, the ship's carpenter was sent to sound the well. He mistook the reading and, in the ensuing hysteria, the crew would have abandoned the ship had Cook not been able to restore calm. In 1919 the schooner *Marion G. Douglas*, which carried a cargo of timber, was abandoned by the crew off the coast of Newfoundland. They had believed their ship to be sinking—but a moment's thought would have reassured them that a ship with a cargo of timber was unlikely to go down. It went on to sail across the Atlantic without them.

The flaw in Deveau's theory is that it means there was a sudden loss of nerve on the part of the captain, and this conflicts with what is known of Briggs' character. Some supporters of this theory have gotten around that point by arguing that Briggs could not exert his leadership because he suffered a heart attack during the panic.

The last of the three most likely theories was the one put forward by Winchester, and it focuses on the nature of the cargo.

Captain Briggs had never before carried crude alcohol, and possibly did not know how it would react on the voyage. The change in temperature from wintry New York to the warmer climes around the Azores would cause the casks to leak and sweat. Then the stormy weather, severely buffeting them, would create vapor, and the pressure that built up could have been enough to blow out the forward hatch cover. The sweating would have been accompanied by rumbling noises that must certainly have sounded ominous to men who did not know the natural explanation for such sounds. Captain Briggs may have ordered the hatches opened to let some vapor escape, and what looked like smoke emerged. One of the casks had been opened, which indicates that it had been inspected. If there had been a naked light in the vicinity, there could well have been a small explosion—too small to leave a trace but enough to start a panic.

In the wake of this threat, the captain's anxiety will have been increased by the presence of his wife and small daughter. Thinking primarily of their safety, he may have ordered everyone into the yawl until they saw whether or not the ship would blow up. There was no explosion—but a great gust of wind filled the

# A Fatal Panic?

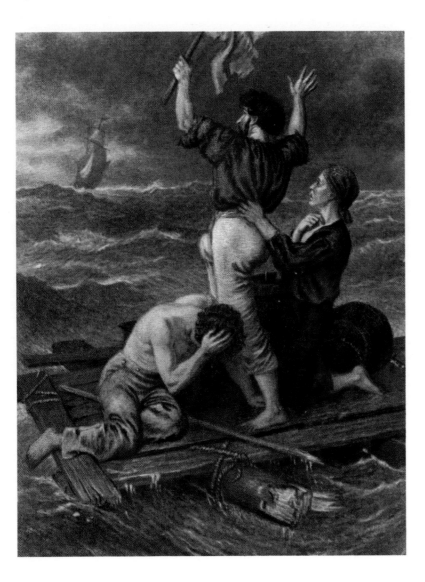

Left: sailors on a raft in mid-ocean signal desperately to a passing ship. Is it possible, as Winchester suggested, that Captain Briggs, not used to a cargo of alcohol, mistook vapor for smoke, ordered the ship to be abandoned in panic, and then watched helplessly as a sudden gust of wind blew the *Mary Celeste* steadily out of reach and out of sight?

# A Macabre Tale

sails, the towline connecting the small boat to the ship snapped, and the *Mary Celeste* inexorably sailed away from them. Their little boat could not withstand the waves and winds of the ocean and finally capsized, drowning all of them.

Was this what happened? No one knows for certain—and probably no one will ever know.

The *Mary Celeste* is the most famous drifter of the sea, but it is only one of many others. Some have the added macabre touch of still being crewed—by corpses. In September 1894, for instance, the British brig *Abbey S. Hart* was found drifting in the Indian Ocean. A boarding party found three seamen dead in their bunks and a fourth man, apparently the captain, delirious or mad. He died an hour later without having uttered one understandable word. The ship had sailed from Java a week previously, and it was assumed that some deadly fever had struck the crew down. It is known that in the days of long voyages under sail, tropical diseases could decimate a crew trapped together far from land.

Other killers at sea are less easy to explain than disease. The Dutch freighter *Ourang Medan* was overwhelmed by an unknown tragedy in February 1948 while steaming through the Straits of Malacca bound for Indonesia. SOS signals from the ship were heard by other vessels in the vicinity, and they hurried to its assistance. The distress calls continued meanwhile, until there came an alarming message: "All officers including captain dead, lying in chartroom and on bridge . . . Probably whole crew dead." This was followed by a series of dots and dashes that made no sense and then the words, "I die." After this—silence.

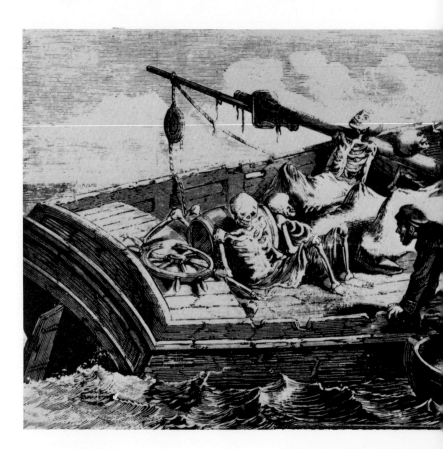

When the *Ourang Medan* was located, it was drifting with the current but a thin ribbon of smoke still issued from the funnel. The captain was found dead on the bridge. Throughout the ship —in the wheelhouse, chartroom, and on the decks—lay the lifeless bodies of the unfortunate crew. The body of the radio operator was found slumped in a chair, his fingers against the transmitter key. Even the ship's dog was found with his lips drawn back in a rictus of death. "Their frozen faces were upturned to the sun," stated the report in the Proceedings of the Merchant Marine Council, "the mouths were gaping open and the eyes staring."

No wounds were discovered on the bodies, and the vessel seemed undamaged. The boarding parties were uncertain what to do next when suddenly flames surged out of the hold and spread rapidly. Everyone hastily returned to their own vessels. Within a short time the boilers of the *Ourang Medan* exploded and the ship sank. Could the crew have been overcome by carbon monoxide or some other poisonous fumes generated within the hold or in the boilers? If so, it is hard to see how that could have killed everyone, even those who were in the open air.

In *Invisible Horizons*, a book of sea tales, Vincent Gaddis cites an even more grisly example of a floating morgue. In the summer of 1913 the British ship *Johnson* caught sight of a sailing vessel drifting off the coast of Chile. As they drew near they could see that the masts and sails were covered with green mold. On the prow, faded with the passing of many years, could still be seen the name *Marlborough*. The timbers of the deck had decayed so greatly that they crumbled as the boarding party picked a

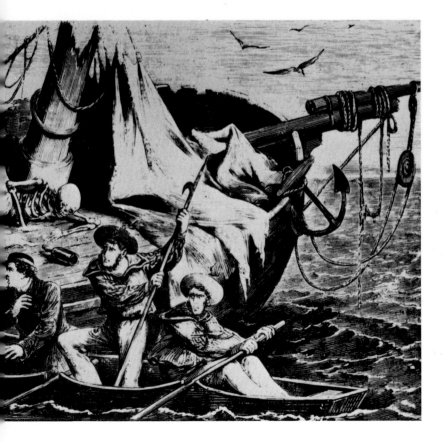

Left: the captain of the schooner *Lancaster*, with three of his crew, finds a gruesome sight on a "deserted" vessel. Another such wreck was the *Abbey S. Hart*, found drifting in the Indian Ocean with its four-man crew struck down by fever. But there have been other, more mysterious tragedies at sea than these.

way across them. A skeleton was discovered beneath the helm, six more were found on the bridge, and 13 others elsewhere in the ship.

It was later learned that the *Marlborough* had left Littleton, New Zealand, 23 years before in January 1890 with a cargo of wool and frozen mutton. There were also several passengers aboard, including one woman. Nothing had been heard of the ship since it had been sighted on the regular course passing through the Straits of Magellan 23 years before. What had happened? Where had the ship been to remain undiscovered for nearly a quarter of a century? Could it have been trapped in an ice ocean like the schooner *Jenny* and others?

The unfortunate *Jenny* was discovered by the whaling schooner *Hope* south of Drake Strait in the Antarctic on September 22, 1860. The towering wall of ice parted abruptly and the *Jenny* emerged, the hull battered and encrusted with ice, snow upon the decks, the rigging fallen, the sails in icy shreds. The cold had preserved the corpses of the crew perfectly, in natural attitudes. The captain's body was seated in a chair, a pen in his hand and leaning backward. Examination of the log revealed that the *Jenny* had been imprisoned in the ice for 37 years. The last entry, signed by the captain, read: "May 4, 1823. No food for 71 days. I am the only one left alive."

The ice of the Arctic Ocean on the other side of the world proved too much for the *Octavius* in 1762. This vessel left England in 1761 bound for China. On the return journey the

Right: an iced-up ship, its rigging clogged and useless, lies helpless in the northern seas. This was the fate of two tragic ships, the *Jenny* and the *Octavius*, both found crewed by corpses in the polar seas.

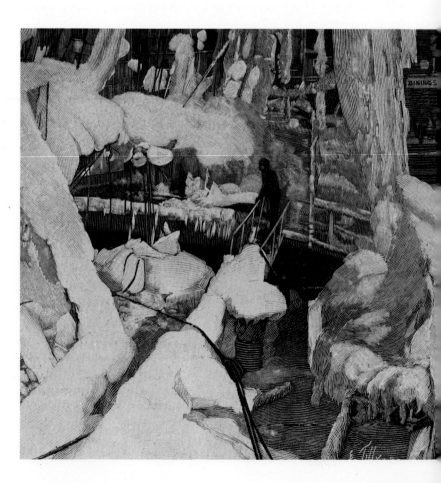

# Ships in the Ice

captain is thought to have decided to look for the elusive North-west Passage rather than to sail all the way around South America. But they got no further than the north coast of Alaska when the ice trapped them. Thirteen years later the whaleship *Herald* caught sight of the *Octavius* drifting into open water between icebergs. The crew of the *Herald* sensed at once that this was a ship of the dead, and they only reluctantly obeyed their captain's order to lower the longboat in preparation for board-ing. Captain Warren led the party.

On the ice-coated deck of the *Octavius* there was no sign of life. Captain Warren made his way to the forecastle, and after kicking away the snow, opened the door. He was met by a heavy musky odor. Stepping inside he saw that every bed, 28 in all, was occupied by a dead seaman, perfectly preserved by the freezing air. The men were heavily wrapped with blankets and clothing, but the Arctic cold had proved too great for them.

In the captain's cabin a dank and mustier smell greeted them. A thin green mold had spread over the dead captain's face although his body was otherwise well preserved. He lay slumped at a table, his hands spread out and a pen beside them. Captain Warren handed the logbook to one of his sailors and stepped into the next cabin. There he found the body of a woman in the bunk covered with blankets. Gaddis writes: "Unlike the captain, her flesh and features were unmarked and lifelike. Her head was resting on her elbow and it appeared as if she had been watching some activity when she died. Following the line of her vision, Captain Warren saw the body of a man cross-legged on the floor and slouched over. In one hand he held a flint and in the other a piece of steel. In front of him was a heap of wood shavings. Apparently he had been attempting to start a fire when death had claimed him. Beside the man was a heavy sailor's jacket. When the captain picked it up, he found the body of a small boy underneath."

Captain Warren's men got panicky and insisted that he let them return to their ship. Back on the *Herald* the captain settled down to read the log, only to find that the sailor entrusted with its care had dropped the center pages into the sea while hastening into the longboat. The surviving front pages gave details of the ship's company and recorded the successful start of the voyage to China. The account of the following 14 months was missing, and the only remaining page was the final one. Dated November 11, 1762 it read: "We have now been enclosed in the ice 17 days, and our approximate position is Longitude 160W, Latitude 75N. The fire went out yesterday, and our master has been trying to rekindle it again but without success. He has handed the steel and flint to the mate. The master's son died this morning and his wife says she no longer feels the terrible cold. The rest of us seem to have no relief from the agony."

The most outstanding feature of the discovery of the *Octavius* is that it occurred in Greenland waters, at the eastern end of the Northwest Passage, even though the ship had been locked in the ice when north of Alaska, at the western end. Only one explana-tion was possible. The ship must have found the Northwest Passage on its own. Season by season it had crept eastward, frozen up each winter and drifting on again during the short

# The "Revenge" of the Unmanned Ship

Below: this photograph of the *Baychimo* was taken in 1931. Caught that year in the arctic ice, the *Baychimo* was abandoned by captain and crew who feared the ice might crush the vessel. The unmanned ship later broke her moorings, and has since been frequently sighted through the years sailing the arctic seas. The last sighting was in March 1962. On this occasion captain and crew escaped safely overland.

summer thaw, until at last it reached the North Atlantic. Ironically, the *Octavius* was the first ship to navigate the Northwest Passage—but the crew and the captain never knew it.

Another ship that went it alone in the Arctic is the *SS Baychimo*. Owned by the Hudson's Bay Company, the *Baychimo* is a trim, steel-clad cargo steamer, considered the finest possible craft for battling the pack ice and the floes. The ship joined the far northern fleet in 1921 and made nine annual visits to the bleak Arctic coasts of Canada, buying furs from the trading posts along the Beaufort Sea and the McClintock Channel. No other vessel had managed to make the perilous trip more than two years in succession.

On July 6, 1931 the *Baychimo* left Vancouver, Canada, with a crew of 36 under the command of Captain John Cornwall. Passing through the Bering Straits, the ship entered the Northwest Passage. The captain spent hundreds of thousands of dollars buying furs along the Victoria Island coast. On the return journey the ship was caught in early winter pack ice during a howling blizzard, and was unable to move. With the vessel in danger of being crushed, Captain Cornwall and his crew established a camp on safer ice closer to shore, and prepared to wait there till the spring. A three-day storm early in November brought a rise in temperature, enabling the men to emerge for a look around. They found that the *Baychimo* had snapped its moorings and disappeared.

Captain Cornwall led his men to the safety of Point Barrow, 50 miles away, where they learned that Eskimos had sighted the

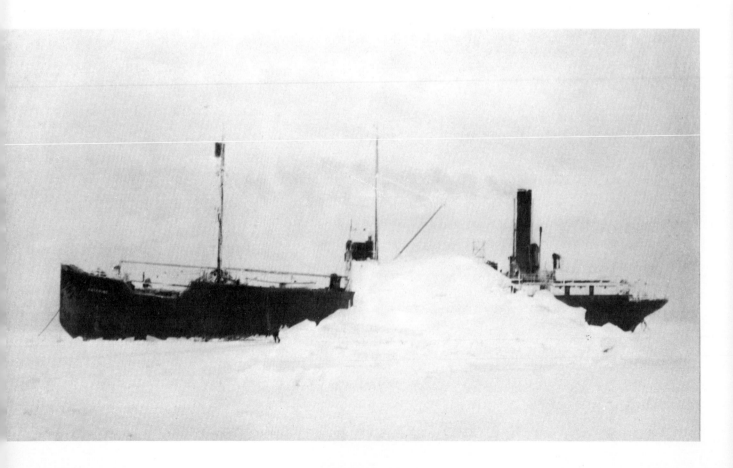

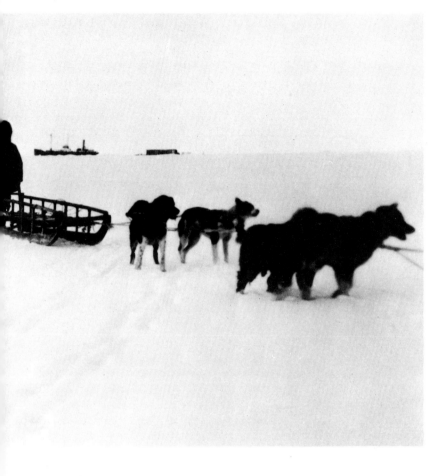

Left: another photograph of the amazing *Baychimo* taken in 1931. The dogsled was used to transport the furs which the ship was collecting. The crew at this time were living in the large hut on the horizon at the right of the ship, which was still firmly stuck in the ice. Shortly after this photograph was taken, the ship set off on its weird and lonely voyage, which has lasted for at least 30 years.

missing ship 45 miles southwest of its former position. The crew and a party of Eskimos managed to reach the ship, and after 15 days of difficult work, removed the bulk of the valuable cargo. Before they could finish, however, the *Baychimo* had vanished again.

The following spring the ship was observed 300 miles further east near Herschel Island. A young trapper and explorer, Leslie Melvin, found the *Baychimo* while on a journey by dog team. He boarded the drifter and reported that it was in excellent condition.

Since then the *SS Baychimo* has been sighted frequently. A party of Eskimos boarded the ship in 1933, but were trapped by a sudden storm and drifted for 10 days before they could make their way to shore on a raft of ice. In June 1934 Isobel Hutchinson, a Scottish botanist, sighted it and went aboard. Year after year reports of sightings have come in from whalers, prospectors, Eskimos, travelers. In November 1939 an attempt to tow the ship into port had to be abandoned in bad weather. Still it survives. After a period of no reports on the *Baychimo*, a party of Eskimos saw it in March 1956, moving north in the Beaufort Sea. In March 1962 fishermen found the still apparently seaworthy ship in the same area. The *Baychimo* seems to have disappeared since then, but may yet turn up again. There is no parallel in modern times for a ship to sail the seas without a crew for so long a time. For over 30 years the *Baychimo* has survived the ice in one of the cruellest seas of the world.

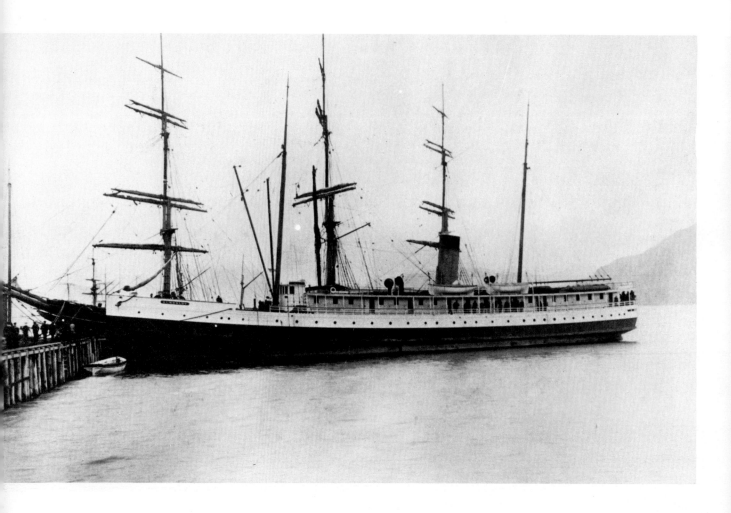

Above: S.S. *Humboldt*, launched in 1898, had a long and useful life under one captain, Elijah G. Baufman. When in 1934 Captain Baufman finally retired, the *Humboldt* was sent to a scrapyard. In 1935 Baufman died, and that same night, in the scrapyard 400 miles down the Californian coast, the old ship broke its moorings and was sailing purposefully for the open sea when a cutter caught up with it and towed the *Humboldt* back. Was it the old ship's final gesture of obedience to its dead captain?

Some ships appear to have a will of their own as well as a sense of survival. Two in particular seem to have been strangely devoted to their owners. One of these was the *SS Humboldt* whose captain, Elijah G. Baufman, was the only master the ship ever knew. The *Humboldt* began its career in 1898 as a passenger and freight carrier between Seattle and Alaska. Captain Baufman reckoned that during the Alaskan Gold Rush it brought back gold valued at over $100 million. Long after those frantic years were over, the *Humboldt* continued to work the Northwest Pacific ports, but in 1934 the time came for Baufman and his beloved vessel to retire. Baufman moved from Seattle to San Francisco and the *Humboldt* was taken farther south to San Pedro, destined for the scrapyard.

On August 8, 1935 Baufman died. That night the crew of the coastguard cutter *Tamaroa* near San Pedro harbor noticed an old steamer making for the open sea. The only light was a red warning light at the stern. No one was aboard, no smoke came from the funnel. It was the *Humboldt*. Somehow the ship had managed to slip its moorings and drift through the harbor, as though determined to sail north to join its former captain. It had done this on the very day its old master died.

Seattle has another tale of mysterious rapport between man and boat. Captain Martin Olsen was a seine fisherman, and for many years he went out in the *Sea-Lion* to net salmon in the deep creeks of Puget Sound. When he retired he beached the *Sea-Lion*

# More Riddles of the Ocean

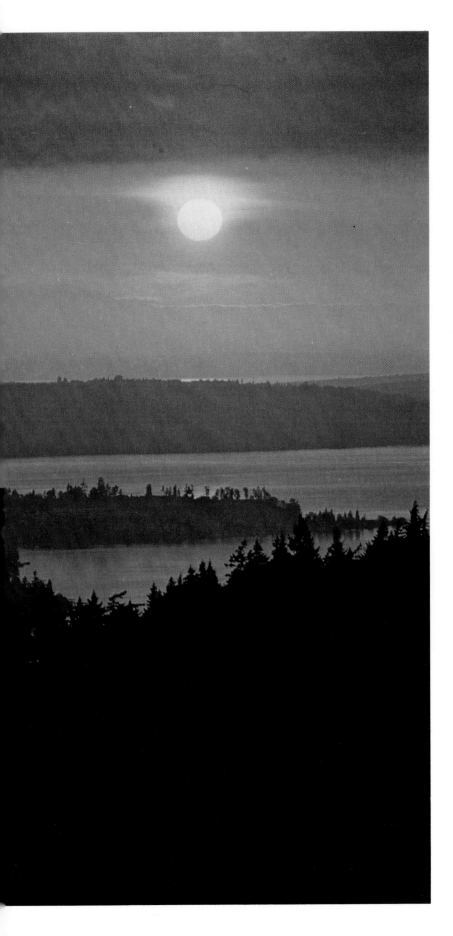

Left: Puget Sound, Washington State. It was in the creeks of this great bay that Captain Martin Olsen sailed his fishing boat *Sea Lion* for many successful years. What happened when he died and was buried is one of the most moving mysteries of the sea.

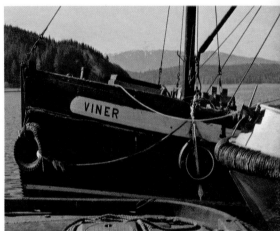

Above: fishing boat of a type similar to the *Sea Lion* which is still used for fishing off the coast of Washington and British Columbia today.

# The Strange Tale of the Baychimo

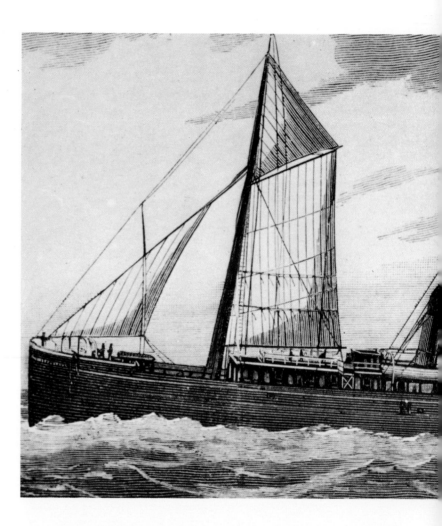

Right: the French ship *Frigorifique*, the first French vessel to carry refrigeration equipment. In March 1884, the *Frigorifique* collided with the British collier *Rumney*. The French captain and 11-man crew abandoned ship and were taken on board the *Rumney*. It was then that one of the most mysterious encounters of sea history took place, when three times the apparently unmanned French ship tried to ram the collier that had first rammed it.

on a sandy point near his home across the sound from Seattle. For 10 years the boat settled deeper into the sand—but on the day Captain Olsen died, a day unmarked by storm or abnormal tides, the boat is said to have floated off the sandspit and begun drifting around the bay. Three days later it attended the captain's funeral, drifting up to the beach on Bainbridge Island at the point closest to the cemetery. After the funeral the *Sea-Lion* drifted away, and a few days later returned to the sandspit on which it had passed the previous 10 years.

Another uncanny tale of a ship seeming to act on its own is the classic story of the *Frigorifique*'s "revenge." This ship was the first French vessel to carry refrigeration equipment, and it enjoyed eight prosperous years bringing frozen meat from Uruguay to France before meeting its doom in a thick fog off the French coast on March 19, 1884. Captain Raoul Lambert heard a siren wail, but could not tell from what direction the sound came. He ordered the engines stopped and blew three warning blasts. Nothing more was heard, so the *Frigorifique* moved forward again at low speed, tolling the bell continuously.

Danger came suddenly. The dark hulk of another ship emerged through the fog to starboard, and though the helm was pulled hard to port there was no escaping the inevitable crash. The rammed *Frigorifique* at once began to list heavily, and the captain ordered his crew of 11 men to abandon ship.

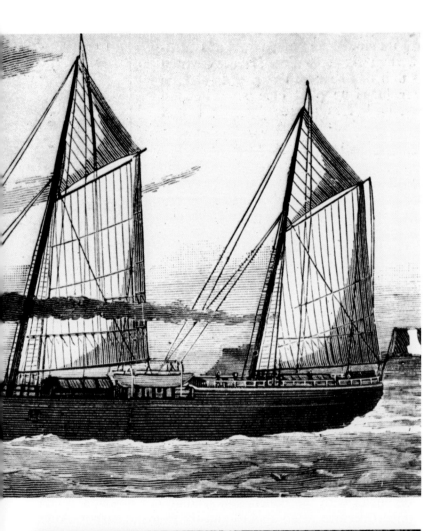

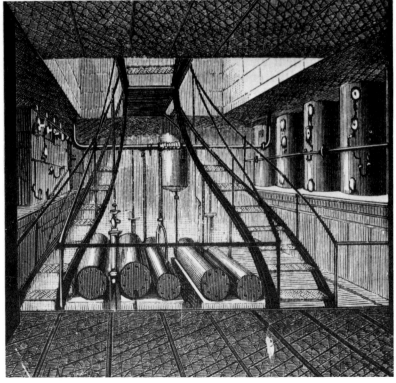

Left: refrigeration equipment aboard the
*Frigorifique*. Both French and British
crews watched with horror as the doomed
ship repeatedly tried to ram the collier.

# The Long Arm of Coincidence?

The other vessel in the accident was the English collier *Rumney*, bound for La Rochelle from Cardiff. The *Rumney* was undamaged and took the crew of the *Frigorifique* aboard. By then the stricken vessel had disappeared in the fog.

Two miles farther on, Captain John Turner of the *Rumney* noticed a ship bearing down on him through the fog. It was the *Frigorifique*, no longer listing, smoke pouring from the stack, and seemingly bent on wreaking vengeance for being rammed. The *Rumney's* helmsman desperately swung the wheel to starboard to put it on a course parallel to the French ship. He acted just in time. The *Rumney* escaped the prow of the *Frigorifique* by just a few inches. Once more the avenging ship vanished into the fog.

The two captains discussed the mystery. Could it have been another ship, resembling the *Frigorifique*? Captain Lambert shook his head. He knew his own ship.

Less than a mile later the *Frigorifique* came at the *Rumney* again, silent, speeding, inexorable, the prow once more aimed to charge.

"Hard to starboard," shouted Captain Turner. Then, "Reverse engines." Neither maneuver worked; this time there was no escape. The *Frigorifique* rammed the collier with a thundering impact, and water began pouring into the hold and engine room. Once more the *Frigorifique* vanished as the *Rumney* began to sink. Two boats, bearing the separate crews, pulled away and watched the English ship go down.

In 15 minutes the lifeboats had rowed out of the fog and sighted the French coast on the horizon. Suddenly, out of the mist behind them they saw the *Frigorifique* yet again, moving in wide circles with the boilers still sending out power. Captain Lambert decided to go aboard and try to make harbor. After some difficulty the two lifeboats managed to pull alongside, and the captain and several volunteers went aboard. There they discovered how the *Frigorifique* had been able to pursue and ram the *Rumney*. The helmsman had left the wheel lashed hard over to starboard, and had forgotten it in the rush of leaving the ship. This made the *Frigorifique* go around in circles after it had been abandoned. Because the *Rumney* was moving in its straight course at reduced speed, one of the *Frigorifique's* circular swings brought it head on into the collier.

Although the first ramming had damaged the *Frigorifique*, the engine room was not flooded. But the second collision had doomed the refrigerated freighter. Water was rising quickly. It seems as though the *Frigorifique* had taken that third circle to avenge itself, and was then ready to sink in peace. For the second time in an hour the French captain gave the order to abandon ship, and the lifeboats rowed away. The *Frigorifique* rolled over onto its side and slowly went down. The honor of the wounded ship had been satisfied.

Other mysteries of the sea have to do with the sea itself playing strange tricks, extending the long arm of coincidence around the globe. Take the case of the *SS Saxilby*, which left Newfoundland in November 1933 bound for South Wales. Somewhere in the North Atlantic it vanished. Twenty-nine men were on board.

Early in 1936 a cocoa can was washed ashore near the Welsh

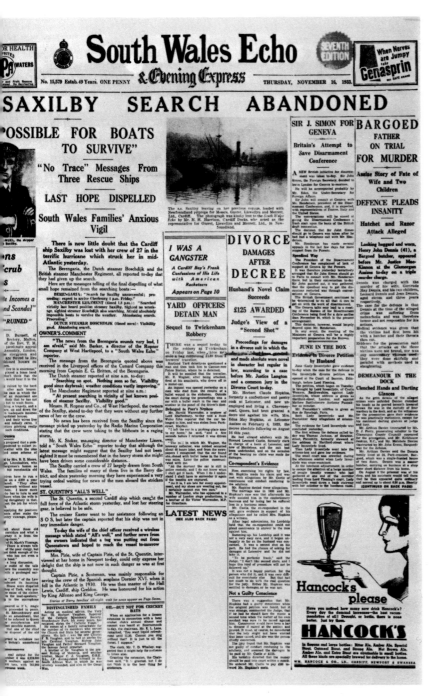

# South Wales Echo
## & Evening Express

SEVENTH EDITION

No. 15,579 Estab. 49 Years. ONE PENNY    THURSDAY, NOVEMBER 16, 1933.

# SAXILBY SEARCH ABANDONED

## "POSSIBLE FOR BOATS TO SURVIVE"

### "No Trace" Messages From Three Rescue Ships

### LAST HOPE DISPELLED

### South Wales Families' Anxious Vigil

There is now little doubt that the Cardiff ship Saxilby was lost with her crew of 27 in the terrific hurricane which struck her in mid-Atlantic yesterday.

The Berengaria, the Dutch steamer Boschdijk and the British steamer Manchester Regiment, all reported to-day that they had given up the search.

Here are the messages telling of the final dispelling of what small hope remained from the searching boats:—

BERENGARIA: "Search for Saxilby unsuccessful; proceeding; expect to arrive Cherbourg 1 p.m. Friday."

MANCHESTER REGIMENT (timed 1.8 p.m.): "Searched vicinity last heard position steamer Saxilby. Sighted no wreckage, sighted steamer Boschdijk also searching. Afraid absolutely impossible boats to survive the weather. Abandoning search. Proceeding."

DUTCH STEAMER BOSCHDIJK (timed noon): Visibility good. Abandoning search.

### OWNER'S COMMENT

"The news from the Berengaria sounds very bad, I am afraid," said Mr. Barker, a director of the Ropner Company at West Hartlepool, to a "South Wales Echo" reporter.

The message from the Berengaria quoted above was received in the Liverpool offices of the Cunard Company this morning from Captain E. G. Britten, of the Berengaria.

The Dutch steamer reported at nine a.m. to-day:

"Searching on spot. Nothing seen so far. Visibility good since daybreak; weather conditions vastly improving."

The Manchester Regiment reported at nine a.m.:

"At present searching in vicinity of last known position of steamer Saxilby. Visibility good."

Messrs. R. Ropner and Co., of West Hartlepool, the owners of the Saxilby, stated to-day that they were without any further news of her or the crew.

No news has been received from the Saxilby since the message picked up yesterday by the Radio Marine Corporation stating that the crew were taking to the lifeboats in a raging storm.

Mr. K. Stoker, managing director of Manchester Liners, told a "South Wales Echo" reporter to-day that although the latest message might suggest that the Saxilby had not been sighted it must be remembered that in the heavy storm she might have been driven some considerable distance.

The Saxilby carried a crew of 27 largely drawn from South Wales. The families of many of them live in the Barry district, and since yesterday morning they have experienced a very trying ordeal waiting for news of the men aboard the stricken vessel.

### ST. QUENTIN'S "ALL'S WELL"

The St. Quentin, a second Cardiff ship which caught the full force of the Atlantic storm yesterday, and lost her steering gear, is believed to be safe.

The cruiser Exeter went to her assistance following an S O S, but later the captain reported that his ship was not in any immediate danger.

To-day the wife of the chief officer received a wireless message which stated "All's well," and further news from the owners indicated that a tug was putting out from Queenstown and hoped to reach the vessel to-morrow morning.

Mrs. Pirie, wife of Captain Pirie, of the St. Quentin, interviewed at her home in Newport to-day, could only express her delight that the ship is not now in such danger as was at first thought.

Captain Pirie, a Scotsman, was mainly responsible for saving the crew of the Spanish seaplane Dornier XVI. when it fell in the Atlantic in 1930. He was then master of the Hall Lewis, Cardiff, ship Greldon. He was honoured for his action by King Alfonso and King George.

### The s.s. Saxilby
The s.s. Saxilby leaving on her previous voyage, loaded with Newfoundland pitprops for Messrs. Gueret, Llewellyn and Merrett, Ltd., Cardiff. The photograph was kindly lent to the South Wales Echo by Mr. H. H. Harrison, Cardiff Docks, who acted as the representative for Gueret, Llewellyn and Merrett, Ltd., in Newfoundland.

### I WAS A GANGSTER
A Cardiff Boy's Frank Confessions of His Life with American Racketeers
Appears on Page 10

### YARD OFFICERS DETAIN MAN
Sequel to Twickenham Robbery

### DIVORCE
DAMAGES AFTER DECREE
Husband's Novel Claim Succeeds
£125 AWARDED
Judge's View of a "Second Shot"

### SIR J. SIMON FOR GENEVA
Britain's Attempt to Save Disarmament Conference

### BARGOED FATHER ON TRIAL FOR MURDER
Assize Story of Fate of Wife and Two Children
### DEFENCE PLEADS INSANITY
Hatchet and Razor Attack Alleged

### LATEST NEWS
(SEE ALSO BACK PAGE)

Left: this newspaper front page gives the news for November 16, 1933, with the headline that the search for the S.S. *Saxilby* has been abandoned. No news had been received from the British cargo ship with 29 men aboard since the message received the previous day that the crew were taking to the boats in a violent storm. Only a pathetic message from a Welsh crewman was washed up on the Welsh coast in 1936. Otherwise the silence was complete.

village of Aberavon. Inside was a message saying, "*SS Saxilby* sinking somewhere off the Irish coast. Love to sister, brothers and Dinah. Joe Okane." Joe Okane, a member of the crew aboard the lost steamer, had lived in Aberavon, the message was addressed to his relatives in Aberavon—and the can had drifted ashore less than a mile from their home.

Another example of a message with a strong homing instinct was one sent by the New Zealander Ross Alexander. In 1952 the troopship he was on ran aground on a reef north of Darwin, Australia, and while awaiting rescue he threw an SOS note overboard in a wine bottle. In 1955 back home in New Zealand, he was walking along the beach one day. There he found the bottle which still contained the message he had entrusted to the sea three years before.

In 1934 Doyle Branscum enclosed a photograph of himself in a bottle and threw it into a river in Arkansas. In 1958 Bill Headstream found the bottle near his home in Largo, Florida. Oddly enough, the two men had been boyhood friends who had not heard from each other for many years. Headstream returned the photograph to Branscum with a letter telling what had happened to him in the 24 years since 1934.

These incidents are astounding enough, but the case of Coghlan's coffin seems to make the impossible come true. Charles Francis Coghlan was an actor. Born on Prince Edward Island, Canada, in 1841 he first appeared on the London stage at the age of 18. Over the years he acquired an international reputation as a Shakespearean actor. On his last tour in the United States, he appeared with Lily Langtry. While they were performing in Galveston, Texas, he died on November 27, 1899. His lead-lined coffin was placed in a granite vault in a Galveston

Below: Charles Francis Coghlan (seated) on stage. Coghlan was born on Prince Edward Island off the east coast of Canada. When he died in Galveston, Texas, in 1899, he had acquired an international reputation as an actor in Shakespearean and other roles.

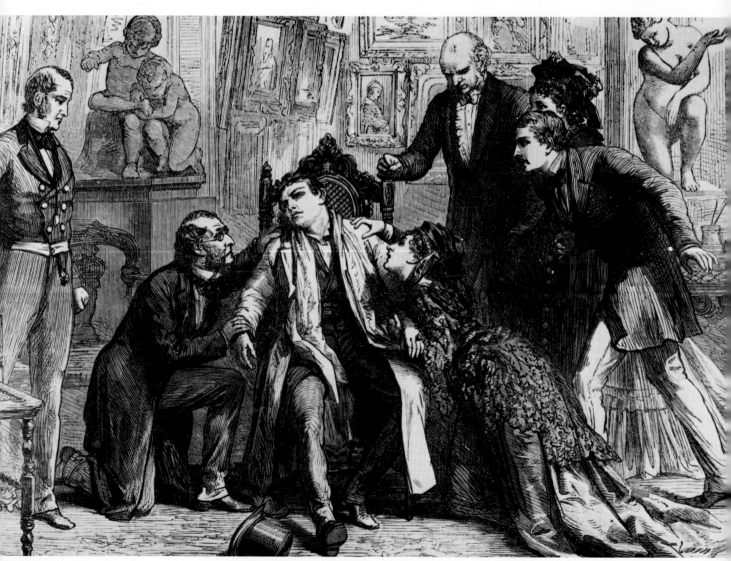

cemetery, many thousands of miles from his birthplace on Prince Edward Island, which he always regarded as his true home though he was so often away from it.

On September 8, 1900 Galveston was struck by a hurricane. Six thousand people were killed and thousands of homes were reduced to rubble. Floodwaters poured into the cemeteries, sweeping coffins out of the graves and shattering vaults. A log jam of coffins floated out into the Gulf of Mexico. Many sank or were washed up on the coast, but Coghlan's coffin must have drifted southeast until it was caught in the West Indian current which carried it northeastward past Florida into the Gulf Stream. In this mighty current the coffin was borne northward until it reached the vicinity of Newfoundland. There a storm must have blown it out of the current because for the next few years it drifted around the eastern Canadian coast.

In October 1908 several fishermen from Prince Edward Island sailed out to set their nets in the Gulf of St. Lawrence. They came upon a large box floating in the waves and towed it back to shore. The wood was encrusted with barnacles, but a silver

# Coghlan's Coffin

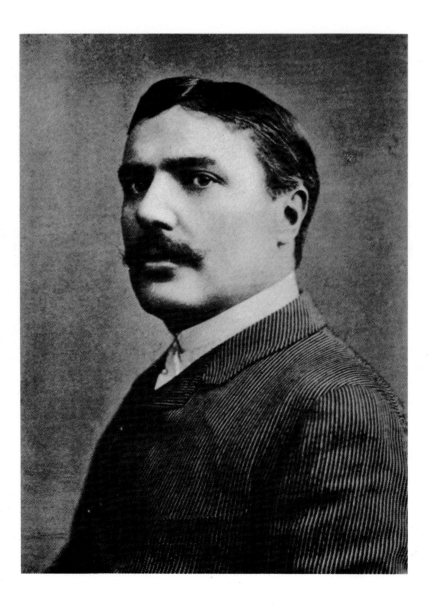

Left: Charles Coghlan in his prime. The legend is that in 1900 a hurricane struck Galveston, killing 6000 people and destroying many buildings. It also washed away numerous coffins from the local cemeteries, including the lead coffin containing the body of Charles Coghlan. If it is indeed true as the legend has it that fishermen from Prince Edward Island picked up the coffin in 1908, then that is surely one of the mysteries of the sea.

# The Joyita Affair

plate on the top told the astonished fishermen that it was the coffin of Charles Coghlan. Only a few miles away stood the village where Coghlan had been born and raised. Also nearby was the home in which he had stayed between his long tours abroad. The actor's body was reburied near the church where he had been baptized. Charles Coghlan had at last reached home to stay.

Not so Thomas "Dusty" Miller, captain of the motorship *Joyita* which has been called the *Mary Celeste* of the Pacific. The *Joyita* was a twin-screw ship that met with disaster in October 1955 some time after leaving Apia in Western Samoa. It was heading for Fakaofo in the Tokelau Islands, a mere 270 miles to the north. On November 10, more than a month after setting out, the *Joyita* was found abandoned and half-foundering. But the ship was cork-lined and therefore practically unsinkable. Captain Miller had known that perfectly well—in fact, he had often boasted of it. His mate "Chuck" Simpson, an American Indian married to a Samoan woman, also knew of the five-inch slabs of cork that lined each of the three holds. Why had they abandoned a ship that should stay afloat indefinitely?

Perhaps they had not, for there were signs that two men had

Right: the motorship *Joyita* has been called the "Mary Celeste of the Pacific." This photograph shows the *Joyita* in trouble in 1957, some two years after this "unsinkable" vessel was found drifting and empty in the Pacific. Nothing was ever found of the 25 missing passengers and crew.

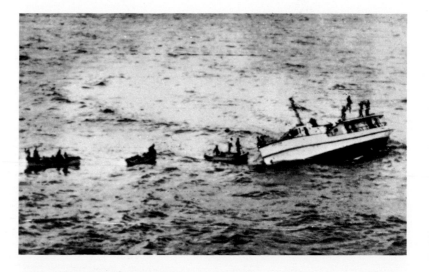

stayed aboard. An awning had been erected either to catch water or to keep off the sun. Where had these men gone?

There could be no doubt whatever that the *Joyita* had been in trouble. Only one of the two engines was working, and the radio was defective. Although the ship could stay afloat, it could not be called seaworthy.

The vessel was taken to Suva, Fiji, where it was drydocked and pumped out. The basic cause of the trouble then became apparent. Under the boiler room floor was a badly corroded section of pipe, which explained why the ship had become waterlogged. Four mattresses were found in the engine room, brought there apparently to block the leak if it could be located. The two bilge pumps were blocked with cotton waste and hardly worked at all. The port engine clutch was partly disconnected, and into a brass T-piece in the port engine's salt water cooling system had

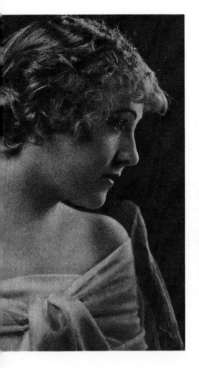

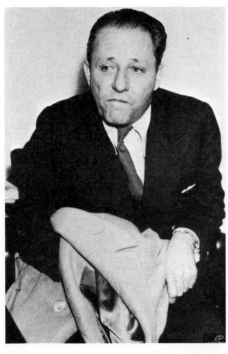

Far left: film star Jewel Carmen, wife of *Joyita*'s first owner, film producer Roland West (left). It was after Jewel Carmen that the *Joyita* (which means "little jewel") was named, in the 1930s. After the war, the ship was made into a fishing boat with cork-lined refrigerated holds.

been threaded a galvanized pipe. This had started the corrosion that results when a ferrous metal is joined to a nonferrous metal.

How had a ship in such bad shape been entrusted with the lives of 25 persons, including children?

The *Joyita* had started out well. It had been built in 1931 for Roland West, a movie director and husband of the movie star Jewel Carmen. Joyita means "Little Jewel." In the war it was used by the United States navy as a patrol ship, and after the war it was converted into a fishing boat with cork-lined refrigerated holds. In 1952 Dusty Miller chartered the *Joyita* and began fishing operations in Hawaii. His first success was followed by consecutive failures. Working in Pago Pago in American Samoa, the ship's refrigerating equipment failed and much of the catch went bad. Miller got into debt and the American authorities seized some of the ship's papers.

Dusty left Pago Pago in March 1955 for Apia in Western Samoa, which is under New Zealand trusteeship. It was there that he met R. D. Pearless, recently appointed District Officer of the Tokelau Islands. Miller took him on a combined fishing trip and tour of the islands, and Pearless suggested to the Western Samoan government that they charter the *Joyita* to provide regular transport of supplies to the Tokelaus. This would have solved Miller's problems completely. Although he was destitute, he would at least have a steady job sailing the ship he loved. The only snag was his inability to provide the papers still held in Pago Pago. For five months the *Joyita* lay at anchor in Apia harbor, and during this period Miller nearly starved, finding food and money where he could. He is described as "good-natured," a colorful character who liked to wear a sarong at sea. He was honest and paid his debts when he had the money, but the long wait from May till September turned him into a desperate man. Personal matters were also troubling him. Back in Wales, the

Below: Captain Miller, who chartered the *Joyita* in 1952, seen here in British naval uniform. Miller was broke when he applied for a charter to run supplies among some of the islands of Western Samoa. Official delays put off his departure on his first trip in October 1955. He and his 24 passengers and crew were never seen or heard from again.

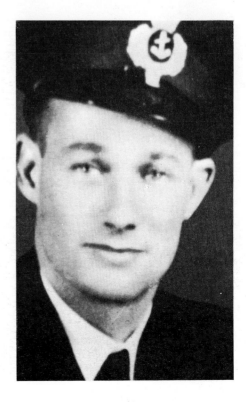

# Why Abandon an Unsinkable Ship?

woman he had married shortly after the war was suing him for divorce on grounds of desertion.

When the *Joyita* was finally given permission to sail it was in poor condition—and Captain Miller knew it. He told the charterers that he would be able to fix the faulty clutch at sea. Even more unwisely, he failed to test the radio transmitter before leaving. A simple check would have revealed a break in the aerial cord above the transmitter that was to prevent the ship's signals from being heard more than two miles away.

Miller saw the journey as his last hope. He hastily found himself a crew that included two Gilbert Islanders, Tokoka, the bosun, and Tanini, the engineer, who had worked for him before. Pearless was impatient to go. The Tokelau Islanders needed medical supplies and there were 70 tons of copra in the islands waiting for collection. Among the other passengers were two doctors and two representatives of the chartering company. One of these, G. K. Williams, carried £1000 in silver and banknotes to buy copra. The remainder of the passengers were local people of the islands.

Before the *Joyita* had left harbor its engine broke down. When Miller finally got it going again at 5 a.m. the following morning, he and his crew had been working through the night and were short of temper. But Miller trusted to luck—the luck that had failed him so often in the past.

Below: Fijian sailors clamber over the waterlogged wreckage of the *Joyita*. The mystery ship was found by aircraft in November 1955, more than a month after setting out on its last disastrous voyage. There was no evidence of fire, explosion, or collision.

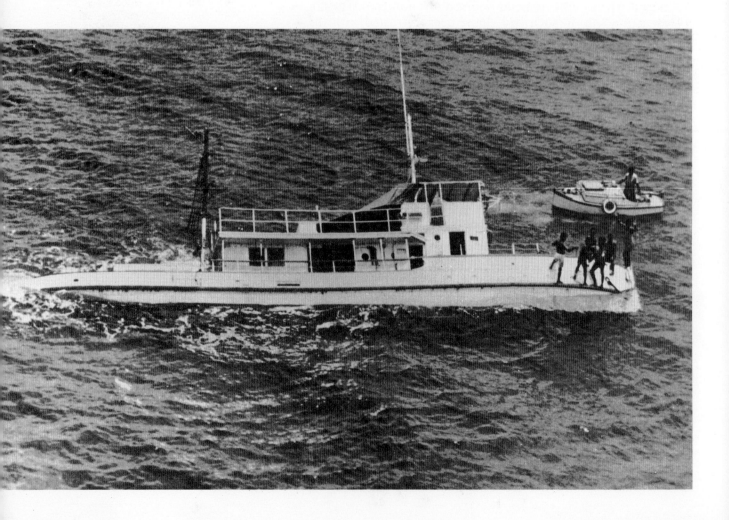

Disaster probably struck the *Joyita* the first night out from Apia. Heavy seas broke the corroded pipe below the boiler room floor and water poured in. The pumps were inadequate because of the blocked suction pipes. The port engine may have already stopped. The starboard engine stopped when water reached a height of 18 inches. All lights would then go out. The radio transmitter was tuned to the distress frequency—where the rescuers found it a month later—but the broken cord failed to carry the signals.

Robin Maugham, the novelist who eventually bought the *Joyita*, guesses that at some stage Miller was incapacitated. In view of what they had been through, it would not be surprising if one of the passengers entered into an argument with him. Miller may have fallen or been pushed from the bridge to the deck, suffering severe head injuries. Maugham's support for this theory comes from the discovery in the scuppers of a doctor's stethoscope, a scalpel, some needles and catgut, and four lengths of bloodstained bandages. One of the doctors may have given Miller first aid. The other passengers either did not know the boat was cork-lined, or with water clearly rising inside, no longer believed it. The *Joyita* carried no dinghy but her floats were hastily launched, the passengers clambered aboard, and drifted away. In the high seas they must soon have capsized.

Someone remained on the vessel and built the awning. Maugham thinks this may have been the Gilbert Islander, Tanini, who was devoted to Captain Miller. But then what happened? At this point another mystery arises. Did some new panic cause Miller and his companion to abandon ship? That is unlikely, since Miller knew his boat was unsinkable. Even if he had died of his wounds, his companion would surely have remained. One theory is that the drifting vessel encountered a pirate ship, and that Miller and his companions were murdered. It is true that some of the cargo was missing but it seems more likely that it was thrown overboard in the original panic to lighten the ship. William's strongbox, which contained £950 in Bank of Samoa banknotes and £50 in silver, was missing. It seems unlikely that he took it on the raft with him, knowing the Bank of Samoa would replace at least the banknotes. The crew of the other vessel may not have come as pirates, but may have been unable to resist temptation after boarding the *Joyita* and finding the money.

Even this explanation leaves questions unanswered. Chuck Simpson also knew the boat was unsinkable and would never have chosen the alternative of a raft in shark-infested seas. What happened to him? Was he also thrown from the bridge and injured?

Dusty Miller's wife had to wait till 1961 before her husband could be declared officially dead. The judge granting her a divorce on grounds of desertion and presumption of death said of him: "Had he reached his destination he might eventually have become a millionaire. But he never got there. Instead he became a corpse."

The exact manner in which he met his untimely death is unknown. It seems unlikely that the full facts will ever come out now to clear up the mystery.

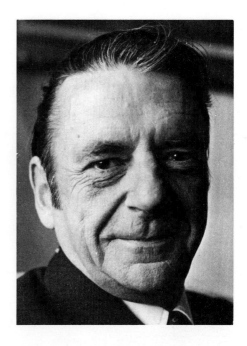

Above: British writer and novelist Robin Maugham. He bought the *Joyita* some time after the tragic voyage under Captain Miller. Maugham's own theory is that the *Joyita* broke down shortly after leaving port, power failed, lights went out, and there was no means of signaling distress. Miller himself fell or was pushed by an angry passenger and was seriously wounded. Not knowing the ship was cork-lined and unsinkable, the rest panicked and took to the rafts, perishing in the waves. The ship was later looted by passing seamen.

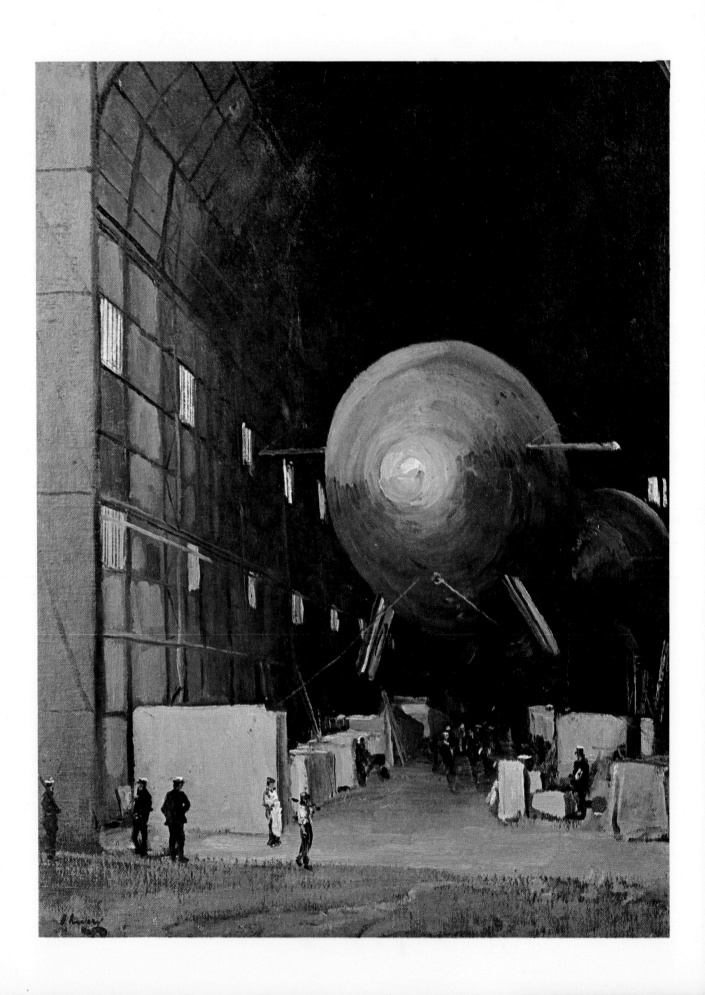

# Chapter 8
# Riddles of the Air

A plane goes down in the South Pacific with a famous woman flier and her navigator aboard. Why did no trace of them ever turn up? The disappearance of Amelia Earhart in 1937 is one of the great unexplained mysteries of aviation history, but there are many others. A plane landed by two corpses . . . the vanishing crew of a blimp in midair . . . the mysterious explosion of the luxury dirigible *Hindenberg* . . . the lost trailblazers of the polar flying route. Will such puzzles be explained some day?

At about 10:45 a.m. on August 16, 1942 a military blimp drifted ashore at Fort Funston, California. The door of its gondola was open; there was no one aboard.

In wartime America on the West Coast, blimps on anti-submarine duty were a common sight, so the hapless airship did not frighten two fishermen on the beach. They simply tried to rescue it. They caught hold of the tie lines in an attempt to pull it down, but a sudden gust of wind forced them to let go after they had been dragged across the sand for 100 yards or so. The derelict blimp raked against a cliff along the beach, at which one of its 300-pound depth charges was released and plummeted onto the earth at the side of the highway below. Lightened by the loss of the charge, the blimp shot up into the air again and drifted southeasterly. About half an hour later, the airship settled to earth in a street in Daly City, just south of San Francisco.

Where was the two-man crew? What had caused them to abandon their vehicle? Why had they failed to complete their mission?

United States military investigators reconstructed the case in an effort to solve the mystery. Blimp L-8 had taken off from Moffett Field at around 6 a.m. that day. Its two officers, Lieutenant Ernest D. Cody and Ensign Charles E. Adams, were experienced and reliable. The weather was cloudy but good, and for nearly two hours the airship made regular radio contacts. At 7:50 a.m. Cody had sent a radio message saying that he had seen

Opposite: a British "blimp," the *Silver Queen*, painted in 1915 by Sir John Lavery. During World War I, British airships were divided into two categories: A-rigid and B-limp. This is the explanation for the word blimp, and it was these "limp" or frameless airships that proved reliable enough to be in use in the United States in the early years of World War II.

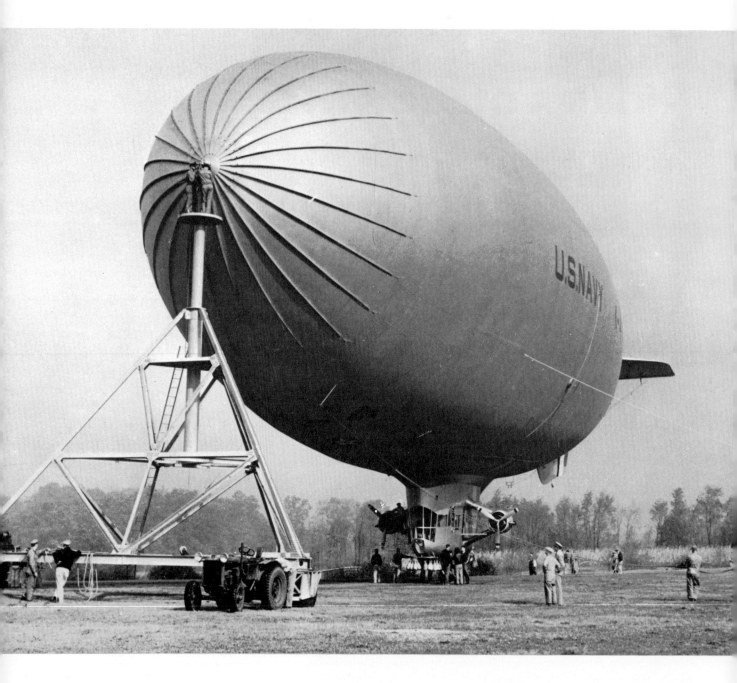

Above: United States Navy airship K.3.
The L.8 which apparently ditched its crew
over the Pacific was of similar type, with
gondola equipped with propellers for
power.

a suspicious oil slick. "I'm taking the ship down to 300 feet for
a closer look," he signaled. "Stand by."

The L-8's position was about five miles east of Farallon
Islands at that point. Two armed patrol boats had been alerted
and were observing the blimp. Two fishing trawlers in the area
also watched the airship circling lower. Guessing that it might be
on the track of a submarine, the fishermen hastily dragged their
nets in and retired to a safe distance in case there was a depth
charge explosion. Instead of making a bombing run, however,
the blimp suddenly shot upward and disappeared into a cloud.

At 8:05 a.m., three hours before the L-8 came to rest in Daly
City, the control tower at Moffett Field had tried to contact the
blimp, but had had no response. After further unsuccessful tries
to get in touch, search planes were sent out. At 10:40 one plane

briefly caught sight of the airship as it rose above the cloud cover and immediately descended into the cover again. Five minutes later the blimp had floated onto the beach where the fishermen who tried to catch it had seen it empty.

When the salvage crew investigated the Blimp L-8's gondola, they found all the equipment in position. Parachutes and rubber raft were properly in place. The only missing items were two bright yellow life jackets, but that was understandable because the crew was required to wear them when in flight over water as Cody and Adams had been. Nothing had been damaged. There was no water in the gondola's lower deck. The motors were turned off, although one throttle was open and the other half open. Ignition switches were still on.

The open door and the sudden ascent of the airship after Cody's last message suggested that the two officers fell into the sea. Perhaps, it was conjectured, one officer fell part way out, and when the second came to his aid, both fell out. But the position of the throttles contradicts this theory, for why would the pilot leave one throttle on full and the other halfway open when he went to help his companion? Besides, no fall or splash was seen by the fishermen or the patrol boat crews who had observed the blimp as it descended for its inspection of the oil slick, even though both men must have had their yellow life jackets on. Finally, no bodies or life jackets were ever recovered after extensive searching.

The absence of water in the gondola's lower deck showed that the blimp had not touched down in the ocean at any time. This countered any idea that Cody and Adams were surprised by a surfacing Japanese submarine and taken prisoner. The intervention of a submarine had always been considered improbable anyway, and Japanese records after the war confirmed that no submarine had been in the area at the time of the Blimp L-8 episode.

To this day no one has any idea what happened to Cody and Adams, and their fate remains an unsolved mystery of the air.

In the less than a century since humans have been flying around the world in airships, planes, and other craft, the air already rivals the sea as a source of mysterious happenings. In the early days odd accidents were only to be expected. Airplanes were light and unstable, airships were difficult to maneuver, and for many years both could be seriously affected by any sudden change of wind. Many crashes were the understandable teething troubles of a new science and could be laid to mechanical faults that were corrected in subsequent designs. But the fate of the Zeppelin L-50 after a bombing raid over England in 1917 is a mystery. Likewise, the cause of the fire that destroyed the *Hindenburg*, last and greatest of the zeppelins, has never been established. Accidents such as these have never been satisfactorily explained to this day.

What are some of the enigmas of the air? Some aircraft have unexpectedly crashed, others have vanished off the face of the earth. Pilots have disappeared in front of witnesses, passengers have stepped out of planes for no clear reason. There may be an explanation for each of these strange events, but so far the answer has eluded everyone. For example, what could have

# What Happened to L-8's Crew?

# The Mystery of "Star Dust"

happened to the British Lancastrian airliner *Star Dust* as it approached the airport in Santiago, Chile on August 12, 1947? A radio message from the apparently doomed plane repeated the word "stendec" rapidly three times at the end of the last call ever heard from the crew. The *Star Dust* vanished utterly in the next three minutes. No trace of it was found. Was "stendec" a warning? Did the strange word contain a clue to what was happening? Would knowing its meaning help to explain the plane's disappearance? Perhaps, but the word has never been deciphered.

World War I gave rise to many puzzles about planes and pilots. One of the oddest events occurred on a fine September morning in 1916 when six German fighter planes were returning from a dawn patrol over the French lines. As the squadron was passing a thick cloud bank over Armentieres, a British two-seater reconnaissance plane suddenly flew out of the cloud toward them. The German planes scattered, just managing to avoid a collision, then darted back to attack, raking the small plane with machine gun fire. To their surprise, the British did not return their fire. Nor did it alter course, but continued in a wide circle to the left. A second attack still failed to down the plane. Cautiously, suspecting a trick, the German squadron leader flew closer until only a few yards separated the two aircraft; then he banked steeply and looked into the open cockpit. A chilling sight met his eyes. Dead but still strapped into their seats sat the pilot and the

Below: the British Lancastrian *Star Trail* in flight. This plane was the sister of the *Star Dust* which in August 1947 vanished completely as it approached Chile's Santiago airport. The last signal received from the plane was the word "stendec" repeated three times. Then silence.

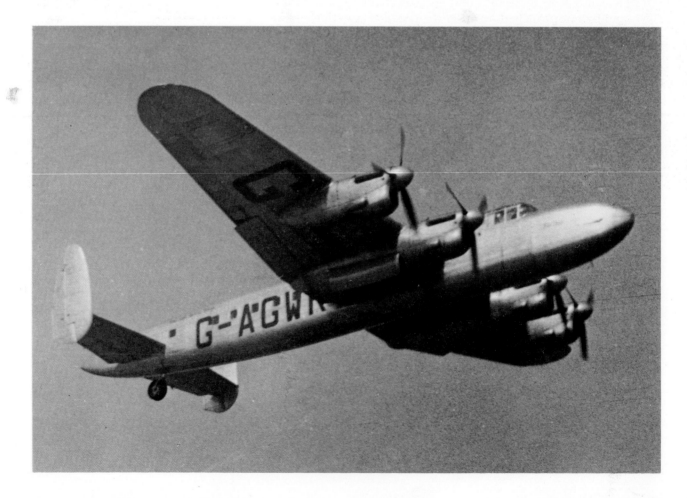

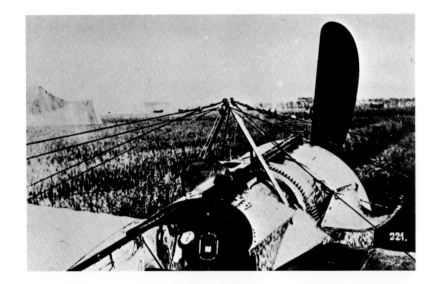

Left: This Fokker E111 flown by German air ace Oswald Boelke during World War I is fitted with the machine gun pioneered by Dutchman Antony Fokker. It enabled German pilots to fire forward without damaging the propeller blades, and proved devastating to Allied pilots. Their machine guns were fitted at either the side or rear of their planes, as shown in the photograph at below left.

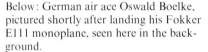

Below: German air ace Oswald Boelke, pictured shortly after landing his Fokker E111 monoplane, seen here in the background.

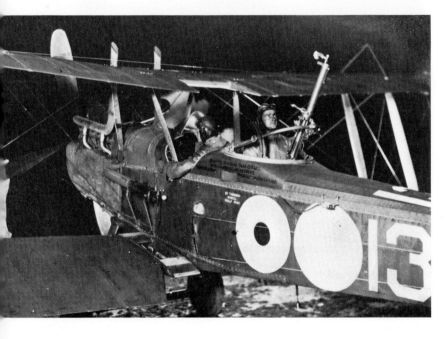

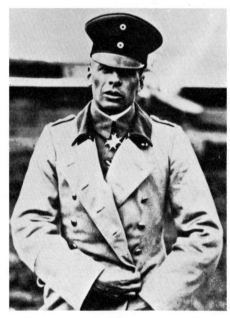

radio operator, their sightless eyes staring ahead, their uniforms smeared with blood from a multitude of wounds. The German pilot dipped his wings in a gesture of respect, and ordered the squadron to return to home base.

The pilotless British plane continued to fly for another 40 minutes until the engine ran out of fuel. Even then it did not crash, but glided smoothly down to a safe landing in an open field. An autopsy on the two fliers revealed that they had been killed by a single bullet that passed through one's left lung and buried itself in the base of the other's brain. Extraordinary as that may seem, it is equalled by the fact that although hundreds of bullet holes were found on the plane, not one of them had struck a vital part—propeller, engine, fuel tanks, and controls were all undamaged. It was as if ghostly hands had brought the plane safely back to land.

In contrast, it was a mysterious crash that killed the German

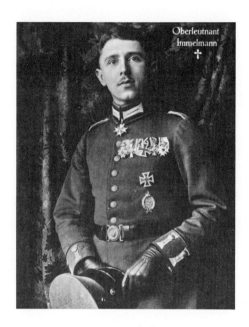

Above: German air ace Max Immelmann, who shot down 16 Allied planes before he was mysteriously shot down himself in June 1916. German and Allied versions of how he died are curiously different. What really happened?

Right: it was in dogfights like this one that men like Boelke and Immelmann made their names. The brown German biplane at right of the picture is a Fokker plane of the type that both German aces flew.

Below: Max Immelmann, the so-called "Eagle of Lille," standing by the wreckage of his seventh victim.

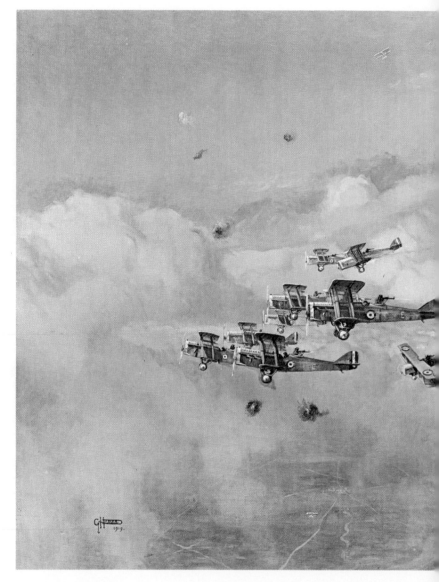

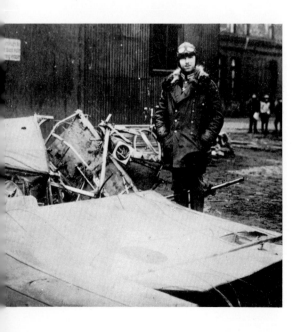

war hero Max Immelmann, the air ace known as *Der Adler von Lille* (the Eagle of Lille). On the morning of June 18, 1916 Immelmann shot down his sixteenth enemy plane. That afternoon he again took off and joined a fierce air battle between four German and seven British aircraft. German ground artillery was effective and shrapnel was whining dangerously close. Suddenly Immelmann's plane was seen to nose upward, whipstall, and fall into a diving spiral. At 8000 feet the plane began to come apart. The tail section twisted free, the rear part of the fuselage ripped away, and finally even the engine tore itself loose and hurtled like a stone to the ground. Buried within the twisted mass of steel, the Eagle of Lille lay dead. The cause of the crash has never been determined.

Wishing to preserve the legend of Immelmann's invincibility, the German High Command gave out that his plane had failed in midair. The designer of Immelmann's fighter plane was not prepared to have his aircraft blamed, however. He examined the wreckage and found evidence that the fuselage had been sliced

# Strange Tales of World War 1

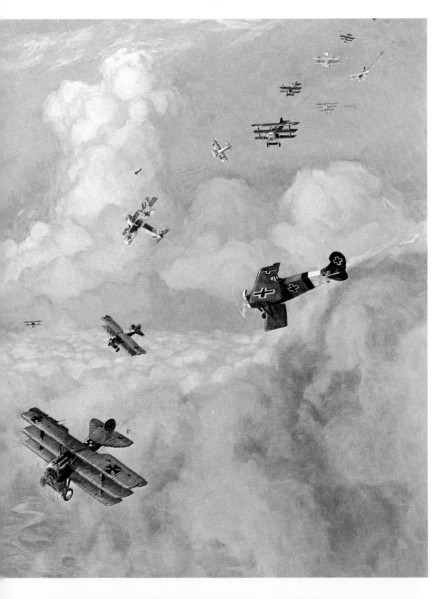

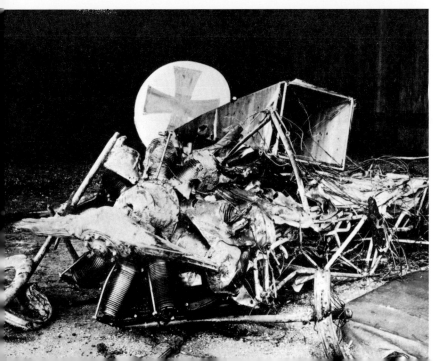

Left: the wreckage of Max Immelmann's own fighter. At least three explanations of how it was shot down and Immelmann killed were produced—by the German authorities, the designer of his plane, and by the British. The truth has never emerged.

# The Air Ace Who Disappeared

in two by shrapnel. A British report provided a third version of events when it announced that an Allied plane had shot down a similar plane at the time and place in question. Which account is correct? It will probably never be known.

Mystery also surrounds the last flight of Georges Guynemer, who by September 1917 was the leading French ace with 54 German planes to his credit. Eight times he had been shot down and escaped unharmed. The French people knew him as "Georges the Miraculous." But his luck came to an end on September 11 when he took to the air over Ypres with two other members of his celebrated *Stork Squadron*. Catching sight of a German two-seater in the distance, he signaled to his companions to stay behind as cover and lookout, then banked his plane into a dive and pursued his adversary. Meanwhile a group of German fighters flew up and Guynemer's companions became occupied in luring them away. Some minutes later one of the French pilots returned to see how Guynemer was faring. His plane was nowhere to be seen. A search up and down the lines and in the sky above the clouds revealed nothing. Guynemer never turned up again.

In the ordinary way of things, Guynemer's death would have been claimed by the Germans, but no announcement was forthcoming. A rumor came filtering through to the effect that

Right: the leading French air ace Georges Guynemer. By September 1917 he was the most successful—and lucky—of the French pilots, with 54 German planes to his credit and 8 amazing escapes. It was then that he mysteriously vanished.

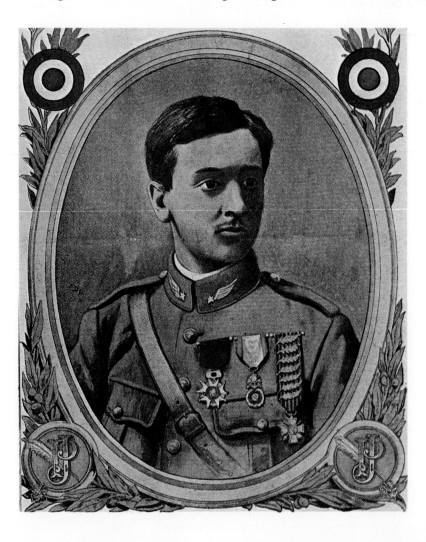

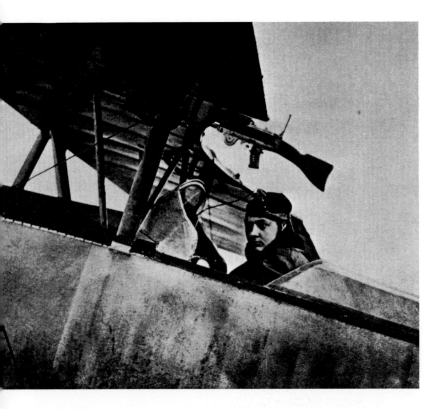

Left: Georges Guynemer in the cockpit of his fighter aircraft shortly before his unexplained disappearance in a dogfight over the front. He was said by the Germans to have been shot down and buried at the Belgian town of Poelcapelle, but a month later, when the French captured the town, they could find no trace of his grave. Could the Red Cross, who confirmed the German report, have made a mistake?
Below: the monument erected by the French to the most successful of their air aces in World War I in the town of Poelcapelle. But where did his body really come to rest?

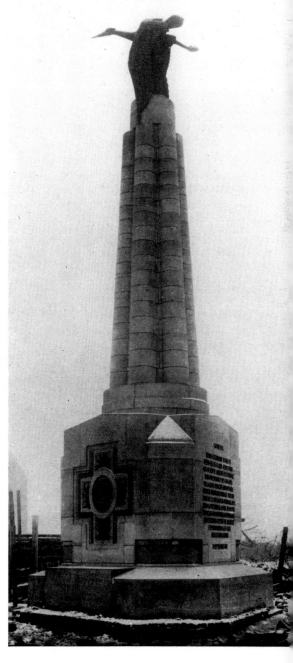

Guynemer had been shot down by a German pilot named Wissemann, and after a longer interval than usual, a German communique was received giving details of his death. But the date given was September 10 instead of 11. The French also received word from the Red Cross that Guynemer had been given a military funeral in Poelcapelle, Flanders.

This news later proved to add to the mystery. When Allied infantry captured Poelcapelle a month afterward, they were unable to find Guynemer's grave. The Germans responded by saying that Guynemer's plane had been brought down near Poelcapelle cemetery, and that the badly wounded pilot had had to be left beside it because an intense Allied bombardment was under way. Guynemer's body and the plane had been shot to pieces in the ensuing barrage.

What this account does not explain is why news of the French ace's death was so long in coming, nor why the Red Cross reported his military funeral at Poelcapelle. If the Red Cross was wrong, whose body was buried in the grave that could not be found? Some believe that Guynemer met a death the Germans thought best to conceal. Perhaps he died in captivity. Whatever the conjectures, no further news concerning him was ever received.

The German prewar development of rigid dirigibles had given them an immense advantage when war came. Zeppelin airships made many bombing raids over England, and if the physical damage they inflicted was slight by the standards of later wars, the psychological effect was great.

On October 19, 1917 a fleet of 11 zeppelins rendezvoused over England for one of the largest bombing raids of the war. They climbed to 16,500 feet, spread out over Hull, Sheffield, and

# The Mysterious "Silent Raid"

Grimsby, dropped their bombs, and turned for home. But though the guns far below were powerless to reach them, the zeppelins soon found themselves at the mercy of the elements. The wind changed. Tailwinds that had been assisting their flight back to Germany became violent, and at high altitudes reached almost hurricane force. Creaking and rolling, the airships made their way across the English Channel where shore batteries shot fire rockets up toward them. Hastily the commanders dropped ballast and rose out of range to 20,000 feet. But they were scarcely better off. Engines and men struggled to keep working in the thin icy air. As the zeppelins came over France the gales scattered them across a wide area. For Zeppelin L-50, commanded by Captain Schwonder, the journey ended in tragedy and mystery.

Seven zeppelins managed to make their way back to base but five were still above France the next day and running low on

Right: the English population were understandably fearful of zeppelin raids, but the authorities were not completely unprepared. Searchlights like the one shown here were quickly set up to pick out the sinister shapes against the night sky, where fighter planes could shoot them down.

Below: damage caused in London by bombs from one of the zeppelins that took part in the German raid on the night of October 19, 1917. In this street, 3 houses were completely demolished, 12 seriously damaged, 10 people killed, and 24 injured.

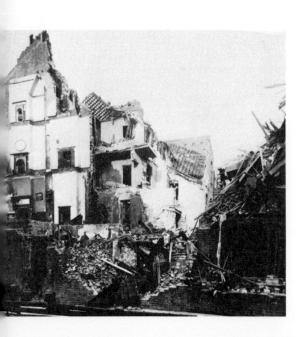

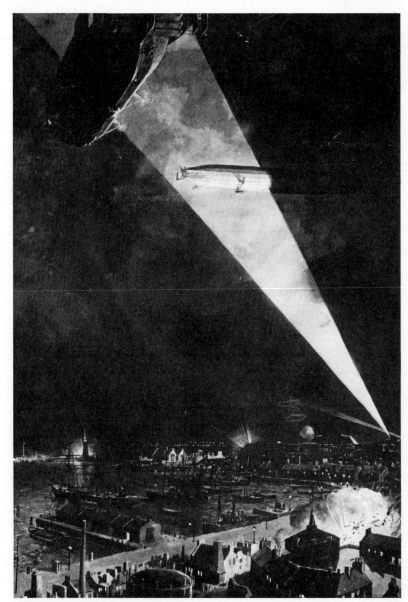

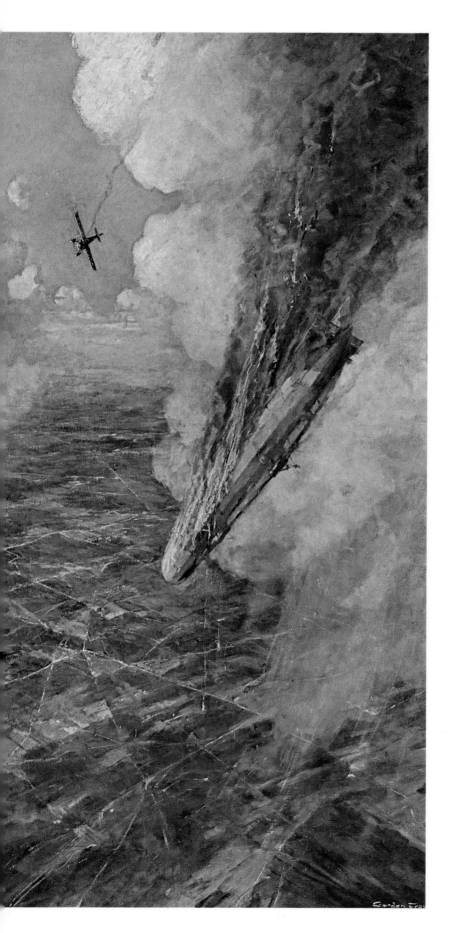

Left: the British were outraged by zeppelin raids on civilian targets, and the first pilot to shoot down a zeppelin single-handed was awarded the VC. He was Flight-Lieutenant R. A. J. Warneford, and the exploit took place over Belgium in June 1915.

Below: the zeppelin L-49, which came down on French soil. The German commander tried to blow up the machine, but was prevented from doing so by a French civilian who happened to be out hunting with his gun and forced the commander and crew to put up their hands and surrender.

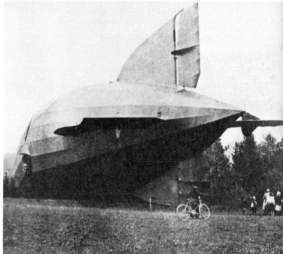

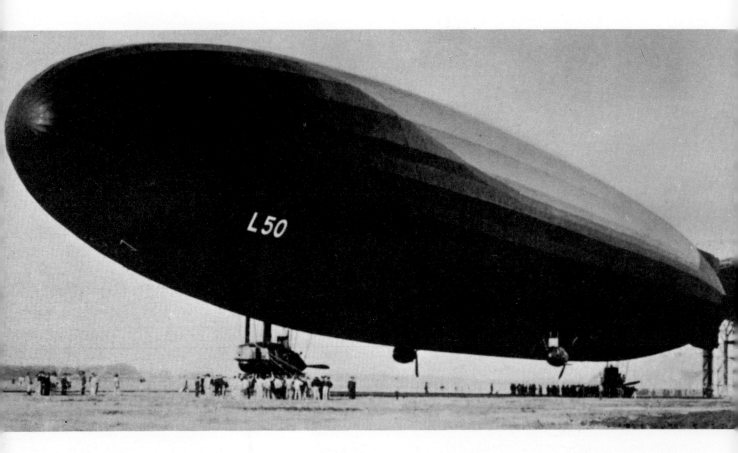

Above: the German zeppelin L-50. All the other zeppelins that took part in the raid on October 19, 1917, were accounted for. Only L-50, under the command of Captain Schwonder, was never traced. It headed for neutral Switzerland but hit the mountains of the French Alps. All but four of the crew, including the commander, managed to get out, but the lightened craft, with four Germans still on board, disappeared up into the foggy sky. It was seen again high over the Mediterranean, then vanished.

fuel. The L-44 was shot down over the French lines. The L-45 managed to get to the Mediterranean coast where it landed on a sandbank; the crew smashed the engines and set fire to the gasbags. The crew of the L-49 tried to do the same when their airship landed, but were too groggy from oxygen starvation to prevent French soldiers from capturing them and the zeppelin. Only the L-50 remained in the air.

Captain Schwonder turned east, hoping to cross the French Alps into neutral Switzerland, but the crew could not function properly as the oxygen supply became shorter. The airship could not even clear the first mountain peak and slumped into it, wiping off the control gondola and one of the engine gondolas. A number of crew members survived the crash, but four unconscious airmen remained in the dirigible when it shot up to 21,000 feet and drifted away.

Schwonder and the other survivors watched it disappear into the Alpine fog. Later that day it floated over the captured crew of the L-45 and out to sea. When last sighted it was far out in the Mediterranean. It then disappeared without trace, and its fate remains a matter for supposition. It may have descended into the sea, or winds may have carried it across to North Africa where it slowly drifted down in some inaccessible and unexplored reach of the Sahara Desert.

After World War I air travel began to establish itself as the modern way of travel. Many wealthy businessmen owned their own planes and hired pilots to chauffeur them. Between England's airport at Croydon and Brussels the flying time was about two hours. It was a route Alfred Loewenstein traveled often. On

July 4, 1928 the plane he had boarded in Croydon reached Belgium, but Loewenstein did not. When he climbed the short flight of steps into the rear of his three-engine Dutch-built Fokker VII, he had embarked on his last journey—leaving an unsolved riddle.

Loewenstein was a well-known international financier who was seldom out of the news. He lived like a prince, making and spending millions in business deals said by some to be dubious. That summer he was under a blackmail threat regarding his financial dealings. Loewenstein certainly had problems on his mind as he climbed into his Fokker at Croydon. But the previous night a private detective had discovered the identity of the blackmailer, and Loewenstein was preparing his counterattack.

Those whom Loewenstein spoke to at Croydon airport that afternoon remembered him as being his usual good-humored self, perhaps only a little tired after a long day in London in the July heat. He gave no indication of depression or despair.

Loewenstein's plane had one unusual feature. When the rear outside door was opened it exposed the toilet and washbasin area, but this compartment could be shut from sight when passengers were boarding by opening the door alongside it that led to the cabin. This was a dual-purpose door, either shutting off the cabin from the toilet and rear of the plane, or shutting off just the toilet to make the whole rear area and the cabin one long continuous space. In flight the door was always closed on the cabin.

In the thickly carpeted cabin Loewenstein took his place at a table toward the front of the plane. His private secretary Arthur Hodgson sat at a table alongside. Behind Loewenstein was his diminutive valet Fred Baxter, and in the fourth corner two typists were busy at their typewriters on the table between them. As the plane reached the channel the copilot glanced back through the window of the cockpit door and saw Loewenstein with his head halfway out of the sliding window next to him, apparently looking down at the sea. The pilot, remembering that high flying gave his employer attacks of breathlessness, thought Loewen-

# The Case of the Lost Financier

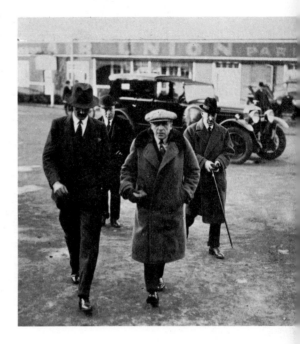

Above: Belgian international financier Alfred Loewenstein (right) walking to his private plane at Croydon, England early in 1928. It was from Croydon on July 4, 1928, that he set out on his last flight, for during the trip the financier disappeared.
Below: Loewenstein's private Fokker aircraft at Croydon airport. In the 1920s, numerous rich individuals ran their own private planes, and hired pilots to fly them around Europe.

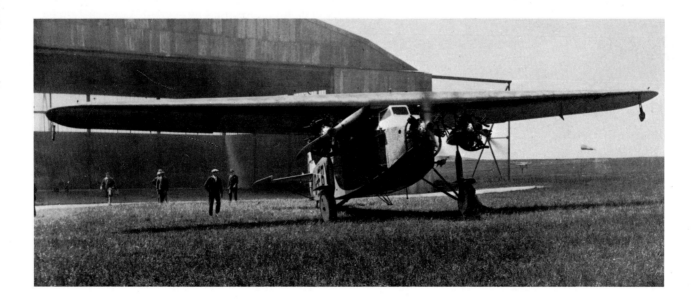

# Did Loewenstein Fall-or Jump?

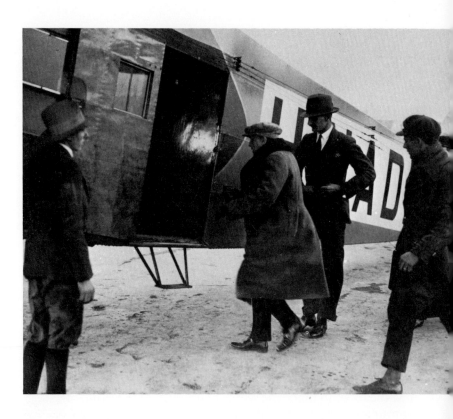

Right: Loewenstein climbing aboard his plane in 1928, the year of his disappearance. At the time of his last and fatal flight Loewenstein was being blackmailed concerning his financial dealings but the previous night a private detective had discovered the identity of the blackmailer. In theory at least Loewenstein had no reason to take his own life on July 4, 1928.

stein might be feeling the need for more air. Although the plane was only 4000 feet above sea level, even the slightly lower oxygen content at that height could make breathing uncomfortable for him.

Halfway over the channel Loewenstein walked down the cabin to the toilet, shutting the door on the cabin after him. It was the last time he was seen alive. Ten minutes later Hodgson became aware of his employer's long absence and spoke to Baxter. The valet knocked on the door to the rear. There was no reply. Hodgson gripped the handle and pushed. The door opened and the two men stared in disbelief. The whole rear area of the plane, including the toilet, was empty. But the outside door was open, shaking slightly. The incredible had happened. Loewenstein had fallen out.

The typists both went into hysterics and the valet collapsed, teeth chattering in fear. Only Hodgson retained some presence of mind. Since the engines were too loud for conversation to be heard, he wrote a brief note to the pilot. The pilot brought the plane down on a stretch of beach north of Dunkirk in order to try to establish what had happened before they faced airport officials and the press.

Was Loewenstein's disappearance accident, suicide, or murder? The first two possibilities seemed to be ruled out when tests on similar planes showed that only by exceptional strength was it possible to open the outside door during flight more than a couple of inches. Murder also seemed unlikely inasmuch as Loewenstein had been in the compartment alone at the time. A fourth possibility was suggested when the announcement of the financier's disappearance led to a sharp fall in the value of shares in his companies. According to this theory, Loewenstein knew that a crash was coming and had laid an ingenious plan for disappearing. It consisted of concealing himself in a secret compartment at the rear of the plane and, on landing on Dunkirk beach by arrangement, slipping away unnoticed by immigration officials.

When Loewenstein's business affairs were examined they were found to be in good shape, and when 15 days later his body was picked up by a channel trawler, all the wilder theories had to be abandoned. The autopsy revealed no evidence of a struggle. Loewenstein had been alive when he struck the water. The impact caused multiple injuries, but his death was by drowning.

How had it happened? Further tests, this time on Loewenstein's own plane, showed that it was possible to push open the outside door to about 18 inches during flight. Although there can be no certainty about what took place in the rear of the plane that day, it does not seem likely that Loewenstein, even if caught by another attack of breathlessness, would have been so unwise as to open the outside door to get more air. The dual-purpose door looms as a likely cause of an accident that may have occurred like this: Loewenstein leaves the toilet to return to the cabin. With his mind preoccupied by thoughts of the man blackmailing him, he ignores the nearer door. It is the door that opens into the cabin, but he thinks of it as the door of the toilet.

Below: this cutaway diagram of Loewenstein's private plane shows the details of the layout which added to the puzzle of how he managed to fall out. Loewenstein's own seat, the seats of the two private secretaries, the door of the lavatory, and the door through which the plane's owner apparently walked to his death are all clearly shown. Tests showed that the door through which Loewenstein walked or fell would open just 18 inches during flight. What really happened?

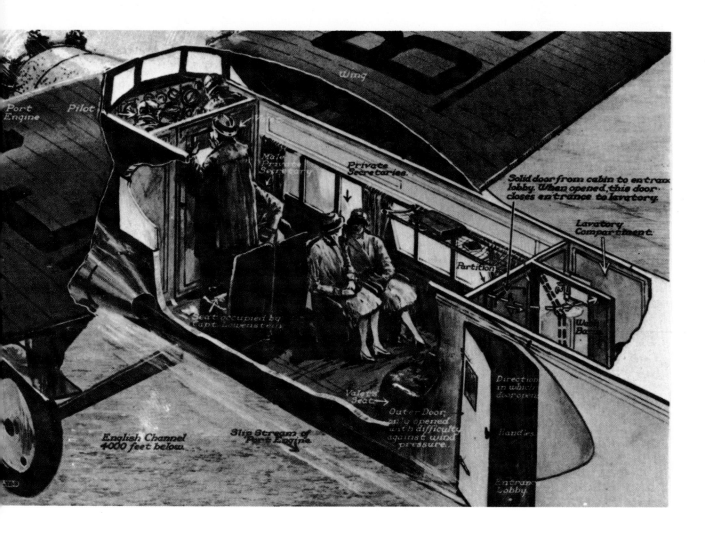

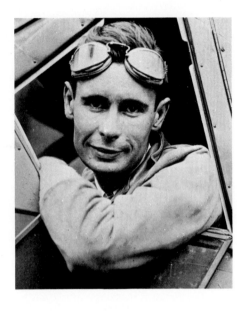

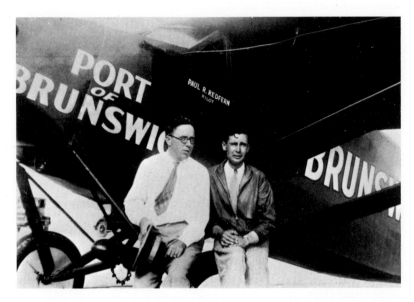

Above: Paul Redfern, the American flyer who in August 1927 climbed into his monoplane *Port of Brunswick* and set off on a solo trip from Brunswick, Georgia to Rio de Janeiro, Brazil. He was last seen flying toward the Amazonian jungle. Then he vanished. Neither Redfern nor the *Port of Brunswick* were seen again.

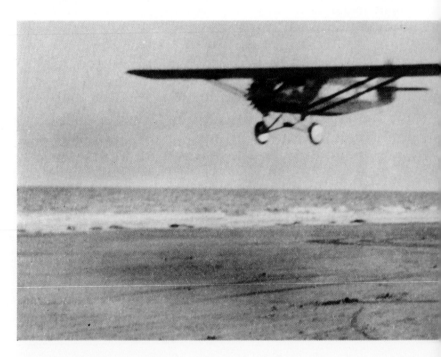

Above right: Redfern is seen here with Paul Varner, chairman of the committee which had sponsored his solo flight to South America.

Right: Redfern taking off in the *Port of Brunswick* on his tragic flight to Brazil.

Instead he turns the handle of the other door, the outside door. As he tries to open it he encounters some resistance, but still he does not realize his mistake. He pushes his body against the stubborn door and it opens—not very far but far enough for the slipstream to drag him out. His cry of alarm is lost in the roar of the engines.

Is that what happened? It is only a guess. There can be no certainty.

The decade of the 1920s was an era in which fame and fortune could be won by pilots who broke speed records or were the first to fly over a given route. Several determined contenders vanished somewhere in the Atlantic in the exciting months before and after Lindbergh's nonstop solo flight in May 1927. One of these was young Paul Redfern, who set off in August 1927 on a solo trip from Brunswick, Georgia, to Rio de Janeiro, Brazil, 4700 miles away. He managed to reach the northern coast of South America in his green and gold Stinton Detroiter *Port of Brunswick*, and was glimpsed flying toward the impenetrable jungle of Guyana and the Amazon. Then he disappeared. Over the next dozen years, several expeditions searched the jungle for some trace of him. Rumors had come back that relics of his lost plane had been seen in the possession of Amerindians. Some fanciful versions of his fate would have it that he was living among the Indians, venerated as a "great white god" who had come out of the skies. In all probability, the *Port of Brunswick* crashed in a tropical storm, killing Redfern instantly. But the facts may never be known.

The same must be said of Amelia Earhart, one of the heroines of early aviation. In 1928 she became the first woman to fly the Atlantic. In 1932 she flew the Atlantic solo and broke the speed record in doing so. In 1937 she set off to fly around the world.

# The Redfern Riddle

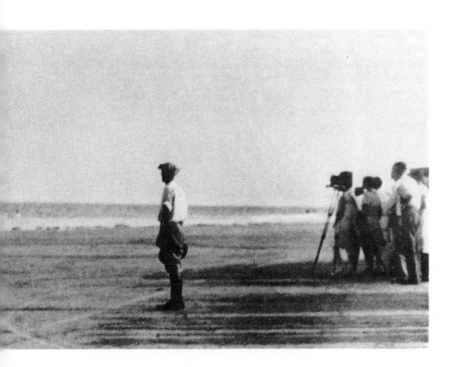

"I feel that I've got one more big flight in me," she said.

She was then 39, and had been married for seven years to a successful New York publisher. Though often in the limelight, she was unprepossessing and unspoiled by fame. This was her second try for an around-the-world flight.

On June 1, 1937 Amelia Earhart took off from Miami, Florida in her twin-engined Lockheed Electra. Her navigator was Frederick Noonan, a man with many years of experience with a commercial airline. Forty gruelling days and 22,000 miles later they reached New Guinea by way of South America, Africa, India, and Southeast Asia. From Lae on the eastern coast of New Guinea they faced the most difficult leg of their journey, the 2556 miles to tiny Howland Island. Howland was a mere speck in the ocean, only $1\frac{1}{2}$ miles long, a half mile wide, and a few feet

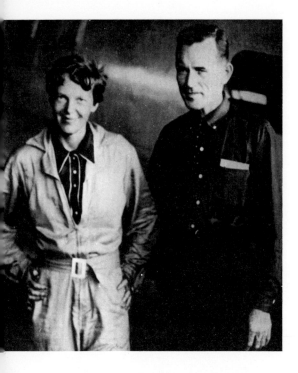

Above: this photograph of experienced flyer Amelia Earhart and her navigator Fred Noonan was taken on one of the stops on her round-the-world flight which began from Miami, Florida on June 1, 1937. Already the first woman to fly the Atlantic solo, she declared "I feel that I've got one more big flight in me" before setting out. She was never to return.

Right: Amelia Earhart and Fred Noonan climb into their Lockheed Electra at San Juan, Puerto Rico on their last disastrous flight.

above sea level. A runway had just been built on the island, and the Electra would be the first plane to land there if the pair managed to reach it. Even the best navigator would be hard put to locate the pinpoint of land, however.

Because of a slight headwind, the Electra's flight time was expected to be 20 hours. The plane carried fuel for 24. The plan was to leave Lae at 10 a.m. and fly all day by dead reckoning, checking their position as they flew over the Solomon Islands. That night Noonan would navigate by the stars, and as they approached Howland Island the next morning, they would home in on radio signals from the United States Coast Guard cutter *Itasca*, anchored off the island for that purpose. The critical section of the journey was the 500 miles in the middle when they would be out of contact both with Lae behind them and the *Itasca* ahead.

Over 1000 people watched the silver plane take off from Lae. For nearly 1200 miles the ground operators at Lae kept track of the Electra's progress through its half-hourly reports. Then, a half-hour after a very faint message, they could hear nothing. The coast guard cutter took over and, as night came on, the operators on the *Itasca* tried to make contact. Static interference was bad, but at 2:45 a.m. they managed to pick up the flier's low voice saying, "Cloudy and overcast," before the static overwhelmed it again. Garbled messages were heard at 3:45 and 4:45. The first clear message did not come through until 6:15, less than two hours before the plane was due to reach Howland Island.

"We are about 100 miles out. Please take a bearing on us and report in half an hour. I will transmit into the microphone."

When the radio operators tried to get a bearing, however, there was no signal.

At 6:45 a.m. Amelia Earhart's voice broke through the static

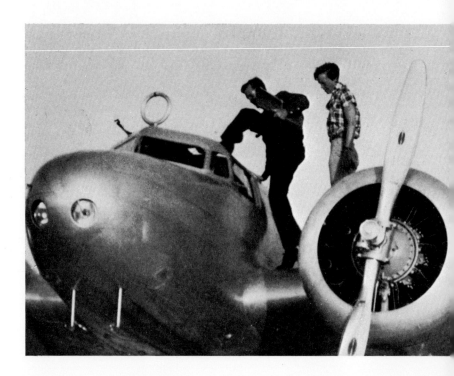

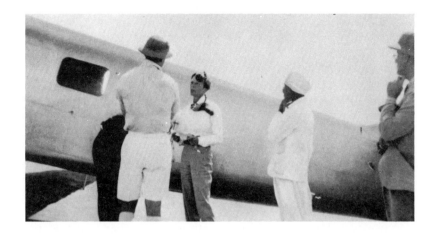

# Amelia Earhart's Final Flight

Left: Amelia Earhart chatting with officials at Khartoum, Sudan on the round-the-world flight.

Below: the United States settlement on the tiny Howland Island, the mere dot in the Pacific Ocean which Amelia Earhart's Electra never reached.

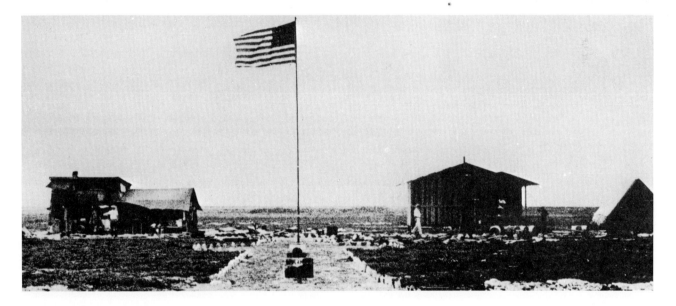

again, urgently asking for a bearing. This try also failed because she had not transmitted long enough for the direction finders to pick up the signals. Not for another hour was her voice heard again.

"We must be right on top of you but we can't see you . . . gas is running low . . . have been unable to reach you by radio . . . we are flying at an altitude of 1000 feet. . . ."

The cutter immediately sent out its homing signal, but when the pilot next made contact it was evident that she had heard none of the *Itasca*'s messages. Something seemed to be wrong with her radio on the very part of the journey that she most had need of it. At 8:00 a.m., however, she spoke again, and her message made the men on the *Itasca* think the worst might be over. She was receiving their signals, she said, but was in urgent need of a bearing. She whistled into the microphone but the sound could hardly be heard above the accompanying static.

One last time the *Itasca* heard Amelia Earhart's voice. "We have only half an hour's fuel left and we cannot see land," she reported. When nothing more was heard it was assumed that the plane had crashed; but this did not necessarily mean that the two occupants were dead. With the tanks empty and the cocks

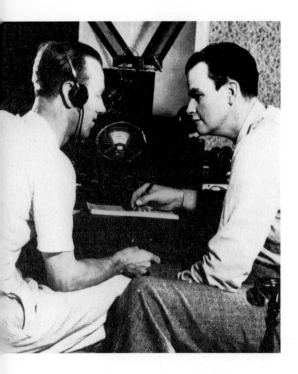

Above: these are two of the amateur radio operators who claimed they picked up signals on Amelia Earhart's agreed frequency some time after her last words were picked up by U.S. Navy radio operators at 8.15 a.m. local time. Then her voice sounded broken, tired, and very worried. The amateurs were not believed.

Below: British cruiser H.M.S. *Achilles*, which was in the Pacific at the time, succeeded in picking up the Electra's last transmission. Then silence.

closed the plane might keep afloat indefinitely in calm weather. Even without a working radio there was still a chance of rescue. For two weeks ships and planes searched a quarter of a million square miles of ocean—and found nothing. Amelia Earhart and Frederick Noonan were missing, presumed drowned.

Later that year a disturbing rumor arose. It was suggested that the United States government had instructed the fliers to spy on Japanese war preparations, probably in the Marshall Islands. Having deliberately flown off course to spy, the story went, they had fallen into the hands of the Japanese and were prisoners. The Japanese indignantly denied this rumor, but when all the Japanese-held islands were captured after the war, an attempt was made to find out if the story had any foundation.

From the Marshall Islands came a report that in 1937 two white fliers, one a woman, had crashed between Jaluit and Ailinglapalap atolls. They had been picked up by a Japanese fishing boat and taken away in another Japanese boat to Saipan, a large island of the Mariana group, which the Japanese were illegally fortifying. From Saipan itself came information that an entire album filled with photographs of Amelia Earhart was discovered.

Other reports from Saipan seemed to contradict those from the Marshall Islands. One said that a plane had been seen to crash in the bay, and a white woman and man had been brought ashore from it. The woman was dressed like a man, and both looked exhausted and pale. Japanese soldiers led them away into the jungle, after which shots were heard.

These reports of the crash and execution, though collected several years after the event, cannot be entirely discounted. But until more conclusive evidence comes to light, the answer to the disappearance of Amelia Earhart and Frederick Noonan lies in the Pacific Ocean's great depths.

Amelia Earhart had once said to her husband, "I don't want to die, but when I do, I want to go in my plane—quickly."

Perhaps her wish was granted.

Surely none of the passengers on the *Hindenburg*, Germany's luxury dirigible, wished to go down with the airship when they boarded it for an Atlantic crossing on May 6, 1937—nor did

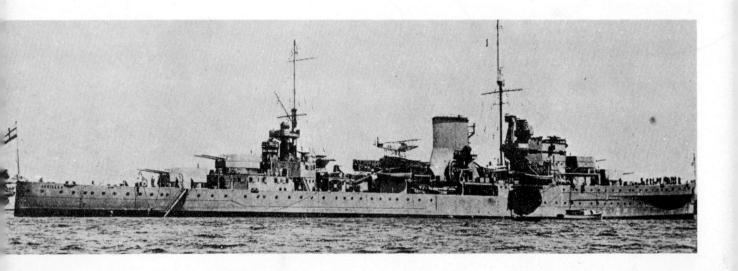

# The Airship Age

they expect to. There had never been a passenger fatality on any of Germany's commercial airships. The *Hindenburg*, largest dirigible ever to fly, was designed for safety as well as beauty and grandeur. There were 70 staterooms, a lounge, a dining room and a bar, all sumptuously decorated. Broad promenades with large windows afforded spectacular views. It was, as it was called, a Great Floating Palace.

The obvious weakness of the *Hindenburg* was its inflammability because of the seven million cubic feet of hydrogen that filled its 16 vast gas cells. This was a flaw created by lack of supply rather than by design, however, since it had been intended to use nonflammable helium. But the only country that produced helium in sufficient quantities was the United States, and with Hitler in power and the danger of war increasing, the Americans refused to supply helium in case it was later used for military purposes.

Fire precautions on board the *Hindenburg* were stringent. The crew members wore antistatic asbestos overalls and hemp-soled shoes. All matches and lighters were removed from the passengers before they boarded. The smoking room was especially insulated, pressurized to prevent hydrogen entering, and fitted

Below: the largest and most luxurious airship ever built, the pride of Nazi Germany, the 240-ton *Hindenburg* is seen here at Frankfurt airfield before taking off on its last flight in May 1937.

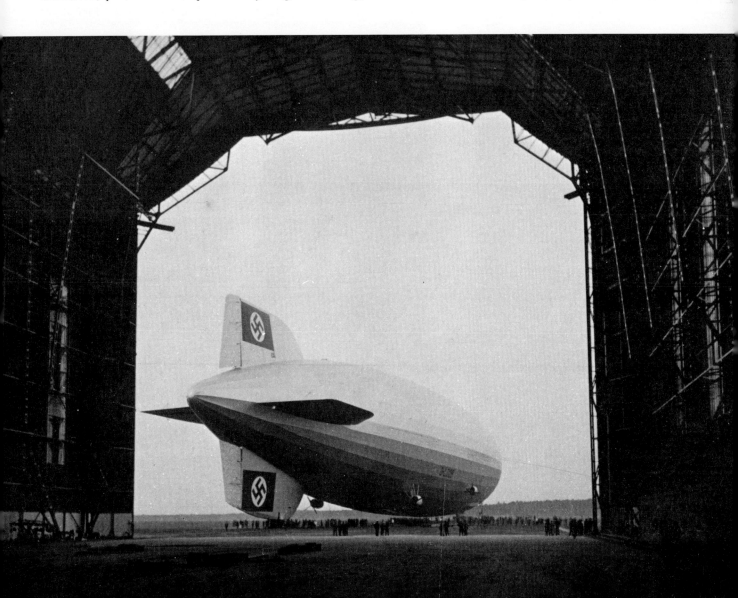

Right: this lavishly appointed lounge on board the *Hindenburg* was even equipped with a light aluminum piano. The lounge was only one of the 70 elaborate staterooms which, together with the decorated staircase leading from one deck to another, made the *Hindenburg* more like an ocean-going liner than any kind of aircraft of the time.

Below: the *Hindenburg*'s dining room. Meals were cooked on board and a magnificent menu offered a wide choice of food and wines. The *Hindenburg* was not called the "Great Floating Palace" without good reason.

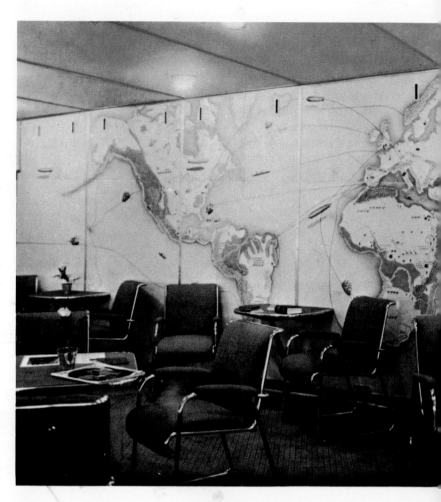

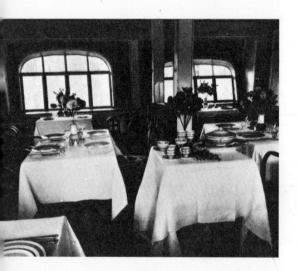

with a double door; a steward lit cigars and cigarettes for smokers, and ensured that no fire left the room.

During 1936 the *Hindenburg* safely cruised back and forth across the Atlantic. Once the captain guided it through a thunderstorm with such ease that many passengers were unaware of the poor weather conditions.

On May 6, 1937 the *Hindenburg* was on another routine crossing. The commander was Captain Max Pruss, an airship officer of long experience, recently commander of the *Graf Zeppelin*. With him in the control gondola was the veteran airship pilot Captain Ernst Lehmann, himself formerly in charge of the *Hindenburg*, who was going to Washington.

When the *Hindenburg* reached the Lakehurst Naval Air Station near Boston, where it was supposed to moor, it was running 10 hours late. Pruss decided to delay the landing still further because of rain, wind, and cloud. He swung over New York, circling the Empire State Building. After waiting another hour, Pruss prepared to land. Darkness was coming on, though the rain and wind had slackened. With the mooring mast 700 feet away, the airship's engines reversed and the Great Floating Palace drifted to a standstill. The mooring ties were dropped 200 feet below where the ground party ran forward to pick them up.

Suddenly the belly of the silver airship glowed red. At the

same time flames broke from the tail, just forward of the upper fin. The crowd below screamed and scattered. In the control gondola Pruss had felt only a slight shock and did not realize what had happened until he glanced out and saw the ground below glowing redly. Within seconds huge flames leaped up, bursting one gasbag after another to feed more hydrogen to the already white hot inferno. Explosions were heard 15 miles away.

Before the blazing zeppelin touched ground, some of the passengers and crew jumped from windows, doors—any opening they could find—and hurtled to the ground. Miraculously there were some survivors. Once on the ground, others were saved.

That anyone at all should have escaped the inferno is a

# White-hot Inferno!

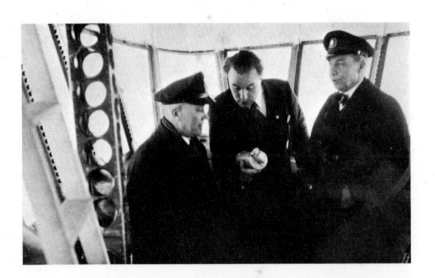

Left: Captain Pruss (left), commander of the ill-fated *Hindenburg* on its fatal crossing of the Atlantic in 1937, together with experienced airship officer Captain Ernst Lehmann (right), who had commanded the *Hindenburg* the previous year, in the control gondola.

Below: "What is it?" asked Captain Pruss when the first small explosion occurred. He thought maybe a landing line had snapped. Then he saw the rosy glow at the tail, the crowd below scattering, and he knew what had happened. This remarkable photograph shows clearly how the explosion and fire began in the rear.

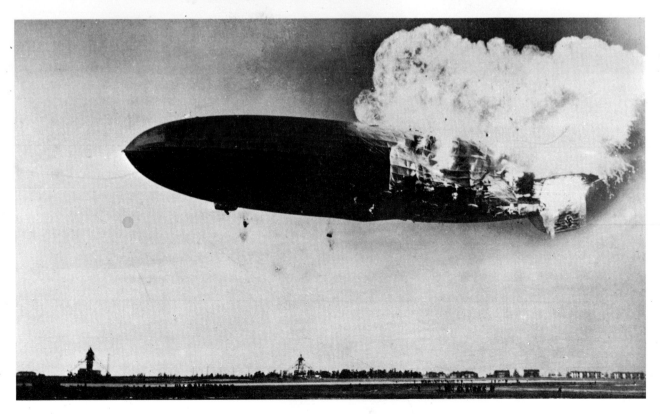

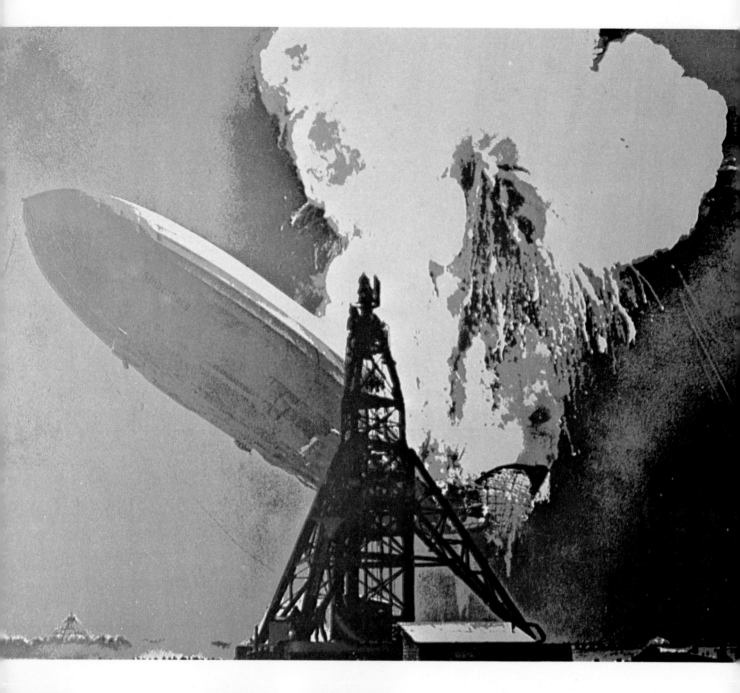

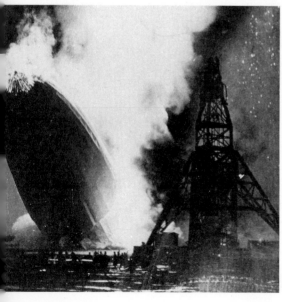

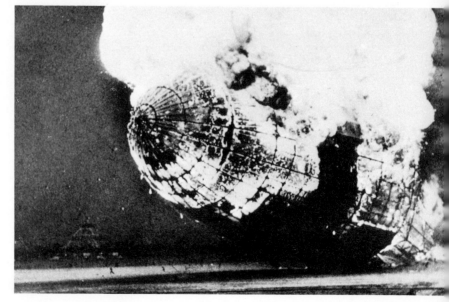

wonder. Only 32 seconds elapsed between the first explosion and the final crash of the melting, white-hot framework. Yet of the 97 passengers and crew aboard, 62 lived through the danger. Captain Pruss repeatedly ran into the glowing wreck to help until he was forcibly prevented from reentering. Captain Lehmann, badly burned, staggered back and forth mumbling, "I don't understand . . . I don't understand. . . ." The following day he died in great pain.

The commission of inquiry set up to discover the cause of the explosion wanted to consider the possibility of sabotage, but crew members well enough to be called to the stand were unhelpful on this point. Other possibilities were examined—a spark from the engine, an electrical fault, a sticking gas valve, structural failure, static electricity—but the crew's evidence convinced the commission that none of these could be responsible. Eventually the commission had to fall lamely back on St. Elmo's Fire, a form of atmospheric static electricity, as "most probably" the cause—even though scientists doubted that St. Elmo's Fire could set light to hydrogen under almost any circumstances.

Not till after the war was it learned that Hermann Goering, chief of the Nazi Luftwaffe, had sent orders to the officers and crew of the *Hindenburg* that "they should not try to find an explanation." The destruction of the *Hindenburg* was a serious enough blow to the pride of Nazi Germany. If it had become known at that time that an enemy saboteur was responsible, the repercussions within Germany might have become uncontrollable. So the crew kept their suspicions to themselves, and only years later did the survivors talk of the frantic passenger who had been pacing up and down the dining saloon 20 minutes before the explosion. "I don't want to go round the field again," he had cried out. "I want to go down!" The FBI discovered that this passenger had claimed in conversation to be an American citizen although he was using a foreign passport.

There is also the puzzling behavior of the tall fair-haired rigger, Erich Spehl. A moody and reserved young man, his hobby

# Was it Sabotage?

Opposite: this extraordinary sequence of photographs shows how the fire gradually engulfed the entire airship in the 30-odd seconds between the first muffled explosion and its final collapse into a heap of white-hot twisted framework. During that brief period a surprising number of those aboard the doomed airship managed to escape with their lives. Of 36 passengers and 61 crew only a total of 35 men and women died on board the *Hindenburg*, together with one member of the ground staff. Fortunately for many, Captain Pruss had already brought the craft down so low that, when the explosion occurred, they were able to jump clear.

Below left: the United States board of inquiry set up to discover the cause of the disastrous explosion which was to end the era of the dirigible airship for ever. The findings of the inquiry were hardly satisfactory. Sabotage, lightning, a spark from an engine, an electrical fault, static electricity—all these were considered and finally rejected in favor of a natural phenomenon known as St Elmo's Fire. Was it really the correct conclusion?

Below: St Elmo's Fire appearing on the spar of a ship at sea. This flamelike light is generally seen in stormy weather or in strong electrical fields. It has been observed on the tips of masts, on tree tops and steeples, along the wings and propeller blades of planes.

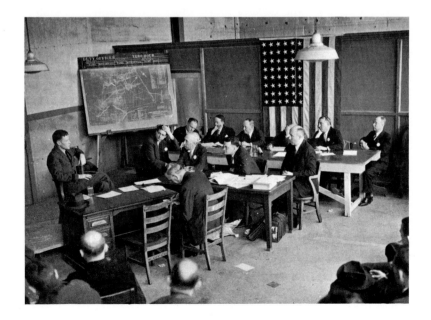

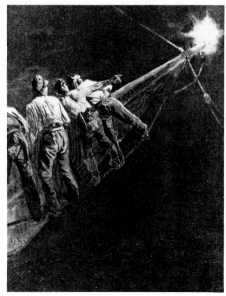

# A Polar Mystery

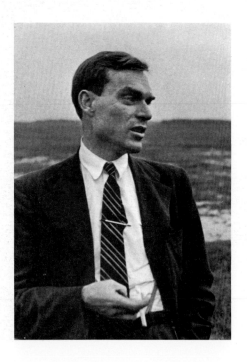

Above: Soviet air ace Captain Levanevsky, who in August 1937 set out with a crew of five to fly nonstop from Moscow in the Soviet Union to Fairbanks, Alaska by flying directly over the North Pole. Shortly after crossing the pole on August 13, Lavenevsky reported that one of his four engines had broken an oil line. This meant the plane had to come down to 13,000 feet, at which height ice formed on the wing surfaces. Shortly after this, the radio operator reported they had to land. There was no further message from the expedition.

was photography. He had full access to the interior of the airship and could have placed an explosive device in the crevices of a gas cell on many occasions. His last watch ended one and a half hours before the explosion, and it is significant that at the time of the blast he was as far away from it as possible, one of the few crew in the foremost part of the nose. Two of the surviving crew members who saw the start of the fire said that it began with the sort of flash that could have been caused by a photoflash bulb.

Before the *Hindenburg* left Frankfurt on its last flight, Spehl had been seen in the company of an older woman believed to have communist sympathies. She called at the zeppelin company's offices three times during the airship's flight to ask about its position. Spehl perished in the tragedy, so his side of the story can never be known. It is always possible that the explosion was timed to occur after the landing, without loss of life, and that the more than 11-hour delay before mooring put the plan awry. Sabotage seems to be the most likely explanation, but there is little chance of this being established beyond doubt.

There seems to be even less chance of ever explaining the disappearance of six Soviet airmen who were trying to establish an air route over the North Pole. Their goal was to fly nonstop from the Soviet Union to Alaska, starting in Moscow and ending in Fairbanks. They set out in early August 1937, a dangerous time of year for polar flight because the summer thaw made a sea of possible emergency landing zones. But three of the crew members were veteran polar fliers, and the other three were exceptionally well qualified. Captain Sigismund Levanevsky was confident of success.

For the first 2000 miles the flight was on schedule, although a headwind cut the plane's speed and the heavy fuel load prevented it from rising above the cloud. Near the pole the plane did manage to climb above the cloud and, after passing the pole, held steady for the next two hours. Then came a distress call. An oil line had burst from the cold, cutting one of the four engines. This meant that the plane had to descend to 13,000 feet, at which level ice was forming on its surface.

Not long after the danger alert, the radio operator signaled that the plane had to land. He gave the location, but the message was too garbled to understand. It turned out to be the last message from the Levanevsky expedition.

The Soviet government, the Explorers Club of New York, and private individuals made intensive searches from the day after the disappearance on August 13, 1937 to the next spring. Only one frail lead turned up: some Eskimos living between Aklavik, Canada, and Point Barrow, Alaska, had heard a plane on August 13. Its engines had died away south and inland, putting it in the hazardous mountain region. Was it the Levanevsky survey plane at all? Even that is not known. Not a trace of the fliers or their plane, and not a clue to the mystery of their end has ever been found by anyone.

If Levanevsky had vanished over the ocean south of Florida instead of over the pole, he would have been one of a statistically improbable number of air disappearances in recent years. The area is known as the Bermuda Triangle—and its mystery has been much plumbed, as the next chapter reveals.

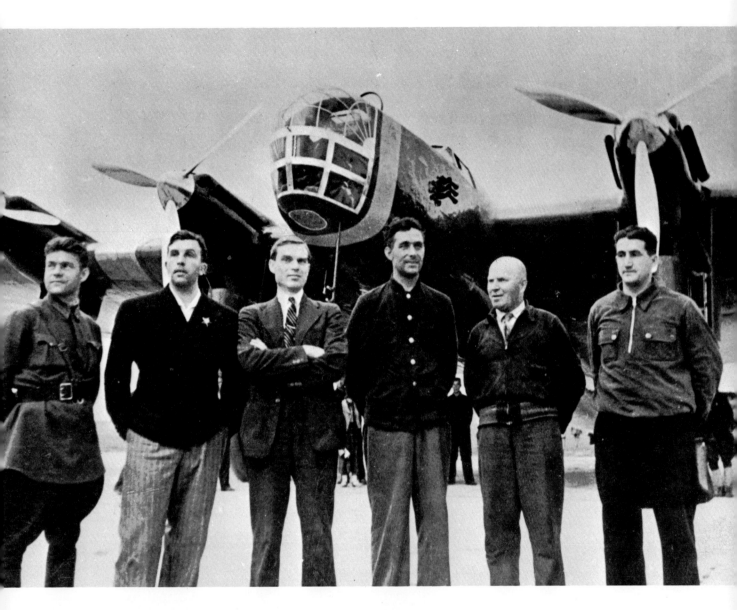

Above: Captain Sigismund Levanevsky (third from left) and the five members of his crew before their attempt to cross the North Pole from Moscow to Alaska. They are standing in front of their giant four-engined H209 plane, one of whose engines was to cut out fatally.

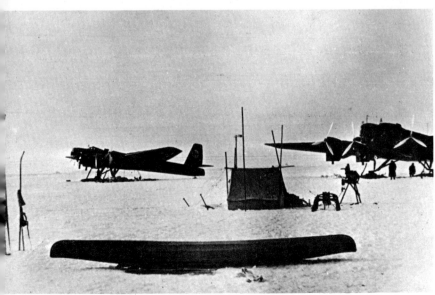

Left: two Soviet planes at the North Pole during the long search operation to find the H209 and its crew. The operation was hampered by fog and the search was finally called off and the men "presumed dead."

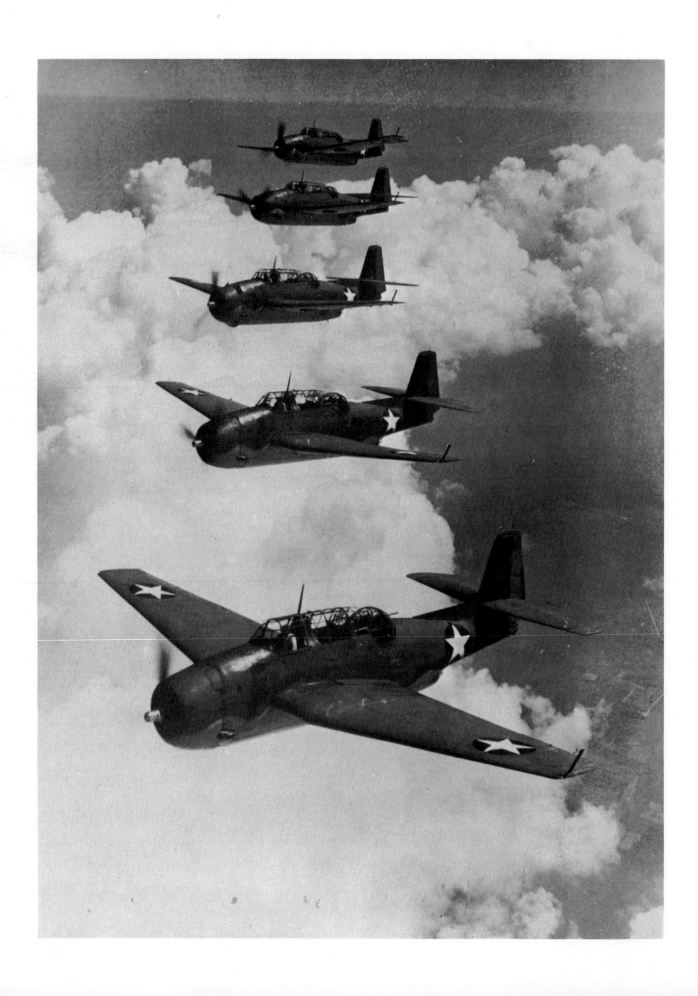

# Chapter 9
# The Bermuda Triangle

Why have so many vessels and aircraft disappeared in that patch of the Atlantic Ocean known as the Bermuda Triangle? Are they swallowed up? Sucked into outer space? Dashed to the bottom of the sea? Why are no bodies or fragments of the ships and planes ever found? For many years the number of unexplained accidents, near accidents, and disappearances in the Triangle has been more than can be laid to mere chance. Will we ever have enough data to understand what happens in this mystery region?

"Calling tower, this is an emergency . . . We seems to be off course . . . We cannot see land . . . Repeat . . . We cannot see land." This was the radio message that alerted the Naval Air Station at Fort Lauderdale, Florida, that something was wrong with Flight 19 somewhere out in the Atlantic between Florida and the island of Bermuda. The speaker was Lieutenant Charles C. Taylor, leader of the five Avenger torpedo bombers making up Flight 19, which had taken off at 2:00 p.m. that afternoon on a routine mission. The date was December 5, 1945 and the time was 3:45 p.m.; the planes should have then been returning to base.

"What is your position?" the tower radioed.

Back came the astounding reply: "We're not sure of our position. We can't be sure just where we are. We seem to be lost."

Lieutenant Taylor was an experienced pilot. It was incredible that he should not know his position. The mission of Flight 19 had been to fly due east from the Florida coastline for 160 miles to the Chicken Shoals in the Bahamas where the planes were to make practice runs on a target hulk. Afterward they were to fly north for 40 miles, and then southwest back to Fort Lauderdale.

At the time of the distress call, the first two legs of the flight had been carried out satisfactorily. Accordingly, the tower instructed him, "Assume bearing due west."

Taylor's reply to this was alarming. "We don't know which

Opposite: five Avenger torpedo bombers. The mysterious disappearance of five such bombers over the Atlantic off the east coast of Florida in 1955 was the first major disaster in the so-called Bermuda Triangle. Later evidence has only increased its reputation for mystery.

Right: the Bermuda Triangle, the area in the Atlantic Ocean where so many strange disappearances of ships and aircraft have occurred. There is a great difference of opinion among investigators as to the exact area of the Triangle. Here the dotted red line shows the traditional area, and the red continuous line incorporates the area that various more recent authors have considered as being part of it.

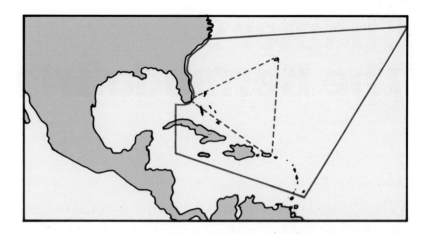

way is west. Everything is wrong . . . strange . . . We can't be sure of any direction. Even the ocean doesn't look as it should."

When the planes had taken off from Fort Lauderdale, flying conditions had been good—sunny with scattered clouds. If the planes were now unable to tell whether or not they were flying west, it must mean the sun was invisible to them. Had weather conditions deteriorated out there? As for the reported "strangeness" of the ocean, this detail was to be the subject of much speculation over the next 30 years. For although the doomed planes of Flight 19 did not know it, they were flying straight into a legend. Many stories, articles, and books were to tell of their last flight, theorizing as to their fate. Films were to reenact their mission to oblivion. They were to become the most celebrated victims of that danger area of the Atlantic known by such names as "The Triangle of Death," "The Hoodoo Sea," "The Graveyard of the Atlantic," but most recently and widely as "The Bermuda Triangle."

Vincent Gaddis, American author of a book on sea mysteries, first coined the phrase in drawing attention to the great number of ships and planes that have disappeared in this relatively small area of the ocean. Most of them leave no trace of wreckage or bodies. They vanish. Gaddis wrote, "Draw a line from Florida to Bermuda, another from Bermuda to Puerto Rico, and a third line back to Florida through the Bahamas. Within this roughly triangular area most of the vanishments have occurred." Others have taken place in adjacent areas to the north and east in the Atlantic, south in the Caribbean, and west in the Gulf of Mexico. But the biggest majority of mysterious disappearances have occurred within the Bermuda–Puerto Rico–Florida triangle.

The Avengers of Flight 19 were well within this triangle when the unknown misfortune overtook them. Apparently they found it increasingly difficult to hear messages from base because of static interference, but Fort Lauderdale was able to hear the messages passing between the five pilots. There were complaints that their instruments had gone wild and that their compasses were spinning. The tone of these radio exchanges moved from bewilderment to fear. Each Avenger usually carried a crew of three—the pilot, a gunner, and a radio operator—but one airman had put in a successful request to be removed from flight duty that day. He was not replaced, so the number involved in this unexpectedly mysterious and fatal journey totaled 14.

The senior flight instructor at Fort Lauderdale picked up a request by one of the pilots to another asking about his compass readings. The reply was, "I don't know where we are. We must have gotten lost after that last turn." The same flight instructor was finally able to contact Taylor who reported back: "Both my compasses are out. I am trying to find Fort Lauderdale . . . I'm sure I'm in the Keys but I don't know how far down."

The senior flight instructor advised him to fly north, keeping the sun on his portside. If Taylor's plane were over the Keys, the chain of low islands strung out like a loose necklace from the southern tip of mainland Florida, the flight north would bring him within sight of the Florida coastline. Then he heard Taylor say, "We have just passed over a small island . . . No other land in sight. . . ." It was clear that Taylor could not have been over the Florida Keys and was totally disoriented.

At 4 p.m. the tower heard Taylor turn over command to one of the other pilots. Since he was the instructor of the flight and the other four pilots were students, this abdication of command was an extraordinary act. It was a terrible confession by Taylor that he could not face up to the hazardous situation. The new flight commander, Captain Stiver of the Marines, sent back a message that Fort Lauderdale managed to hear through the static:

"We are not sure where we are . . . We must have passed over Florida and we must be in the Gulf of Mexico."

The flight turned east, and at once the voices of the pilots

# "The Hoodoo Sea"

Below: Avenger bombers of the type that disappeared in extraordinary circumstances in the Bermuda Triangle in 1955. One theory is that the flight instructor was disorientated and simply led the planes east in the firm belief that he was leading them west toward the Florida Keys. Will we ever know the truth?

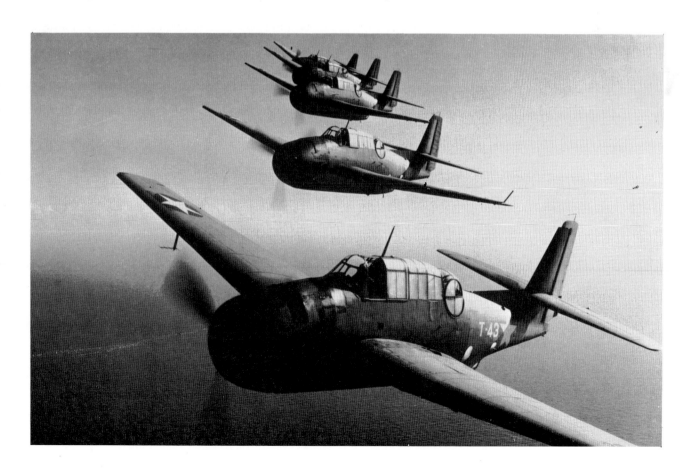

# An Unsolved Riddle

began to fade. They were evidently on the Atlantic side of Florida rather than the Gulf side, heading for the open sea again.

Faint messages between the planes were still heard for a time. Once they turned and flew west, a change of direction that would have brought them home if their fuel had lasted. But within a few minutes they were flying east once more, farther and farther from land. Some reports claim that the last words heard from the flight was the mysterious phrase, "We are entering white water. . . ." After that came silence.

The disappearance of five planes and 14 men produced consternation at Fort Lauderdale. Worse was to follow. A Martin Mariner flying boat, with a crew of 13, was dispatched on a

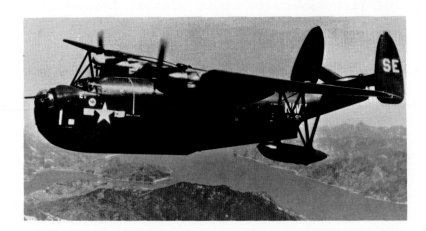

Right: a Martin Mariner of the type that went in search of the lost Avengers. A seaplane of this type with 13 crewmen aboard took off as part of the search operation. Like the five bombers it was hunting, it vanished completely. Nothing was ever found of the plane or its unfortunate crew.

rescue mission. The huge and powerful Mariner, 77 feet long with a wingspan of 124 feet, was fully equipped with rescue and survival gear, and its specially reinforced hull enabled it to make rough landings at sea. It flew northeast toward the area where the Avengers were presumed to have been. A message received soon after takeoff from one of its officers reported strong winds above 6000 feet. Twenty minutes after the Mariner left the base, the tower sent out a message to check its position. There was no reply. Anxiously the tower continued its call while apprehension mounted among the officers present. The Mariner never answered. It had vanished as completely as the Avengers it had set off to find.

Darkness fell, but throughout the night Coast Guard vessels watched for signal flares that might indicate survivors. The next morning a massive rescue operation got under way. There were eight Coast Guard vessels, four destroyers, several submarines, and hundreds of private yachts and boats for the surface search. The aircraft carrier *Solomons* moved into the area and added 60 planes to the 240 land-based planes for the air reconnaissance. They meticulously crisscrossed the area, flying in grid search formation. The Royal Air Force dispatched all available planes from the Bahamas and the West Indies to assist in the operation. Land parties combed the shore line of Florida. Low-flying planes checked the swamps and the Everglades. Not a scrap of wreckage was found, not a hint that there had been a single survivor from any of the six lost planes.

The Avengers were capable of staying afloat for 90 seconds, and the crew had been trained to abandon the plane in 60 seconds. They could have obtained life rafts from outside the plane. Yet no wreckage was discovered, despite the long search over 280,000 square miles of water.

It is this absence of wreckage that gives the Bermuda Triangle its special strangeness. There are several other areas of the world notoriously dangerous for shipping. But the vessels that go down at Cape Horn, the Cape of Good Hope, the Great Australian Bight, or Sable Island produce wrecks and wreckage. The Bermuda Triangle sometimes yields up identifiable wreckage, but the number of ships and planes that disappear without trace has created a yet unsolved riddle.

The report of the Naval Board of Inquiry that investigated the disappearance of Flight 19 stated in part: "A radio message intercepted indicated that the planes were lost and that they were experiencing malfunctioning of their compasses." The instrument officer at Fort Lauderdale was exonerated of possible blame, however, when it was established that all the instruments had been fully checked before takeoff. What went wrong for Flight 19? An Air Force information officer had to admit in a press interview that, "Members of the Board of Inquiry were not able to make even a good guess as to what happened." But theories abounded. One had it that all five planes had collided in midair, simultaneously killing all the crew members. Another maintained that a freak waterspout had destroyed the planes. One officer remarked, "They vanished as completely as if they had flown to Mars." His comment was hardly intended to be taken seriously, but it foreshadowed many later theories that some power unnatural to the earth, possibly involving UFOs, must be operating within the Bermuda Triangle.

Curiously, the area in which the planes disappeared was not at first considered significant. Not until the 1960s did such writers as Gaddis and Charles Berlitz, author of *The Bermuda Triangle*, draw attention to the long list of disasters associated with this part of the Atlantic Ocean. Among his writings, Berlitz has listed 61 known disappearances that occurred before 1945, and 80 other instances in the 31 years between then and 1976.

For example, in December 1947 a United States Army C-54 Superfortress carrying a crew of six disappeared 100 miles southwest of Bermuda on a routine flight to Palm Beach, Florida. The intense air and sea search covered over 100,000 square miles of sea. Apart from some seat cushions and an oxygen bottle that were not identified as equipment from the lost plane, no wreckage, no survivors, no oil slick was sighted. Some authorities suggested that "a tremendous current of rising air in a cumulo-nimbus cloud might have disintegrated the bomber." It is accepted that such clouds can produce turbulence capable of destroying aircraft, particularly jets, but the disintegration of a plane invariably produces debris in the sea.

The next incident, coming a few weeks later, involved a British Tudor IV passenger plane on the Azores–Bermuda run. At 10:30 on the night of January 29, 1948 the *Star Tiger*, carrying 29 people on board, radioed its position as 400 miles northeast

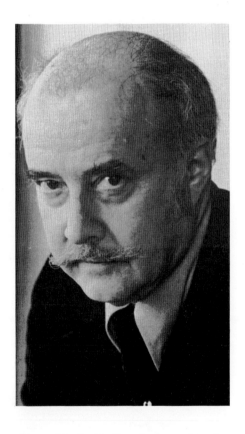

Above: Charles Berlitz, who has written the bestselling account of the peculiarities of the Bermuda Triangle. The grandson of the man who founded the Berlitz language schools, he is an accomplished linguistic expert himself.

# Lost Without a Trace

Below: this is the actual *Star Tiger* that completely disappeared with its 29 crew and passengers on January 29, 1948. The plane radioed its position as 400 miles northeast of Bermuda. Final message was "Expect to arrive on schedule" which was followed by the kind of inexplicable silence that experts on the Triangle have become accustomed to over the years.

of Bermuda. The message commented on the favorable wind and the excellent performance of the plane's engines. The final words were, "Expect to arrive on schedule." There was no further word.

About a year later, and seeming to establish a pattern that disappearances occurred in the few weeks either side of Christmas, the *Star Tiger*'s sister plane, *Star Ariel*, vanished in the middle of the Bermuda Triangle. The *Star Ariel* left Bermuda for Jamaica on the morning of January 17, 1949 climbing into a clear tropical sky. Fifty-five minutes later the pilot sent Bermuda a radio message on weather conditions ending, "All's well." He changed radio frequency to pick up Kingston, Jamaica—but neither Kingston nor anyone else heard from the *Star Ariel* again.

The British Court of Inquiry on the case commented: "It may truly be said that no more baffling problem has ever been presented for investigation." Did both planes suddenly, without any warning and given no time to send an SOS, dive into the sea and sink to the bottom? Could they so crash without leaving a trace of debris? The Court of Inquiry experimented with exact replicas of the vanished planes, sending them crashing into deep water; in all cases fragments escaped to litter the surface. The British investigators remained baffled by the problem.

About three weeks before the disappearance of the *Star Ariel*, the Bermuda jinx had struck at a DC-3 passenger plane chartered for a night flight from Puerto Rico to Miami. The 32 passengers,

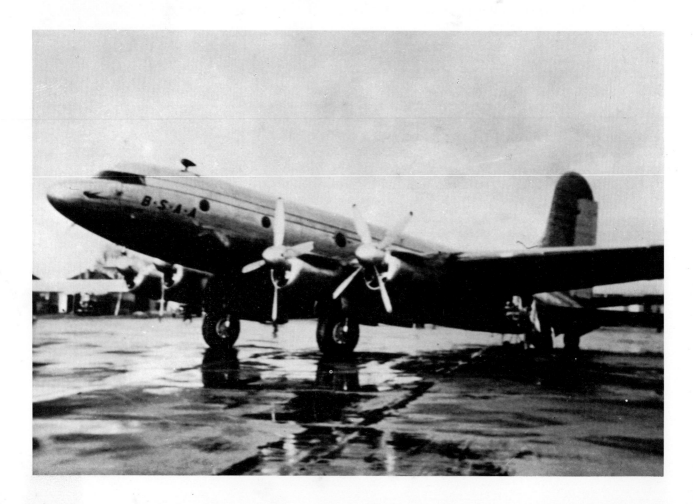

including two babies, had been spending Christmas on the island and the atmosphere on the plane was happy.

"What do you know?" Captain Robert Linquist reported by radio at an early stage of the flight, "We're all singing Christmas carols."

The time was 4:13 a.m. on December 28, 1948 when the DC-3 approached the end of its 1000-mile flight. Captain Linquist could see the lights of Miami ahead. "We are approaching the field . . . One fifty miles out to the south. All's well. Will stand by for landing instructions."

Whether he heard those instructions will never be known. Nothing more was heard from him or his plane. If it vanished into the water, which is clear and shallow around the Keys toward which he had been flying, his plane left no trace. Search planes would have been able to see an object as large as a DC-3 through the clear water. But though they watched for debris and scanned the sea for telltale groups of sharks and barracuda, nothing was ever found.

In the years following the loss of the *Star Ariel*, a succession of aircraft—one or more each year—have vanished in the same mysterious way. In March 1950 a United States Globemaster disappeared on a flight to Ireland while on the northern edge of the Bermuda Triangle. In February 1952 a British York transport carrying 33 passengers and crew vanished at about the same area on a flight to Jamaica. On October 30, 1954 a United States

Below: sister plane of the *Star Tiger*, this is the *Star Ariel*, which simply disappeared over the Bermuda Triangle on the morning of January 17, 1949 on a flight from Bermuda to Jamaica. The pilot commented "All's well" before changing radio frequencies—but no more was heard, and no identifiable wreckage of the *Star Ariel* was ever found.

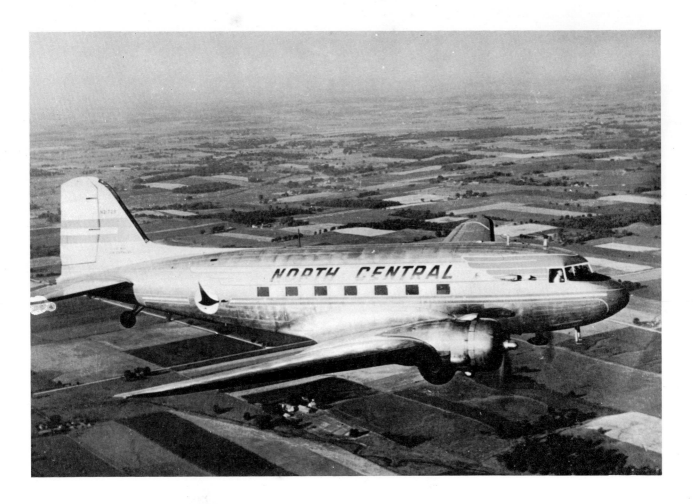

Navy Constellation flying from Maryland to the Azores was lost in the Triangle, never to be heard of again. There were 42 on board, the highest number lost in the mystery area so far. Aircraft of all kinds, light planes and jets, cargo and passenger, vanish abruptly. On two occasions an SOS message is thought to have been heard, but neither gave a clue to the disaster that had overwhelmed the planes. What power is it that, in Gaddis' dramatic words, "snatches planes from the sky?"

Some have suggested that the planes fall instant victims to the disintegrating rays emerging from a subterranean power source placed on the seabed by former inhabitants of the earth. Others suggest that unknown forces operating within the Triangle create space warps, or time warps, that convey the planes into another dimension from which they cannot return. It has also been suggested that the planes are not forced down into the water but up into space, either through a reversal of gravity or through capture by extraterrestrial beings. The mother of one of the young pilots of Flight 19 stated at the time of the inquiry that she had received the impression that her son "was still alive somewhere in space." Manson Valentine, a Miami doctor whose

Below: artist's impression of pilot Church Wakely's experience in November 1964 on a solo flight from Nassau to Miami. First his wing tips glowed, then his instruments failed. The glow from his wing tips became blinding, then began to fade. Then the instruments began to function normally, and Wakely returned safely to Miami. Wakely was one of the lucky ones.

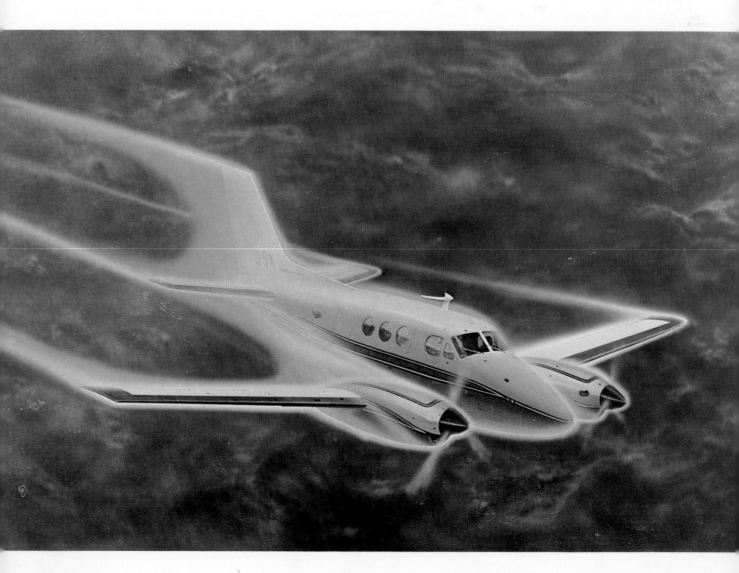

interest in the subject goes back many years, has said: "They are still here, but in a different dimension of a magnetic phenomenon that could have been set up by a UFO."

These are modern attempts to provide an answer, but the problem goes back long before anyone would have been discussing UFOs and multidimensional space. The area of the ocean now called the Bermuda Triangle has been a place of disaster for centuries.

Soon after its discovery in 1515 Bermuda became known as "the Isle of Devils" because of the numerous ships that sank around its shores—some without survivors. In Shakespeare's play *The Tempest*, the sprite Ariel recalls the island's sinister reputation when he says: "Thou call'dst me up at midnight to fetch dew / From the still-vexed Bermoothes [Bermuda] . . ." And vexed they have remained to this day.

A large part of the Bermuda Triangle falls within that area of the West Atlantic known as the Sargasso Sea, a slow-moving tract of water many hundreds of miles wide, named after the seaweed *Sargassum* that floats in enormous masses throughout the area and particularly around its borders. A sea within a sea, it

# A Magnetic Phenomenon?

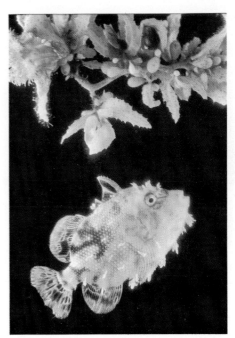

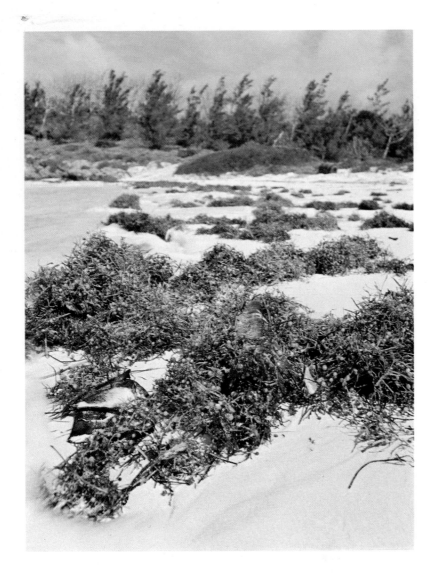

Left: sargassum weed washed up on the east coast of the United States. Berlitz suggests that the Sargasso Sea, characterized by its deadly calm, has helped to create a sailor's legend of a great Atlantic "sea of lost ships," "graveyard of lost ships," or "sea of fear."

Above: a young trigger fish, which lives close to the sargassum weed, taking refuge in it when in danger. It is conveniently camouflaged by the deceptive coloring of the weed's growth.

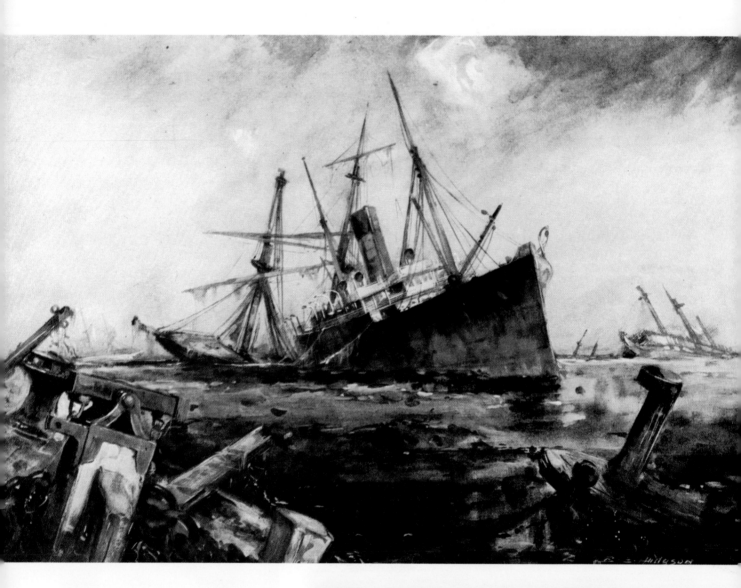

Above: lurid mariners' stories of the Sargasso Sea and its perils, colored by the area's lack of currents, in addition to the sinister weed that drifts around it, began in the time of Columbus. There must, argue the 20th-century experts, be some foundation for them. But, in spite of the picture above, recent exploration of the region has failed to find any real evidence for the trapping of vessels in the weed.

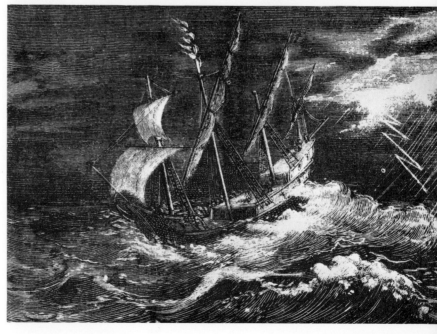

Right: St Elmo's Fire glowing on the rigging of Columbus' ship, the *Santa Maria*. Columbus himself reported seeing the strange glowing fires in this mysterious region.

is bounded by the Gulf Stream and other strong ocean currents, but it itself is nearly stagnant and largely without currents. This seaweed sea was held in dread by mariners in the days of sail. Their ships could be immobilized by the weeds and becalmed for weeks—perhaps forever—by the deadly lack of winds. "The Graveyard of Lost Ships" and "The Sea of Fear" are only two of the many names applied by sailors to this accursed sea.

There are other curious phenomena associated with the Bermuda Triangle region, and one of the first seamen to take note of them was Christopher Columbus. On the eve of his discovery of the New World, a bolt of fire shot across the sky to plunge into the ocean, terrifying his already fearful and mutinous crew. As his ships neared the Bahamas he observed an inexplic-

# The Mystery of the "White Water"

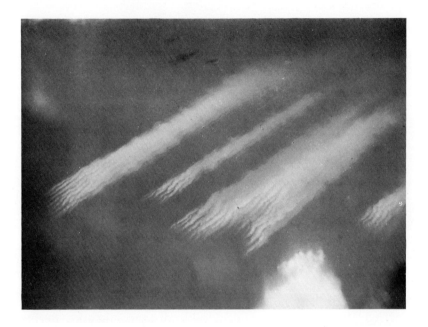

Left: the so-called phenomenon of "white water" as seen by the astronauts of the Apollo 12 mission. This strange phenomenon of streaks of apparently white water in the area of the Bermuda Triangle has also been seen from aircraft, chiefly near the Bahamas.

able glowing in the sea two hours after sunset. This is now a well-known phenomenon in the area. Interestingly, the Apollo 12 astronauts reported that these same luminous streaks were the last light visible to them from earth. The cause of this luminosity is not precisely known, but possible explanations include the movement of fish, fine particles of marl stirred up by fish, or the movement of organic matter. At sea level the phenomenon presents itself as a wide-spreading luminosity in the water, but from the air it appears strikingly as regular white banding.

The Sargasso Sea was a death trap because of being nearly without currents. In contrast, the area around the Bahamas, where wide banks slope abruptly into abyssal depths, is dangerous and unpredictable—a death trap because of wild currents. Divers exploring the underwater limestone formations of the banks have discovered extensive cave systems called "blue holes." Stalactites and stalagmites can be seen in some of these caves, evidence that they were formed when the seabed was dry land. The holes penetrate the substratum for enormous distances, branching into smaller passages of bewildering complexity.

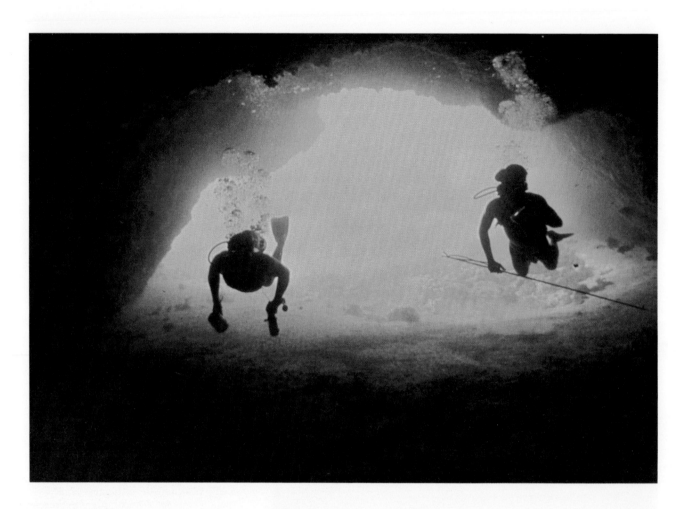

Above: two skin divers explore one of the "blue holes," the strange underwater caves found in the Bahama Banks. Berlitz points out that strong currents sweep through these passageways and the wreckage of some small boats has been found wedged inside them.

Divers have reported that even the fish seem confused, and can be found swimming upside down. Extremely powerful currents flow through these holes, funneled by the tides, and fish can be carried along them for considerable distances inland. Berlitz reports that a 20-foot shark once made a sensational appearance in a quiet inland pond 20 miles from the shore, creating great agitation among the local inhabitants.

The currents of the Bahamas waters form such strong whirlpools at the surface of the sea that they are capable of sinking a small boat, and dinghies and fishing boats have been found wedged far within the blue holes at depths of up to 80 feet. It is natural hazards, then, that have been responsible for the majority of ships lost in the area.

Certain disappearances, however, have never been satisfactorily explained. When the British frigate *Atalanta* left Bermuda for England in January 1880 there was a crew of 290 aboard, mostly young naval cadets in training. The large ship was never seen again, and no identifiable debris was ever found. The British Navy conducted a long search during which six ships from the Channel Fleet advanced in a line, separated from one another by a few miles, over the area in which the *Atalanta* was presumed lost. The search continued until May without success.

The first strange disappearance of a ship within the Triangle in the 20th century occurred in 1918. This ship was the USS *Cyclops*, considered at the time it was launched in 1910 to be the last word in marine construction. Its displacement was 19,500 tons, and the special superstructure that gave the ship a rather odd silhouette enabled it to deliver coal to other vessels at sea. On March 4, 1918 the *Cyclops* sailed from Barbados in the British West Indies for Norfolk, Virginia, carrying a valuable cargo of manganese ore. There were 57 passengers on board and a crew of 221. The weather was calm. The *Cyclops* had excellent radio equipment, but no radio messages were received. No vestige of the ship was ever found.

Because World War I was still in progress, first thoughts were that the American ship had struck a German mine or met a

# Inexplicable Disappearances

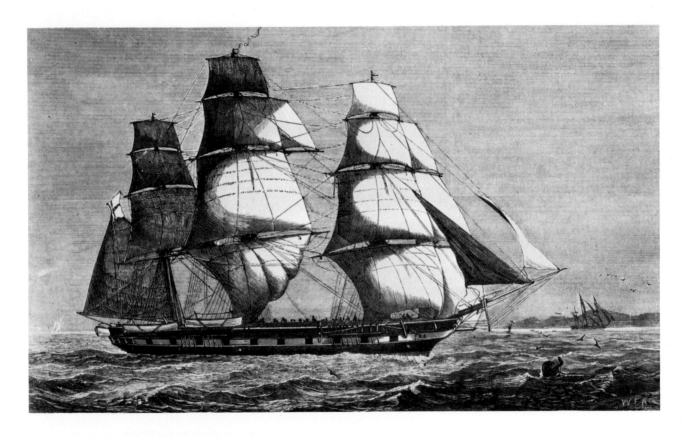

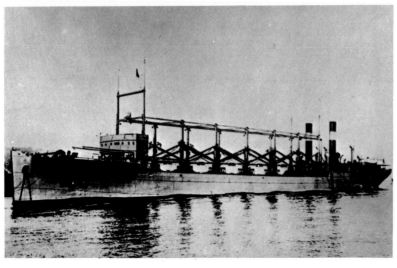

Above: the British sailing ship *Atalanta* which with a crew of over 200, most of them naval cadets, went down in the area of the Bermuda Triangle in early 1880.

Left: the first victim of the Bermuda Triangle in the 20th century was the USS *Cyclops*, a vast 19,500-ton coal carrier with a spectacular silhouette. The ship left Norfolk, Virginia in March 1918 and was never seen again. What happened to it?

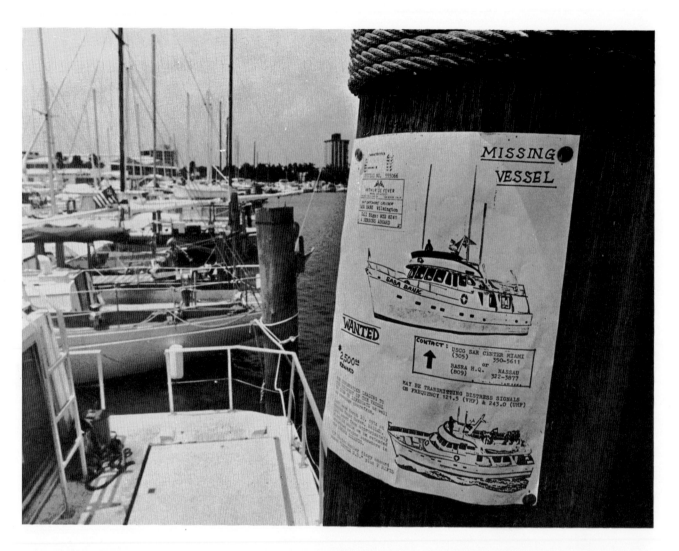

Above: this poster offers a reward to anyone producing information about the missing yacht *Saba Bank*, one of the many small boats that have disappeared in the area of the Bermuda Triangle since 1945.

German submarine, but examination of German records after the war showed that no mines were laid and no submarine had been in the area at that time. Another theory cast suspicion on the German-born captain of the ship, who had changed his name to Warley from Wichmann, and who had sold his house in Norfolk before leaving on his last journey. It was suggested that he had steered the *Cyclops* with her valuable cargo to a sympathetic neutral port, or perhaps sailed to Germany. Some initial support for this idea came from the fact that on leaving Barbados the *Cyclops* had turned south instead of north. Another possibility was that the crew had mutinied against their captain. He was undeniably eccentric and may even have been mad, one of his weird habits being to walk the bridge wearing long underwear and a derby hat.

Another and more plausible explanation of the disappearance was based on the ship's high superstructure which, with a shifting of the cargo, may have caused the boat to turn turtle and sink almost immediately. The British battleship *Captain* had sunk in just this manner. However, the Naval Board of Inquiry rejected this theory, arguing that the *Cyclops* had proved its seaworthiness in eight years of service. As for the cargo shifting, it was of the sort that could only have shifted in extremely rough weather.

During the time the *Cyclops* was at sea, the weather had been fair and the winds no more than light to moderate.

"The disappearance of the ship," stated a Navy fact sheet, "has been one of the most baffling mysteries in the annals of the Navy, all attempts to locate her have proved unsuccessful . . . Many theories have been advanced, but none that satisfactorily accounts for her disappearance."

So the loss of the *Cyclops* remains an enigma. Forty years later it has been joined by an unusual number of similar enigmas.

What happened to the *Cotopaxi*, an American freighter bound for Havana from Charleston that vanished in January 1925? The cargo tramp *Suduffco*, sailing south from Newark to Puerto Rico in May 1926? The Norwegian freighter *Stavanger*, carrying a crew of 43, lost in October 1931 somewhere south of Cat Island in the Bahamas? What was the fate of the United States frigate *Sandra*? It left Savannah, Georgia, in June 1950 with a cargo of insecticide. It was seen passing St. Augustine, Florida. Then contact was lost, never reestablished, and the ship was never seen again.

John Godwin, an author who was one of the first to gather together details of The Hoodoo Sea, points out that all these vessels varied greatly in age, tonnage, cargo, and equipment. "The only similarity about them was the manner of their disappearance," he writes. "Although all carried radios, none sounded a distress call. Not one of these ships had encountered serious storm conditions. In spite of wide search sweeps, nothing associated with any of them was ever found. The case of the *Cyclops* was repeated over and over again."

One ship that did send out a brief and tantalizing last message was the Japanese freighter *Raifuku Maru*. It disappeared between the Bahamas and Cuba during the winter of 1924, and the last

# The Navy Baffled!

Below: the 20,000-ton Norwegian cargo ship *Anita*, yet another of the ships to disappear mysteriously in the Triangle.

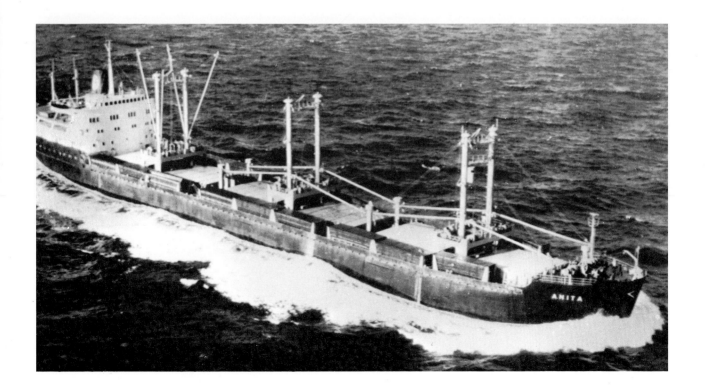

# The Case of the Vanished Tanker

words heard are reported to have been, "Danger like a dagger now . . . Come quickly . . . We cannot escape. . . ." The nature of the danger remained unspecified. A ship that steamed toward the *Raifuku Maru* on hearing the SOS found no wreckage, no survivors.

One of the most recent ships that disappeared sent no distress signals, but did leave three scraps of wreckage consisting of one life jacket, one life belt, and one man's shirt—not much to survive from a 425-foot long freighter with a crew of 39. The ship was the *Marine Sulphur Queen*, and it left the port of Beaumont, Texas, on the morning of February 2, 1963. It carried a cargo of 15,000 long tons of molten sulfur in specially designed steel tanks. The destination was Norfolk, Virginia, and the route lay through the Gulf of Mexico, past Florida, and north through the Triangle.

The weather was good, the sea calm. On February 3 the ship reported its position near Key West in the Straits of Florida. No more was heard. Berlitz reports that the ship was first missed not by her owners but by a brokerage house. One of the seamen aboard the *Marine Sulphur Queen* had been speculating in wheat future on the stock market and had placed an order to buy before the ship left Beaumont. The brokerage house carried out his instructions and cabled him confirmation. Receiving no reply, they informed the owners and the alarm went out. From February 6 to February 15 Coast Guard cutters searched the waters from Virginia to Key West. Five days after the search was called off a life jacket from the ship was found bobbing in a calm sea between Florida and Cuba. A new search was begun and this brought in the other two items. Nothing more. Did the ship

Below: the *Marine Sulphur Queen*, a tanker that left the port of Beaumont, Texas on the morning of February 2, 1963. A perfectly normal radio message was received from the ship the next day, but after that nothing was ever heard of her again.

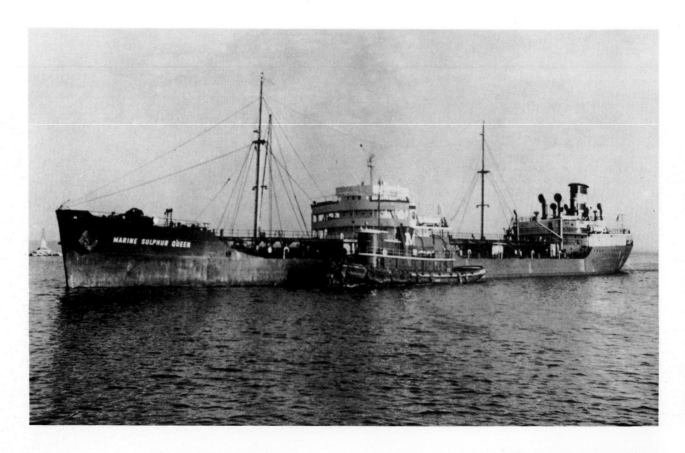

capsize? Had she struck a mine or been sunk by Cubans? Did the sulfur explode? The investigation could offer neither theory on nor solution to the disappearance.

As much as anything else it is the absence of bodies that has puzzled investigators of the Bermuda Triangle disappearances. In other cases of shipwreck in other localities, a few bodies are usually washed up on nearby beaches even though the floating corpses become the prey of sharks and barracuda. Since many of the ships that have disappeared in the vicinity of the Triangle have done so almost within sight of land, the complete absence of corpses on the beaches is hard to explain.

Cases of total disappearance are only one aspect of the many sea mysteries on record. Perhaps equally perplexing are the numerous discoveries of drifting ships from which all passengers and crew have vanished. The earliest recorded example is the French ship *Rosalie*, bound for Havana in 1866. When discovered, its sails were mostly set and its cargo was intact—but the only living thing on board was a half-starved canary in a cage. If everyone had abandoned the ship, they had left no message explaining why. If they had been forced off, it was by someone or something unknown with more interest in human beings than in the ship or its cargo.

In August 1881 a schooner was found drifting west of the Azores by the American schooner *Ellen Austin*. The abandoned boat was boarded and found to be shipshape, with sails furled and rigging intact. The captain of the *Ellen Austin* decided to take advantage of this seeming piece of good fortune by claiming the derelict ship as a prize and putting a crew aboard her. Almost

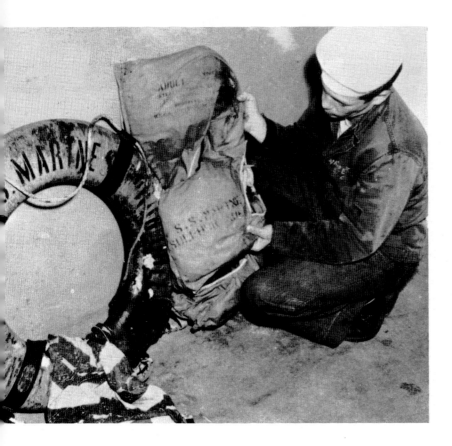

Left: three days after the last radio message was received from the *Marine Sulphur Queen*, rescue planes and cutters took part in an extensive search which managed to come up with the few bits of equipment pictured—a life jacket, a life belt, a man's shirt. It was all that has ever been found of the ship and the 39 men that sailed in her. No oil spots, no drifting boats, no other pieces of the missing ship. It was as if the 7240-ton tanker had never existed.

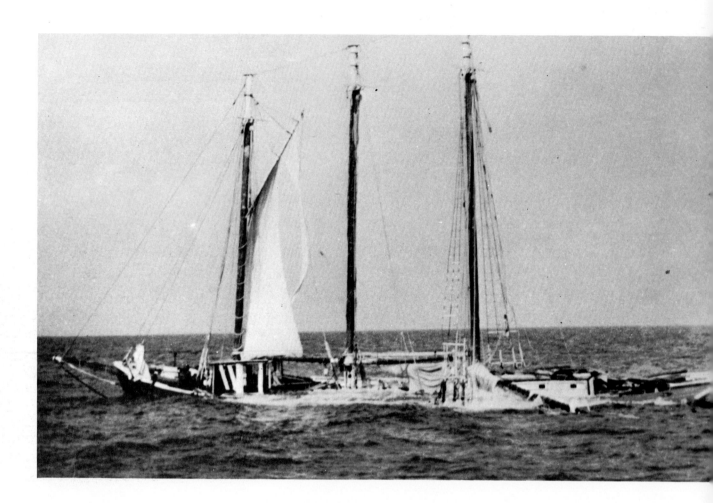

Above: the British schooner *Gloria Colite* as it was found apparently abandoned in the Gulf of Mexico in February 1940. The authorities assumed that her crew of nine and her deck cargo were simply swept into the sea in a storm. Is this a feasible explanation in the context of other similar disappearances in the same area?

immediately a sudden squall caused the two ships to lose sight of each other, and it was two days before the *Ellen Austin* sighted the other boat again. Oddly enough, it was drifting once more. On investigation it was discovered that the prize crew had disappeared, leaving nothing to indicate what had happened or where they had gone. It was a strange repeat of the first encounter.

The captain was not to be thwarted of his prize, though he had to use all his powers of persuasion to get a new prize crew aboard the mysterious and possibly dangerous ship. Unbelievable as it may seem, another squall blew up, contact between the ships was lost once more—and this time neither the vessel nor its second prize crew was ever seen again.

It was not stormy when the German boat *Freya* vanished in the early part of the 20th century. The *Freya* sailed from Manzanilla, Cuba, on October 3, 1902, and was discovered 17 days later partly dismasted, listing, and with no one aboard. The date on a calendar in the captain's cabin was October 4, so the mysterious fate of the crew had been decided on the ship's second day out. Between the 3rd and the 5th only light winds had been reported in the area.

The list of Triangle victims goes on. In April 1932 the two-masted schooner *John and Mary* was found 50 miles south of Bermuda, its sails furled, its hull newly painted—but not a soul on board. The *Gloria Colite*, a 125-foot schooner from St. Vincent, British West Indies, was found abandoned in February

1940. Fourteen months before the disappearance of Flight 19, the Cuban freighter *Rubicon* was discovered drifting off the coast of Florida. A dog was the only living thing aboard.

The late Ivan Sanderson, naturalist and writer, was a supporter of the theory that the unexplained disappearance of planes and ships was the result of kidnapping by extraterrestrial beings. He found special significance in the fact that animals have been left behind on ghost ships. He pointed out that when a crew has to abandon ship it is most unusual for them to leave their mascot or their pets. From this he argued that the crew must have been forcibly removed, and suggested this was done by entities who only wanted creatures able to communicate by words. Sanderson made the point that whereas cats, dogs, and a canary have been left behind on ships from which the crews have vanished, ". . . parrots seem to vanish with the humans. . . ." In his view, this confirms the fact that the ability to talk—even parrot-fashion—is the decisive factor in abductions by outer space creatures.

Berlitz was not the first person to write about the Bermuda Triangle, but he was the first to assemble reports from people who had narrowly escaped its strange perils. One of these was Captain Don Henry, owner of a salvage company in Florida. He described how in 1966 he was aboard the tug *Good News* towing an empty petroleum nitrate barge from Puerto Rico to Fort Lauderdale. The tug had reached that area of the Bahamas known as the Tongue of the Ocean, a very deep and precipitous trench immediately to the east of Andros Island, and the site of many disappearances. The weather was good, the sky clear.

# Sanderson's Theory

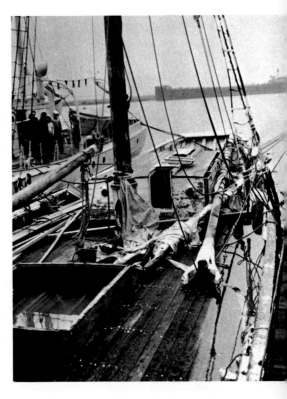

Above: the schooner *Gloria Colite* when it was taken under tow in February 1940. The 125-foot schooner was found adrift and abandoned.

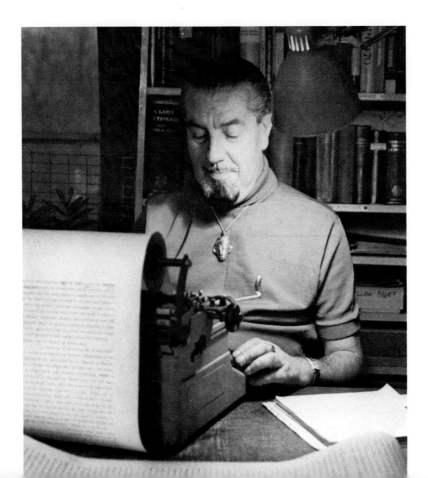

Left: Ivan Sanderson, the late naturalist and writer, investigated many unexplained phenomena. It was his suggestion that the Bermuda Triangle was just one of those areas of the world's oceans known as "devil's graveyards," more notorious because within its area are found some of the busiest of the world's shipping lanes—a plausible theory.

# The "Devil's Graveyards"

Below: this map shows, in simplified form, Sanderson's placing of the 12 "devil's graveyards" (the dark green spots). Two of them, the North and South Poles, are not shown. Each is centered at 36° north or south of the Equator, producing five in the Northern Hemisphere and five in the Southern, plus the two Poles. It is interesting that only two of these points fall in land areas.

Suddenly the tug's compass began to spin clockwise. The sea became turbulent. "We couldn't see where the horizon was," Captain Henry recalled. "The water, sky, and horizon all blended together." All electrical apparatus stopped working. The generators continued to run but produced no electricity. "I was worried about the tow. It was tight but I couldn't see it. It seemed to be covered by a cloud, and around it the waves seemed more choppy than in other areas." Henry signaled full speed ahead, but had the feeling that something was holding the tug back. Slowly it moved forward with the emerging 1000-foot towline sticking out straight behind her "like the Indian rope trick." Nothing was visible at the end, where it was covered by a concentration of fog, although there was no fog anywhere else and visibility ahead was 11 miles. After further effort on the part of the tug, the barge came out of the mist. In the clouded area where the barge had been the water continued to be choppy, but Captain Henry had no wish to go back and find out what was causing it. The generators of the *Good News* began to work normally again, though all the batteries were dead.

Berlitz also quotes the experience of Joe Talley, captain of the *Wild Goose*, a 65-foot shark fishing vessel being towed south in the Tongue of the Ocean by the 104-foot tug *Caicos Trader*. It was night and Captain Talley was asleep in his bunk below decks on the *Wild Goose*. He awoke to find a flood of water pouring over him. Grabbing a life jacket, he fought his way out through an open porthole. Once outside he discovered he was still under

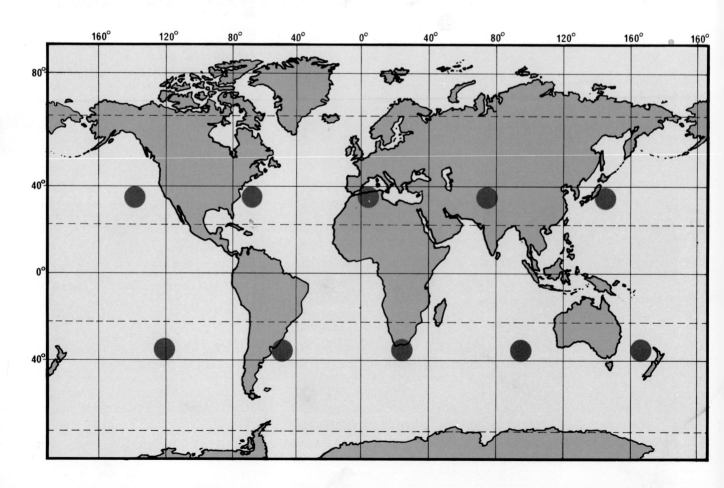

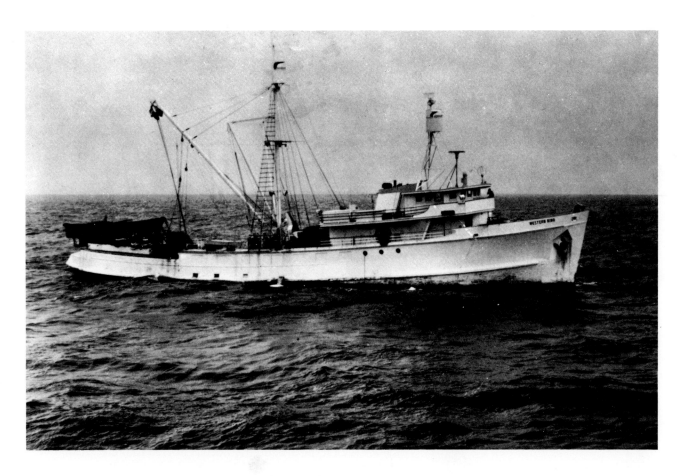

water but he found a line and followed it to the surface, a distance he estimated to be between 50 and 80 feet. The *Wild Goose* had been submerged about 50 feet when he managed to escape from her.

When he reached the surface he found that the *Caicos Trader* was nowhere to be seen. After a worried half hour, he was relieved to hear his name being called through a megaphone. He was told that the crew of the *Caicos Trader* had seen the *Wild Goose* sink straight down "as if in a whirlpool." The force dragging the boat down to the bottom was so powerful that it threatened to capsize the *Caicos Trader* as well. The crew therefore had cut the towline and hastily left the area. They had returned just in case Talley had managed to escape.

Both the *Good News* and the *Caicos Trader* crews talked about a powerful force exerting a tremendous pull. Was this sensation of fighting an unknown power felt by all the ships that sailed into oblivion? It is impossible to know in cases in which no tug crews were present as witnesses.

The reports of individual survivors, however, may lead to a clearer understanding of what happened to those who did not survive. For example, the Avengers of Flight 19 were not the first planes to report malfunction of instruments. In 1928 Charles Lindbergh, flying the *Spirit of St. Louis* from Havana to Florida, recorded in his log: "Both compasses malfunctioned over Florida Strait, at night. The earth indicator needle wobbled back and forth. The liquid compass card rotated without stopping. Could recognize no stars through heavy haze. Located

Above: "the water, sky, and horizon all blended together." That was the mystifying message from the captain of the tug *Good News*, the sister ship of which is shown here. The *Good News* simply lost its way temporarily. The barge it was towing also came out of the mist, and all was well, but the tug's batteries were dead.

# Submarines Are Not Immune

Right: Charles Lindbergh unloading mail at Miami, Florida at the completion of the first trip of the newly opened Pan American Airline route between the United States and Panama. It was on this same trip in February 1928 that he noted "Both compasses malfunctioned over Florida Strait at night. . . . Located position at daybreak over Bahama Islands, nearly 300 miles off course."

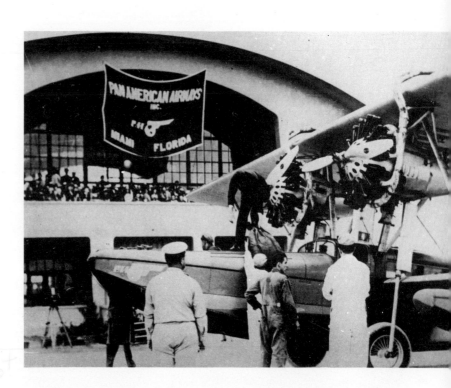

position, at daybreak, over Bahama Islands, nearly 300 miles off course. Liquid compass card kept rotating until the Spirit of St. Louis reached the Florida Coast."

Since then it has frequently been reported that electromagnetic instruments "go crazy" in the area. In 1944 a B-24 piloted by Lieutenant Robert Ulmer was flying at 9000 feet in the same locality east of the Bahamas where Flight 19 disappeared the following year. Suddenly the plane went out of control, shook as if it were about to fall to pieces, and lost 4000 feet of altitude in an instant. Since the plane would not respond to any of the controls and was clearly heading for the water, the crew bailed out. The crewless plane then righted itself and flew off in a southeasterly direction for about 2500 miles before crashing into a mountain in Mexico. All but two of the crew survived, one of them the navigator. Thirty years afterward, that lucky survivor summed up his recollection of the incident with the words: "There is just no logical explanation for what happened."

Electromagnetic malfunction has also been known to occur underwater in the region. When in February 1955 the submarine USS Tigrone crashed into an underwater peak between Puerto Rico and the Virgin Islands, the only such obstacle in the area, its bow was crushed. The vessel would undoubtedly have sunk had it not been the only submarine in the Atlantic Fleet equipped with an icebreaker bow. Despite sophisticated radar and sonar guidance through gyro and compass backup systems that worked perfectly before and after, the submarine was four miles off course when it struck the reef. Numerous smaller craft have had comparable experiences.

The phenomenon affecting instruments has found its way into jokes. One of these is about a group of airline executives on a flight between Florida and Bermuda. Just for fun they send the captain a jerkily handwritten message saying, "Do you know we

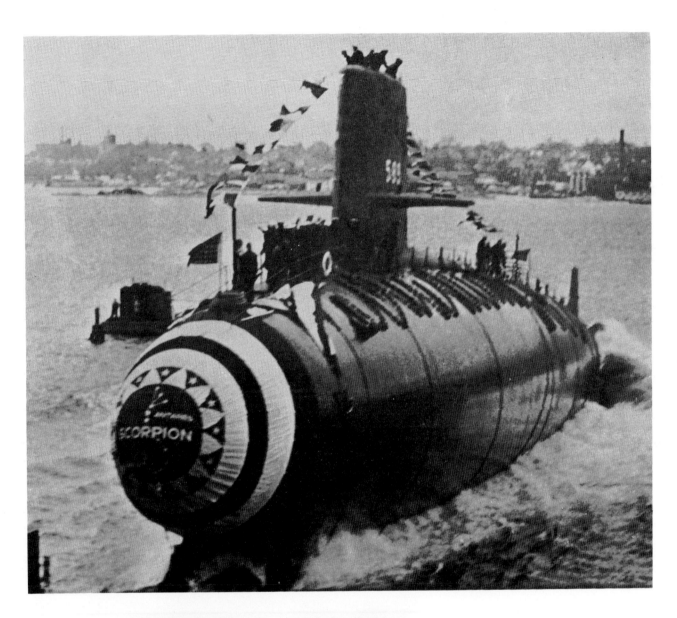

Above: the US Navy nuclear submarine *Scorpion* at its launch ceremony in December 1959. In May 1968 it made a routine message to its base at Norfolk, Virginia from a position 250 miles west of the Azores. Nothing more was heard from the submarine and its 99-man crew.

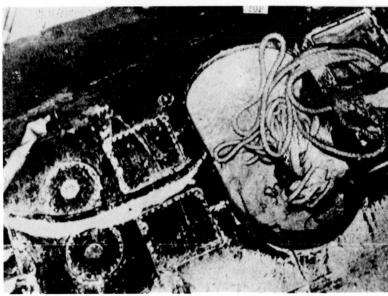

Left: wreckage of the sunken *Scorpion* photographed lying on the seabed at a depth of more than 10,000 feet. A US Navy research ship located the wreckage about 460 miles south of the Azores, on the edge of the Sargasso Sea. The reason for the loss of the nuclear submarine has never been established.

# The Scientists Investigate- and Vanish!

are in the Bermuda Triangle?" The captain replies, "I can't worry about that now. All my instruments are off and my compass is spinning."

The late Wilbert B. Smith, who headed a magnetic and gravity project for the Canadian government, claimed to have found certain locations in which normal magnetic forces did not apply. He called these "areas of reduced binding." The locations were only about 1000 feet in diameter, but extended upward to an undetermined height. Smith's discovery has not been confirmed, but if such areas do exist, a plane, ship, or submarine would have no advance notice of an approach to one until all its instruments suddenly "went crazy."

Professor Wayne Meshejian, a physicist who has plotted satellite pictures for several years, is reported to have observed that polar orbited satellites at an altitude of 800 miles frequently began to malfunction when above the Bermuda Triangle. The official explanation for these failures is that they are due to tape rewinding, and without further information it is hard to draw any reliable conclusion from Professor Meshejian's findings. Could it not be, however, that the magnetic field above the Triangle is as peculiar as the sea within it? It is worth remembering that the area of the Bermuda Triangle is one of two places on the earth where a magnetic compass points true north. In all other places it points toward the magnetic north, and the difference between the two can vary as much as 20° in the course of circumnavigating the earth. The Seventh Coast Guard District, which commands the Florida coastline, points out that, "If the compass variation or error is not compensated for, a navigator

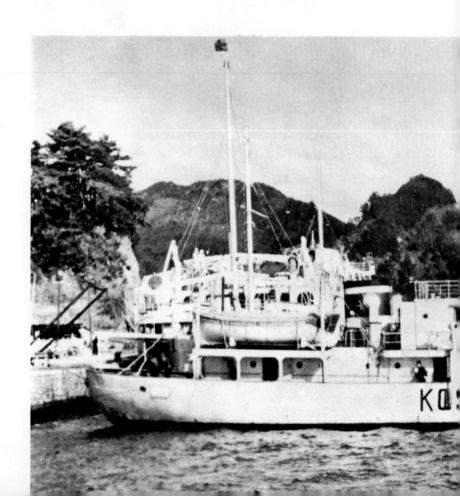

could find himself far off course and in deep trouble." To take that further, no compensation at all could be made if instruments go awry as they seem to over or in the Triangle. That means trouble for certain.

The other place on the earth where compasses point due north is off the southeast coast of Japan. Known to Japanese and Filipino seamen as the "Devil's Sea," it exhibits many of the same characteristics as the Bermuda Triangle. Ships unaccountably disappear there without apparent reason, and have been doing so for at least a century. Between 1950 and 1954 no less than nine ships vanished without trace. No wreckage, no lifeboats, no bodies. The Japanese government declared the area a danger zone, and early in 1955 sponsored an expedition to survey weather and water conditions in the area. A group of scientists set sail aboard the *Kaiyo Maru 5*. The *Kaiyo Maru* itself vanished.

Since there seems to be a parallel between the two danger areas, this works against what believers in the Bermuda Triangle call its "special and unique danger." The Seventh Coast Guard District has never minimized the danger of the Atlantic area—it cannot since it annually receives about 10,000 calls for help. But the experienced and qualified seamen of the Coast Guard feel that the so-called baffling disappearances all have a natural explanation. In their view, it may never be known exactly why the *Cyclops*, the *Marine Sulphur Queen*, and others vanished, but enough natural hazards exist to have been the cause.

The coastguards point to the unpredictable Caribbean–Atlantic weather pattern that brings sudden thunderstorms and

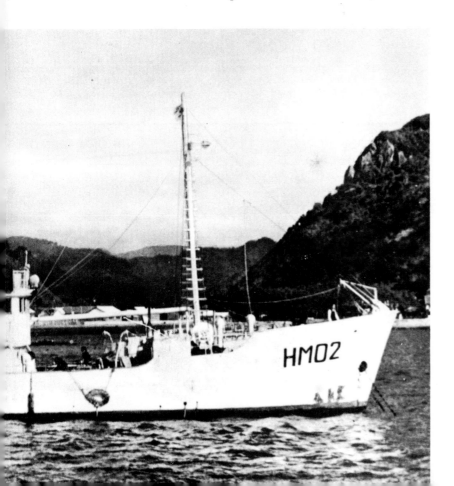

Left: the *Kaiyo Maru 5*, which vanished in 1955 in the so-called "Devil's Sea"—another mystery area located in the Pacific Ocean southeast of Japan. The ship was on an investigatory mission sponsored by the Japanese government when it disappeared, scientists and all. The Devil's Sea is one of Sanderson's 12 "devil's graveyards."

# More Theories

waterspouts; to the complex submarine topography of the area, varying from extensive shoals to deep trenches; and to the swift and turbulent Gulf Stream. They also draw attention to the general lack of seamanship of many who own or use small private boats.

Mrs. Athley Gamber, president of Red Airways in Fort Lauderdale, is of the same opinion. The widow of a pilot who disappeared on a flight to the Bahamas, she has had ample opportunity to watch the search operations for lost planes. She does not believe that there is anything mysteriously sinister about the Bermuda Triangle. In her estimation, as many as half of the disappearances are due to simple pilot error.

This is also the opinion of Lawrence Kusche, author of *The Bermuda Triangle Mystery—Solved*. Kusche has compiled an exhaustive bibliography of articles and books dealing with the Bermuda Triangle, and makes some telling points about the incident that really started it all—the disappearance of Flight 19. He argues that the tragedy came about because Captain Taylor, who had just been transferred to Fort Lauderdale from a station in southern Florida, made a crucial error of observation. When Taylor said, "I'm sure I'm in the Keys but I don't know how far down," he assumed he was over the Florida chain of islets. Kusche maintains that he was in fact over the Bahamas, based on Taylor's words that, "We cannot see land." Both sets of islets have a similar appearance, but those in the Bahamas do not connect with nearby land as they do in Florida.

Supporters of the mystery theory argue that Taylor must have seen something out of the ordinary when he remarked, "Even the ocean does not look as it should." According to Kusche, Taylor was desperately trying to make the sea around the Bahamas fit his memory of the sea around the Florida Keys,

which was impossible. Disbelieving what his instruments were telling him, Taylor altered his course to head in the direction he thought Florida would be. This only took Flight 19 farther away, eastward over the Atlantic toward Africa. After Taylor, by then completely disoriented, had handed over command, one of the other student pilots was heard to say, "Dammit, if we flew west we'd get home."

It may have been his misfortune to be led by a commander who, according to Kusche, mistook his position and trusted to his intuition rather than his instruments.

As for the Mariner flying boat sent out to rescue the Avengers, Kusche points out that to keep them flying a long time, the Mariners were so heavily laden with fuel that they were popularly known as "flying gas tanks." Kusche thinks it possible that some member of the crew, affected by the aura of alarm surrounding the disappearance of Flight 19, in his nervousness disregarded the safety instructions and lit a cigarette. That could have meant the destruction of the fuel-laden aircraft. The merchant ship SS *Gaines Mills* observed an explosion high in the sky at 7:30 p.m., but this fact is not emphasized by Gaddis and Berlitz who both imply that the Mariner left "within a few moments" of the last words heard from Flight 19 at 4:25. In fact the Mariner took off at 7:27 p.m., a few minutes before the explosion seen by the crew of the merchant ship.

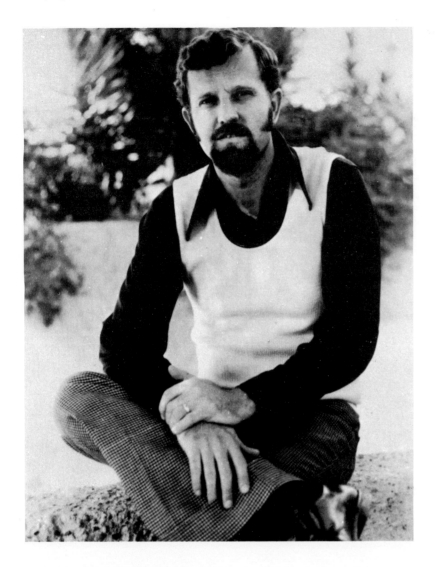

Left: American writer Lawrence Kusche, who wrote *The Bermuda Triangle Mystery— Solved*. In it he debunks the whole idea of there being anything sinister or even mysterious about the Bermuda Triangle. Nevertheless, the controversy continues. What is the truth?

If there is less mystery to Flight 19 than many writers infer, the absence of bodies from the mission's planes and other planes and ships remains unexplained. The disappearance of the British Tudors, particularly the *Star Ariel* in 1949, is also a genuine mystery. The *Star Ariel* was sound, fully equipped with every navigational device, and carried life-saving equipment. It was moreover lightly loaded with passengers, carried more than enough fuel for the $5\frac{1}{2}$-hour flight, and manned by a skilled and experienced crew. When it took off the weather was almost perfect for flying, and it sent three routine signals all suggesting a perfectly normal flight ahead. Then it vanished.

The messages from the pilots of Flight 19, properly interpreted, give an idea of what must have happened. But no further messages were heard from the *Star Ariel* in the four hours that elapsed before the station at Kingston began to wonder at its long silence. Isaac Asimov, scientist and science fiction author, has said he does not "think that anything is essentially un-explainable. There are things that are unexplained. They may never be explained because we may have no data to explain them with." Is this not true of the Bermuda Triangle? Where there is insufficient data, a mystery may always be a mystery.

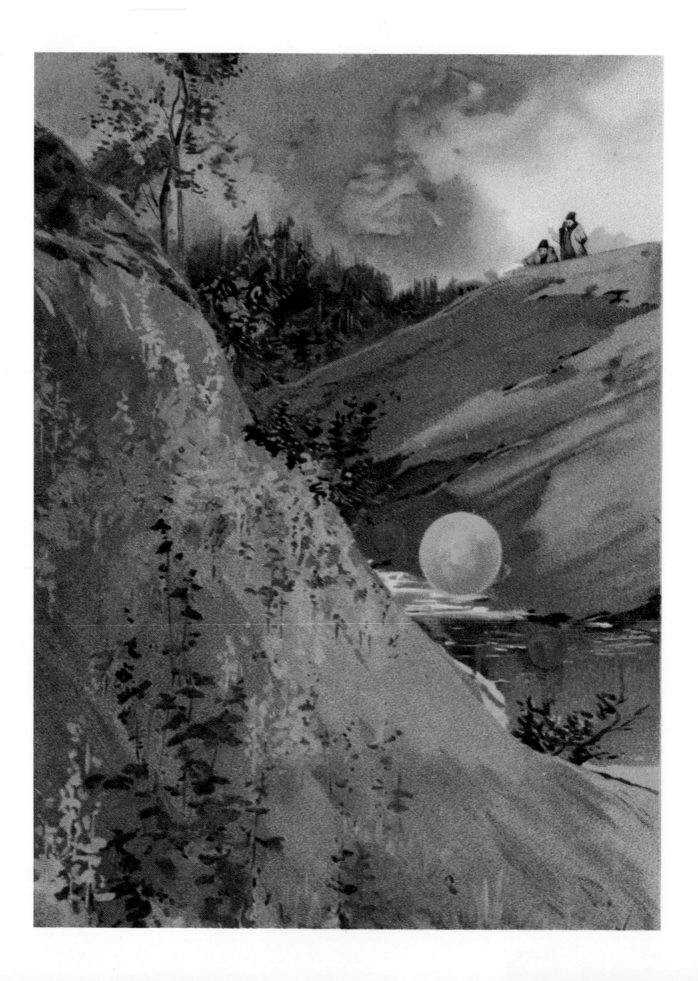

# Chapter 10
# Fires from Nowhere

There have been many reports of ball lightning during electrical storms, and some of them have a strange twist: the phenomenon seems to have a mind of its own. It also seems to act in a friendly way towards humans. This is in contrast to fireballs, which appear to attack people. Can there be a force that causes fires from nowhere? Is there such a thing as spontaneous human combustion? Do halos and other cases of glowing arise from internal fires? Perhaps all of these are tied in with the still mysterious relationship of mind to matter.

In the summer of 1921 the Reverend John Henry Lehn, then a young man of 24, had a strange experience during an electrical storm. He saw a ball of lightning enter his bathroom, roll around his feet, and jump up into the wash basin before it soundlessly disappeared.

"It was about the size of a grapefruit and yellow in color, similar in hue to sodium flame, though it did not dazzle my eyes," he later wrote of this odd event. "It made no sound at any time."

The ball lightning had somehow managed to get through the wire screen of the open window without losing its form and without damaging the screen in any discernable way. But that was not all that was surprising about its behavior. It also melted the steel chain holding the rubber stopper of the drain, leaving it in two parts. The whole mysterious episode lasted only several seconds, and the young man was left guessing where the bright ball had gone. He thought it must have disappeared "down the drain."

A few weeks later during another electrical storm, almost exactly the same thing happened in the same bathroom. The lightning globe entered through the window without melting the screen and circled Lehn's feet as before. Then it again melted a chain holding a rubber drain stopper—this time the one in the bathtub!

Is the phenomenon called ball lightning explainable as a

Opposite: these examples of ball lightning were seen near St Petersburg (now called Leningrad) in the 19th century. According to reports, they grew smaller and smaller and finally vanished.

# Ball Lightning Phenomena

natural happening? Scientists do not even agree that these floating balls of fire are lightning at all in the strict sense of the word. Although ball lightning is always reported as luminous, it is variously described as to size and color—from a few inches to several feet in diameter, and from a dull white to a fiery red. Sometimes the lightning balls disappear with a loud bang, suddenly, and sometimes they merely fade away in silence. Ball lightning does not act like lightning, in fact. It moves more slowly, lasts much longer, and disregards conductors. It does not seem to harm humans, even when it vanishes with a blast. Most curious of all, it seems to display an independent will. For as John Henry Lehn remarked with good humor, "maybe the second sphere wanted a chain of its own to melt in two—at any rate, that's what it did."

Other reports appear to support the theory, formulated by

Right: a photograph of ball lightning taken in England in August 1961. The ball lightning on this occasion appeared to cause a small explosion. A case described by British scientist Dr Alexander Russell sounds similar. "I saw two globes of lightning. They were reddish-yellow in color, and appeared to be rotating. One of them struck a building and burst with a loud report." This description was published in the British science journal *Nature* in November 1930.

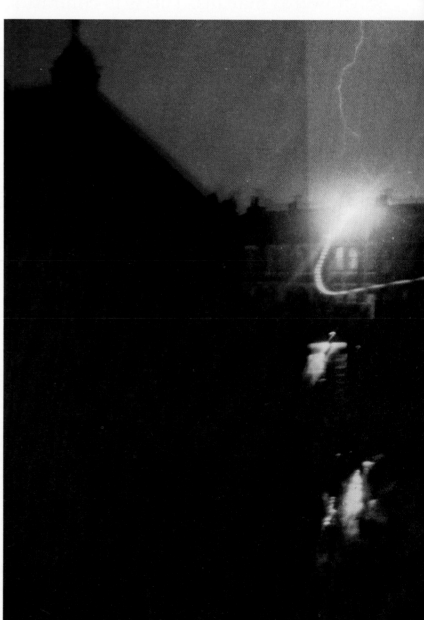

Vincent Gaddis in his book *Mysterious Fires and Lights* (1967), that ball lightning has a definite will of its own, and that it is benevolent toward humans. Gaddis cites several examples of what he calls "socially minded lightning balls" from the collection of incidents recorded by the French astronomer Camille Flammarion. In one of these, a fiery globe actually pushed open the door in order to get into the house it invaded. Another time, a ball of light stopped at the top of a tree, went down it slowly from branch to branch, and moved carefully across a farmyard. When it arrived at the door of the stable, one of two children standing there kicked it. The ball lightning exploded with a deafening noise, but left the children unhurt. Not so the animals inside the barn. Several of them were killed.

Flammarion recounts another instance in which animals suffered death from contact with a lightning ball that did no

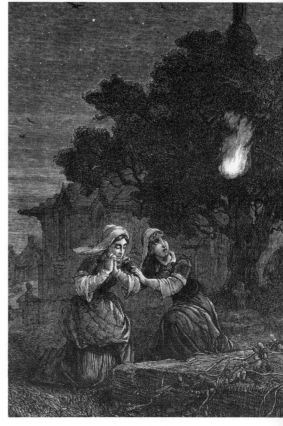

Above: a will-o'-the-wisp frightens two girls in a churchyard. While ball lightning is an electrical phenomenon, the will-o'-the-wisp is a wandering shadowy fire produced by hydrogen gases rising out of places where vegetable and animal substances are decomposing. The gases become spontaneously inflamed when combined with the oxygen in the air. Their appearance in graveyards naturally led to belief that they were the spirits of the dead.

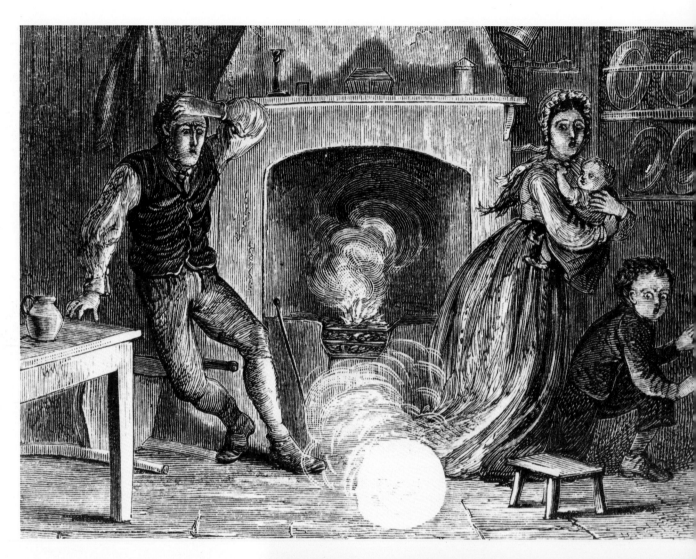

Above: an early 19th-century illustration of
ball lightning descending the chimney of an
English family, to their understandable
terror. The history of ball lightning
phenomena suggests that, when these globes
of light touch the ground, their movements
are extremely capricious and irregular.
Frequently they roll about, divide into
smaller globes, and finally explode with a
terrifying noise.

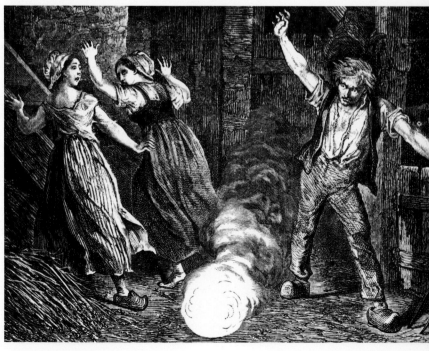

Right: a ball lightning experience in France
in the 18th century. The ball came down the
chimney of a farmhouse, through two
rooms, and finally entered a small stable.
After passing some straw without setting it
alight, it touched a pig, killing it, before
disappearing.

# "Will-o'-the-Wisp"

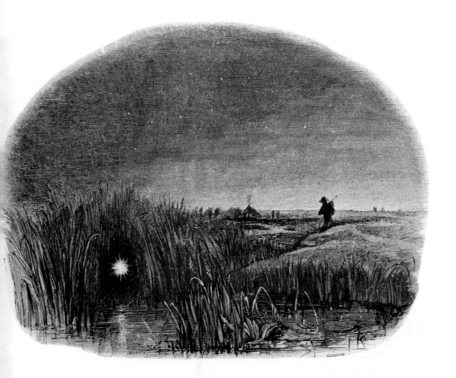

Left: a will-o'-the-wisp seen hovering over a swamp. Also known as *ignis fatuus* (from the Latin for "foolish fire") and jack-o'-lantern, it is caused by marsh gases spontaneously igniting in contact with oxygen in the air around.

injury to people. It happened in a village in southwest France. A burning sphere came down the chimney of a farmhouse and, passing through a room with a woman and three children in it, entered the adjoining kitchen. During its progress through the kitchen, it nearly touched the feet of a young farmer, who was not harmed. The ball lightning ended up in a small stable that was part of the house. There, as though it was its intent, it touched a pig as it vanished—and left the animal dead.

No cases have been reported of people being killed by ball lightning. But there is another fiery phenomenon that seems to be malevolent toward human beings. This is the fireball. Unlike ball lightning, fireballs are not connected with electrical storms. They fall suddenly, move quickly, and cause intense heat in their vicinity. Something of the power possessed by these strange objects can be seen from the experience of Richard Vogt of Eagle Bend, Minnesota. Driving home on the night of May 10, 1961 he saw what looked like "a ball of fog, about three feet in diameter and slightly elongated." It was heading for his car at about a 45-degree angle, and came so rapidly that he could not hope to avoid it. Indeed, he did not. The bright ball struck his car just in front of the windshield, exploding as it did. At this, the car became so hot that Vogt had to jump out as quickly as he could. When he touched the windshield, which had been cracked by the impact, he could not leave his fingers on it for more than a second. Asked to give an opinion on the incident, scientists from the University of Minnesota could not offer much help. They were as baffled as anyone that the object fell out of a perfectly clear sky.

The sky was also clear on May 29, 1938 when a fiery object dropped to earth and burned nine men in a town in England. They described the mysterious menace as "a ball of fire." When the barn on a Massachusetts farm was burned down on April 29,

# Spontaneous Combustionof Human Beings!

Right: "Oh! Law! There's Pa's boots—but where's Pa?" is the caption to this satirical drawing of spontaneous human combustion. It appeared during the controversy that followed Charles Dickens' description of the apparently spontaneous burning of the villainous Mr Krook in *Bleak House*, first published in November 1853. It seems likely that Dickens based his account on reports of a case of spontaneous human combustion in Germany in 1847.

Below: the scene of the death by apparently spontaneous combustion of 92-year-old Dr. J. Irving Bentley in Coudersport, Pennsylvania in December 1966. Reports said at the time that the fire consumed over 90 per cent of his body, causing minimal damage to surrounding objects.

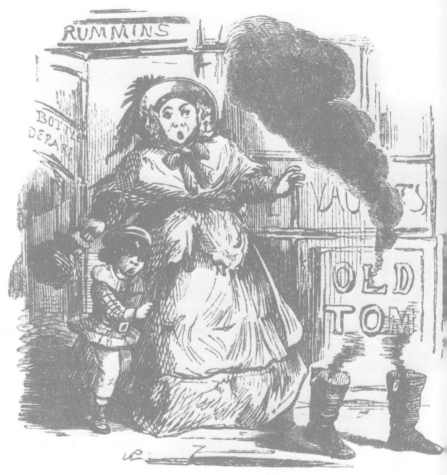

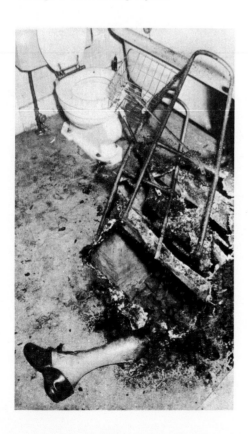

1965, more than one witness said that they saw a sphere that looked like a "flaming basketball" fall near the barn just before the outbreak of the fire. The local fire chief said that he did not think the fire could have started from a natural cause.

Perhaps the strangest and least understood of all kinds of burning from a seemingly unnatural cause is that in which the human body is consumed by a heat so great as to turn bones to ash. Some cases of death by burning have been so baffling that the only answer seems to be an impossible one: spontaneous human combustion. How else to explain a body burned to ashes when nothing—or very little—around it has been in any way touched by flames?

The classic case supporting the idea of spontaneous human combustion is that of Mary Hardy Reeser, who died on July 1, 1951 under circumstances that have never been explained. When found in her apartment, almost nothing remained of the 170-pound woman—only her liver still attached to a piece of back-bone, her skull, her ankle and foot encased in a black satin slipper, and a little heap of ashes. These gruesome remains lay inside a blackened circle about four feet in diameter, which also contained a few coiled seat springs. Nothing outside the four-foot circle had been burned. No flames had been seen to alarm her landlady or neighbors. The landlady had suspected nothing when she went to deliver a telegram to the widow at eight o'clock in the morning. Having found the doorknob too hot to handle, however, she had sought help in getting into the apartment and, with the two workmen who came to her aid, had made the appalling discovery. She remembered that she had looked in on her tenant about nine o'clock the night before and had seen her seated in her armchair, ready for bed but smoking a last cigarette.

Could the cigarette have ignited Mary Reeser's rayon night-gown and burned her and the chair? No fire started in this way could possibly have consumed flesh and bone so completely. In crematories, for example, a temperature of 2500°F or more, sustained for three or four hours, is required to cremate a body; sometimes pulverization is still necessary to reduce the bones to a powder. After long and intensive investigations, no one could come up with a reasonable solution—not firemen, not detectives, not outside experts, including a leading pathologist specializing in deaths by fire. A year after Mary Reeser's death, the detective on the case admitted, "Our investigation has turned up nothing that could be singled out as proving, beyond a doubt, what actually happened." The police chief agreed, saying, "As far as logical explanations go, this is one of those things that just couldn't have happened, but it did."

Is it possible that spontaneous combustion is the logical explanation, little as people want to believe it? Spontaneous combustion is fully accepted as a natural occurrence in the vegetable and the mineral kingdoms. Haystacks and ricks of corn have frequently been consumed by the heat generated during the fermentation produced from moisture within them.

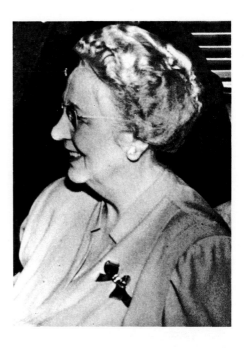

Above: Mrs. Mary Hardy Reeser, a cheerful 67-year-old widow who was inexplicably burned to death in her apartment on the night of July 1, 1951. Once again, as in the case of Dr. Bentley, nothing outside a circle about four feet in diameter had been burned.

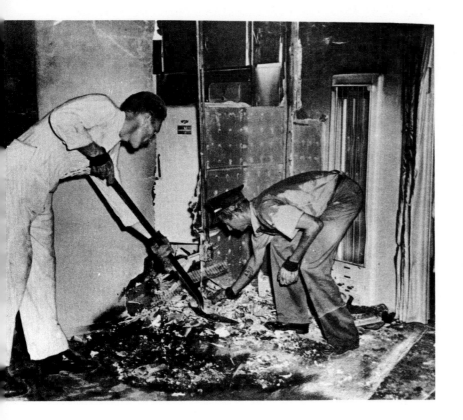

Left: fire officials examine the few remains of the unfortunate Mrs. Reeser. "I've never seen or heard anything like it. There is no clue," said one arson expert. The coroner's verdict was "Accidental death by fire of unknown origin," and no satisfactory explanation was ever found.

# Mystery Fires

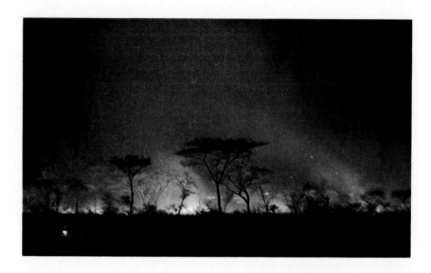

Right: a grass fire at night in Tanzania. Spontaneous combustion is fully accepted as the cause of bush and grass fires around the world.

Below: burning cliffs at Weymouth, England, in the early 19th century. These cliffs still burn regularly and apparently spontaneously, a phenomenon probably due to the presence of oil shales in the clay which forms them.

Barns, paper mills, stores of explosives, all have gone up in flames from the same causes. In certain circumstances a mass of powdered charcoal will heat up as it absorbs air and spontaneously ignite. Bird droppings can produce the same effect; it has even been suggested that some church fires have been caused by the spontaneous ignition of bird droppings accumulated over the centuries on the roof.

The surface of the earth can also burn, usually because of the presence beneath the topsoil of oil-bearing shale or coal. The so-called Burning Cliff near Weymouth, England periodically burns for days, and in past centuries did so for years. Around the English village of Bradley, a thick bed of coal lying eight feet below the surface began burning in the 1750s, and continued to do so for at least 60 years.

Though doctors and scientists accepted these forms of spontaneous combustion, however, they remained largely blind to any evidence that the same phenomenon could occur in humans. Dr. Alfred Swaine Taylor, author of the influential *Principles*

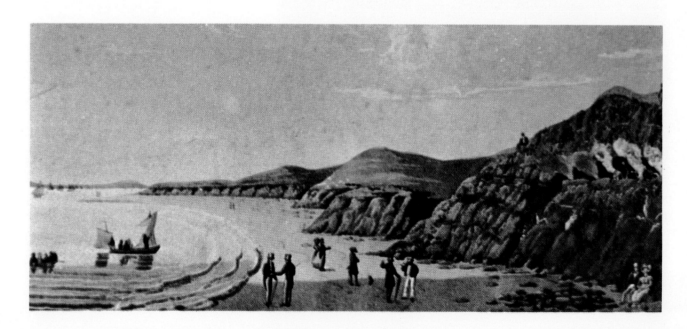

*and Practice of Medical Jurisprudence*, wrote in 1873: "The hypothesis of such a mode of destruction of the human body is not only unsupported by any credible facts, but is wholly inconsistent with all that science has revealed." Ignoring the possibility that science had not by 1873 revealed all the facts of the universe, he went on to say, "In the instances reported which are worthy of any credit, a candle, a fire, or some other ignited body has been at hand, and the accidental kindling of the clothes of the deceased was highly probable."

It is interesting to follow in successive editions of Taylor's great work a modification of this denunciatory attitude. The editor of the 8th (1928) edition, while still "absolutely rejecting any doctrine of spontaneous combustion," thereupon adds, "it must be admitted, on the other hand, that there are cases recorded by credible authorities which require some explanation to account for the unusual amount of destruction (burning) which has been produced in a human body by what are at first sight very inadequate means."

Doctors of an earlier century found no difficulty in accepting the fact of death by spontaneous combustion, although in nearly all the cases they considered the deaths to be the result of too much drinking. Thomas Bartholin, a 17th-century Danish medical writer, described the case of a poor woman of Paris who "used to drink spirit of wine [brandy] plentifully for the space of three years, so as to take nothing else. Her body contracted such a combustible disposition, that one night, when she lay down on a straw couch, she was all burned to ashes except her skull and the extremities of her fingers."

A celebrated murder case in 18th-century France brought about a more scientific study of spontaneous human combustion in Europe. The lawyer in the case got his client acquitted by producing evidence to support the idea of spontaneous combustion of the victim rather than murder. The fact that the dead woman was an habitual drunkard led to a connection being made between deaths by unexplained burning and alcohol. In 1763 a book dealing with "the spontaneous burnings of the human body" was published in France. Medical writers in the Netherlands, Germany, and elsewhere followed with their studies. One book of 1832 cited a case of 100 years before in Italy. It had happened in Cesena in 1731 when the 62-year-old Countess Cornelia Bandi died under mysterious circumstances. What was left of her body was found about four feet from her bed—her legs, her half-burned head, and a pile of ashes. No other signs of fire were present.

The authorities laid the cause of death to "internal combustion"—and gossip added that the Countess often washed her body with "camphorated spirit of wine" when "she felt herself indisposed." So alcohol makes its appearance again, if in a discreet way. It would not do to suggest that a countess went to bed drunk, but alcohol had to be introduced in some manner. Doctors began to warn their drinking patients to steer clear of flames—and no doubt similarly warned them against cooling themselves with camphorated spirit of wine.

It was not hard to find examples of those who had disregarded such warnings. In 1744 a woman in Ipswich, England, who "had

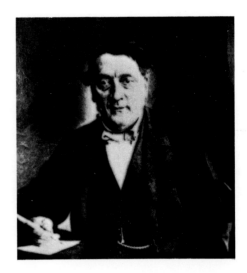

Above: Dr. Alfred Swaine Taylor, British forensic expert, who in 1873 published an influential book debunking any idea of spontaneous combustion. He said that there was a natural, scientific explanation for all causes of such deaths.

Below: this illustration taken from an 1879 temperance pamphlet published in The Netherlands. Titled "The Triumph of Bacchus," it shows how the belief was fostered in the popular mind that there was some connection between the drinking of spirits such as gin and death by fire.

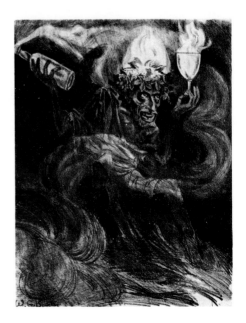

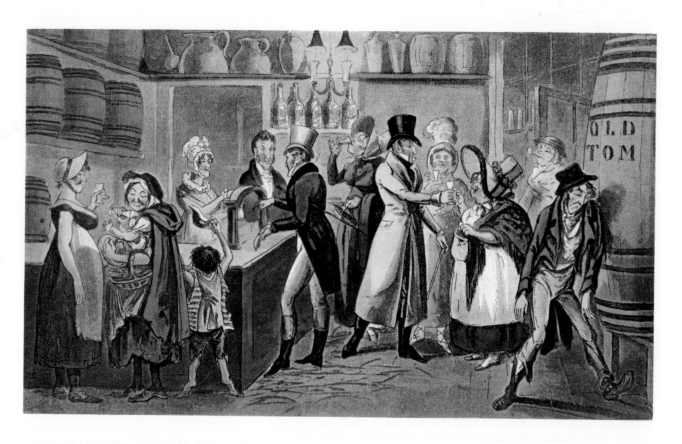

Above: a London gin shop in the early 19th century. The consumption of strong spirits such as gin and brandy grew enormously in Britain during the previous century, especially among poor people. The various attempts by authority to check it were helped by the link with spontaneous combustion among heavy drinkers.
Below: an illustration of the death of Mr Krook. Dickens' account did much to encourage the belief in the phenomenon.

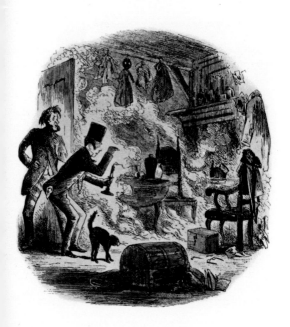

drunk plentifully of gin,'' was found burning like a log near the grate—but there was no fire going. A few years later a woman "much addicted to drinking" was found dead in similar circumstances in Coventry, England. John Anderson of Nairn, Scotland, a carter known for his indulgence in whisky, was found "smoldering" and dying by the roadside outside his hometown.

Deaths like this were ammunition for the rising Temperance Movement. The abstainers warned of the horror of dying from an inner, self-started fire. It was said that water could not extinguish these particular flames; that they burned from within and destroyed nothing but the drunken victim; even that the smoke which issued from the bodies was unlike other smoke, depositing an oily, sticky soot on whatever it touched.

It was also as the consequence of—and sometimes the punishment for—drunkenness that spontaneous human combustion entered the novels of the 19th century. The best known incident of spontaneous combustion in the fiction of the period occurs in Charles Dickens' *Bleak House*, in which the old miser Krook meets this repulsive death. The build-up to the discovery is vivid with horrifying details—the smell like burning chops in the air outside the room, the soot that smears "like black fat," the "thick yellow liquor" that drips from the corner of a window sill to lie in a "nauseous pool." Once inside Krook's room: "There is a very little fire left in the grate, but there is a smoldering suffocating vapor in the room, and a dark greasy coating on the walls and ceiling." And so to the discovery between the chairs: "Is it the cinder of a small charred and broken log of wood sprinkled with white ashes . . .?" It is not. It is all that remains of old Krook—a man "continually in liquor."

Dickens received many letters from readers who found this death incredible, and who took him to task for "giving currency to a vulgar error." But Dickens was not merely a sensationalist. He had attended an inquest on just such a case when he was a cub reporter 20 years before, and he had followed later developments in the subject.

Searching for a pattern in human deaths by mysterious burning, Michael Harrison in his book *Fire from Heaven* considers the possibility that the better educated are spared from seemingly malicious attacks by fire. He cites the case of James Hamilton, who was a professor of mathematics at the University of Nashville, Tennessee. In January 1835 Hamilton was standing outside his house when he felt a stabbing pain in his left leg—"a steady pain like a hornet sting, accompanied by a sensation of heat."

When he looked down, he saw a bright flame, several inches long, "about the size of a dime in diameter, and somewhat flattened at the tip." It was shooting out from his trousered leg. He tried to beat it out with his hands but this had no effect. He did not give way to panic, however. Although what he was seeing was clearly impossible, he accepted that it was taking place. Possibly without consciously recalling the fact, he knew that combustion requires oxygen. He cupped his hands around the flame, cutting off the supply of oxygen, and the flame went out.

Hamilton's quick-wittedness saved him from a fiery attack,

# Fiery Deaths- and Immunity

Below left: a 19th-century illustration of the University of Nashville, Tennessee. It was a professor of mathematics at this seat of learning, James Hamilton, who in January 1835 had a narrow escape from being killed by spontaneous combustion.

Below: the uppermost image on this early Christian cross represents Shadrach, Meshach, and Abednego. Like James Hamilton, they seem to have avoided almost certain death by fire.

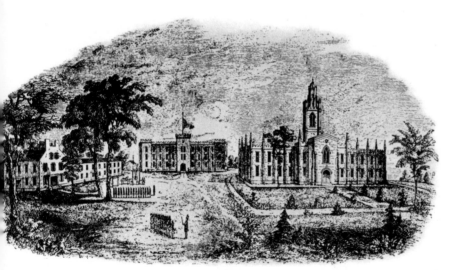

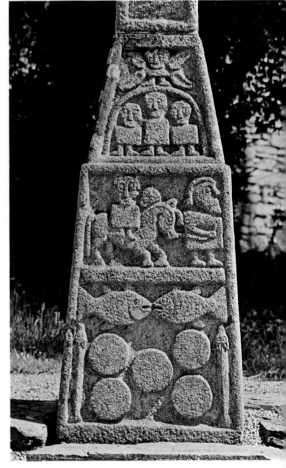

and perhaps even death. But how can some people's apparently natural immunity to fire be explained? The well-known Bible story in which Shadrach, Meshach, and Abednego walk around in a fiery furnace without getting a single mark on them or their clothes depends on a divine agency for protection. What about the many recorded cases of mystics and shamans who walk unscathed across red-hot beds of coal or lava? How can certain people control fire so that it does not burn them?

In Paris in the 18th century, two young women demonstrated remarkable ability to submit themselves to what would be torture by fire for others. Gabrielle Moler and Marie Sonet were *convulsionnaires*, the name given to those who claimed

Right: the Frenchwoman Gabrielle Molet being tested after she experienced a series of religiously inspired convulsions. After this experience she astonished witnesses by placing her feet and even her face in fire without being burned or scarred.

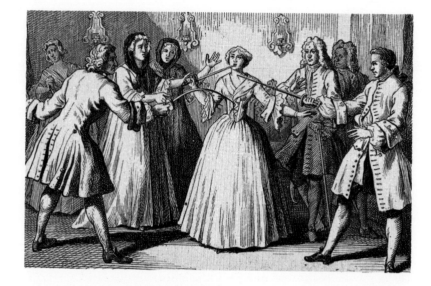

Below: Daniel Dunglas Home, the great 19th-century medium, who on several occasions showed an apparent immunity to the effects of fire.

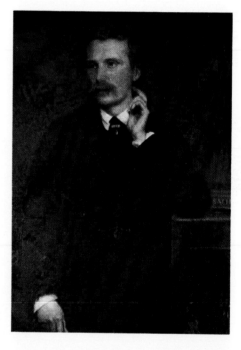

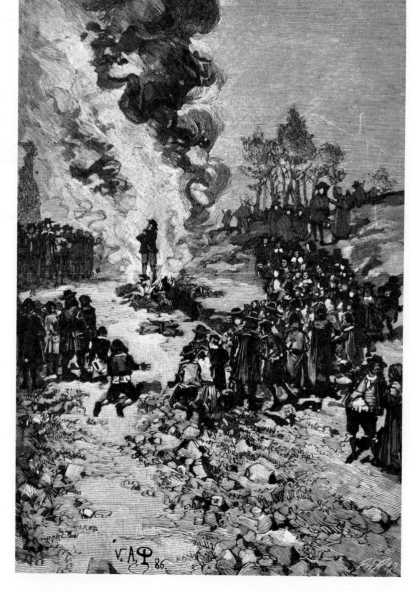

Right: a crowd watches in amazement as the 17th-century French Huguenot leader Claris survives being burned to death on a pyre. The flames rose above his head, all the wood was consumed, but he was completely unhurt. There was not even a mark on his clothes.

miraculous cures after experiencing convulsions at the tomb of a highly esteemed local deacon known for his kindness and humility. Gabrielle Molet astounded onlookers by thrusting her face into a blazing fire and withdrawing it unburned. She would also leave her feet in the fire until her shoes and socks were burned away—and come out without a burn on her flesh. Marie Sonet went even further. She exposed her whole body except her head and feet to a raging fire by lying over it supported on stools at each end. Wrapped only in a sheet, she remained rigid over the flames for hours.

The 19th-century medium Daniel Dunglas Home also exhibited feats of daring with fire. While in a trance or semi-trance, he could handle scorching hot coals as though he had asbestos gloves on. Once he was reported to have picked up a glass lampshade, touching a match against it. The glass was hot enough to ignite the match. Home then put the shade between his lips, which showed no ill effects from the intense heat. This medium, who was never caught in fraud throughout his exceptional career, also had the added quality of being able to transfer his own immunity to fire to other people and to objects. For example, it was said that he could hand searingly hot coals to someone else without that person feeling any pain or burning. He also put such coals against handkerchiefs or clothing without so much as singeing the cloth.

It is an accepted fact that an increase in body temperature is one of the physical changes sometimes associated with trances and other unusual states. The most celebrated 20th-century case is that of Padre Pio, a saintly Capuchin friar who lived in the southern Italian town of Foggia and was known for performing miracle cures. His normal body temperature was slightly below normal, but during one of the ecstatic states he experienced, it would soar beyond the reach of an ordinary clinical thermometer to the extraordinary figure of 118.4°F. During his trancelike states, it was observed that Padre Pio seemed to glow. This phenomenon is frequently mentioned in the lives of saints and other holy figures. Saint Philip Neri, Saint Ignatius Loyola, and Saint Francis de Sales are among the many who are said to have been seen surrounded by a bright light when preaching or saying mass. When Moses came down from Mount Sinai "the skin of his face shone," and in the presence of other people he had to wear a veil. In Christian religious art God and Christ are represented as being surrounded by a shining nimbus or glory. The golden haloes shown encircling the heads of saints are stylized expressions of this same glow. Travelers who have climbed to the summits of mountains in stormy weather have sometimes observed sparks shooting from their clothes and hair. Their heads can even be surrounded by an electric aureole very like that of a medieval saint, and it is possible that some people can unconsciously produce a similar effect at ordinary altitudes.

Is there, then, such a thing as a human firefly? Take the case of Anna Monaro, whose strange glowing hit headlines all over the world in May 1934. An asthma patient in the hospital at Pirano, Italy, Mrs. Monaro emitted a blue glow from her breasts as she slept. This emanation lasted for several seconds at a time, occurred several times a night, and continued for a period of

# Unharmed by Blazing Fire

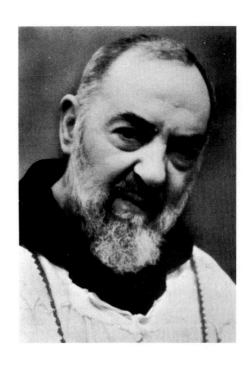

Above: Padre Pio da Pietralcini, the Italian Capuchin friar who performed numerous miracles before his death in 1968. His body temperature apparently rose abruptly during his frequent ecstatic experiences and witnesses said that he also seemed to glow.

Right: Saint Philip Neri, the 16th-century Italian saint. It was said of him that, like Padre Pio, he appeared to be surrounded by a bright light when preaching or saying Mass.

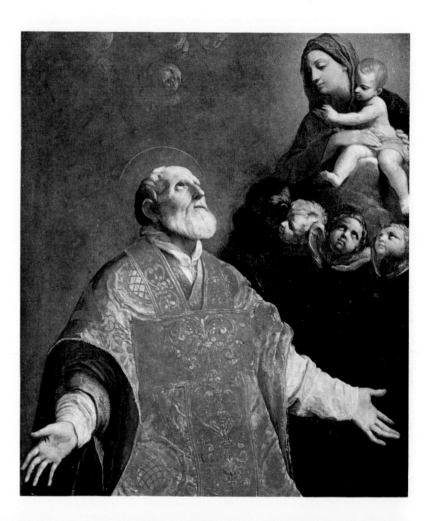

Below: Saint Ignatius, the Spanish founder of the Jesuit Order, shown on his deathbed. He too emitted a bright aura on occasions, according to reports.

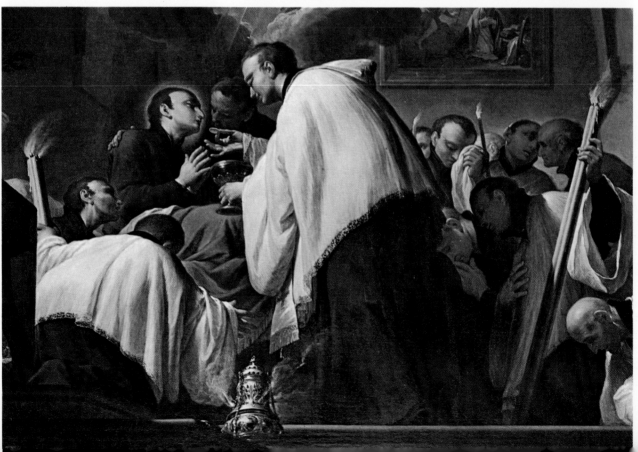

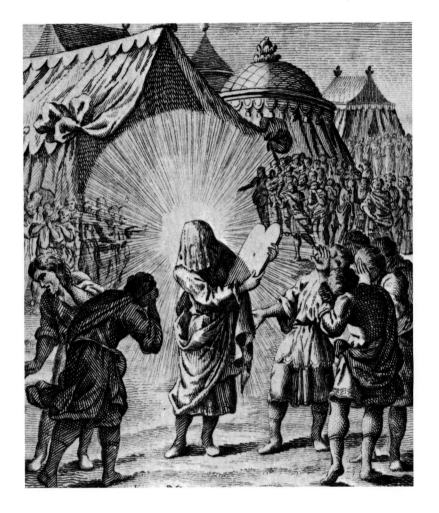

# The Mysterious Haloes of Fire

Left: Moses presents the Israelites with the two tablets of the Ten Commandments. According to the Book of Exodus: "When Aaron and all the children of Israel saw Moses, behold, the skin of his face shone. . . . . And till Moses had done speaking with them, he put a veil on his face."

Below: this illustration of a haloed man standing on a mountain top represents a phenomenon that sometimes occurs on high peaks. It appears when the head or other part of the body is surrounded by a glow caused by electricity in the stormy surrounding atmosphere.

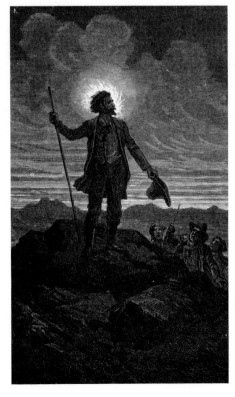

weeks. Many doctors and psychiatrists observed the phenomenon. None could explain it.

Can some of the mysterious fires and lights be connected with the poltergeist phenomenon? There are many well-attested and recent reports of poltergeist activity involving fire, including self-destructive attacks as well as assaults on others. Harrison in *Fire from Heaven* also sees in this an unconscious suicide bid—and most cases of spontaneous combustion as an unconscious suicide bid that succeeded. He theorizes that in a trancelike state, or when half-sleeping, intoxicated, or in some other manner "outside themselves," the victims were able to call forth fires or flameless heat because they were possessed of an unconscious wish to die. Can the mind influence matter so much?

It seems only fitting that this book should end as it began, with the undefined relationship between mind and matter. Just as incomprehensible powers exerted by the one upon the other seem to lie at the roots of coincidence, and to give a reality to our beliefs in jinxes and curses, so the mystery of the "fires from nowhere" may eventually be understood in similar terms. Until this understanding is forthcoming, many phenomena must remain *mysterious*—a word that in the Ancient World meant "a secret known only to initiates." At some future time, mankind may be initiated into those secrets—and mysteries will be mysteries no more.

# Index

# Picture Credits

*Key to picture positions: (T) top (C) center (B) bottom; and in combinations, e.g. (TR) top right (BL) bottom left.*

Agence Top 24; Aldus Archives 35, 38(T), 48(L), 70, 75, 78, 106, 112, 113, 139(B), 154, 157, 162–163, 191(R), 195, 240, 242(T), 245(T), 246(B), 247(L); © Aldus Books 17(T), 210, 229, (Christopher Foss) 216, (John Webb) 67; Archiv Gerstenberg 32(T), 36, 37(R); Courtesy of *Ablaze! The Case for, and Cases of, Spontaneous Human Combustions*, by Larry E. Arnold, Vol. I of *Earth in Transition, Revised Planetary Perspectives* 242(B); Associated Press 21(L), 176, 177(TR)(B), 178, 179(B), 221(B), 231; The Barbados Museum and Historical Society 146; Charles F. Berlitz 219, 228, (Photo Frances McLaughlin-Gill) 213; The Bettmann Archive Inc. 100(L), 205(R); Bildarchiv Preussischer Kulturbesitz 33, 46, 92, 93(B), 94(TR), 97, 127, 128(R), 186(TL), 202(L), 204(B); Bilderdienst Süddeutscher-Verlag 25, 26(L), 52, 69, 90, 94(B), 95, 96(T), 98(B), 114(B), 203(B), 205(L); Photos Eileen Tweedy © Aldus Books, courtesy Viscount Bledisloe 62–63; British Museum/Photos Michael Holford © Aldus Books 28, 98(T); Bulloz 11(T), 13, 41; California Historical Society 51; Canadian Press photo 88(B); Harold Wilkins, *Captain Kidd's Treasure Island*, Cassell & Co. Ltd., London, 1935 83; Archives de Documentation Photographique Cauboue 20(B), 104, 108(L); Photo courtesy Chambre de Commerce et d'Industrie de Marseille 170–171(T); J.-L. Charmet 14, 20(T), 96(B), 100(R), 111, 115, 128(L), 188, 189(L); C. J. Lambert, *Together We Wandered*, Chatto and Windus Ltd., London 1953 120; Bruce Coleman Ltd. 217(L), (David C. Houston) 244(T), (R. K. Pilsbury) 34(R); Compix, New York 23(B), 87, 124, 126, 167, 196, 197, 198(B), 199(B), 200, 207(T), 208, 215, 222–226, 227(T), 235; *Daily Telegraph* Colour Library 65; C. M. Dixon 247(R); Mary Evans Picture Library 18(R), 30(T), 31, 39, 40, 44(B), 101(R), 138, 140, 141, 143, 144, 164, 221(T), 236, 239(R), 248(R), 251; Photo Meteorological Office © Dermot P. Fitzgerald 38(B); Fortean Picture Library 27(R); Giraudon 8; Ronald Grant 177(TL); Robert Harding Picture Library 169(R); W. G. Lucas/Hebridean Press Service, Stornoway 54–57; Reproduced by Gracious Permission of Her Majesty Queen Elizabeth II 15; *The Herald and Weekly Times*, Melbourne 45; The Historical Picture Service, Brentwood 68(L), 84(T), 88(T), 102, 139(T), 148, 218(T); A. C. Doyle, *The Poison Belt*, Hodder & Stoughton Ltd., London, 1913 44(T); IBA Internationale Bilderagentur, Zürich 43, 49(L), 99(B); Imperial War Museum, London 50, 185, 186(BL), 187(B), 190(L), 192, (Photos Eileen Tweedy © Aldus Books) 49(R), 180, 187(T), 191(R); The Reverend Canon A. Irwin Johnson, M.B.E. 145; Jupiter Books 30(B); Keystone 150–152; Charles and Nancy Knight, National Center for Atmospheric Research (NCAR), Boulder, Colorado 37(L); Kunsthistorisches Museum, Wien/Photo Erwin Meyer 158–159(B); Kyodo News Service 232–233; Roy Jennings/Frank W. Lane 238; Local History Library, Taunton/Photo © Aldus Books 60; The Mansell Collection, London 64, 101(L), 103(B), 137(L), 142, 153, 158(T), 161, 201, 202(R), 245(B), 246(T); Middle East Archive, London 42; From the Rex Nan Kivell Collection, National Library of Australia, Canberra 160; National Maritime Museum, London/Photo Michael Holford 125; Nova Scotia Communications & Information Center photos 73, 82, 86, 89; Photo Alan Smith/*The Oklahoma Journal* 17(B); Earl Roberge/Photo Researchers Inc. 169(L); Photri 48(R), 58, 132, 135, 204(T); Picturepoint 18(L), 248(L); Courtesy Pitt Rivers Museum 137(R); Popperfoto 22, 85, 114(T), 129(B), 133(L), 134, 179(T), 182, 184, 206, 207(B), 249; Press Association 214; Public Archives, Nova Scotia/Photos Steve Zwerling © Aldus Books 74, 76, 79–81; *Radio Times* Hulton Picture Library 32(L), 34(L), 53, 66, 68(R), 84(B), 93(T), 116(T), 117(L), 131, 133(R), 147, 155, 174, 175, 198(T), 199(T), 230; George Rainbird Ltd./Photo Derek Witty 118; Roger-Viollet 10, 21(R), 103(T), 189(R); Ann Ronan Picture Library 218(B), 241; Photos Eileen Tweedy © Aldus Books, courtesy of the Principal, St. Hugh's College, Oxford 11(B), 12(L); *St. Petersburg Times and Evening Independent* 243; Photo Martin Dain/courtesy Mrs. Ivan Sanderson 227(B); Scala 136, 250; Dr. Helmut Schmidt, The Mind Science Foundation, San Antonio 23(T); Peter David/Seaphot 217(R); Seattle Historical Society 168; Snark International 12(R), 19, 105, 107, 108(R), 109, 110, 116(B), 171(B); Städtische Kunsthalle Mannheim/Photo Hans Bergerhausen 130; Loren McIntyre/*Sunday Times* Colour Library 26–27(C); Photo Aaron Sussman 16; Syndication International Limited, London, 193, 194; Paul J. Tzimoulis 220; Ullstein Bilderdienst 94(TL), 117(R), 190(L), 203(T); U.S. Navy photos 211, 212; Vancouver City Archives 166; Photothèque Vautier 121, 122; Martin von Wagner Museum der Universität Wurzburg/Foto-Verlag Gundermann 99(T); Western Mail and Echo Ltd., Cardiff/Photo John Webb © Aldus Books 173; Weymouth and Portland Museum Service 244(B); J. H. Winchester & Co., Inc./Photo George Adams, New York © Aldus Books 156; G. Berone/ZEFA 129(T).